LIFE
AFTER MEDICAL SCHOOL
A Physician's Guide To Survival

A Humorous, Inside Look
At Balancing Family With Career

by Bill Truels, MD, FACS

Treasure every moment
Heed the children's pleas
Take time each and every day
To count your memories!

This book is dedicated to
St. Jude Children's Research Hospital

Donations may be made at www.stjude.org

FOREWARD

William P. Truels, M.D., surgeon par excellence, continues to demonstrate his literary excellence, and has once again succeeded in bringing literary relief to our often-routine existence. This time the author, alias Dr. Truewater, has presented us with a brilliant, passionate selection of short stories and poems that comprise many of life's major issues. The pertinence and relevance of this work far exceeds in my opinion that which has preceded it – which appears to be a natural progression of Bill's enormous talent.

My student once again has addressed in a direct, succinct fashion the "slings and arrows" of our existence! I have personally delivered, with great apparent success, his story, "Graduation Day" at a recent Tulane University Medical School Graduation. His ability to capture important issues and human emotions appears to be key to his talent! Evolution of this God-given talent will undoubtedly continue in the future, offering all of us further food for thought concerning issues pertaining to our existence.

In my opinion, my talented friend and colleague has now traveled to lands visited many years ago in Kahlil Gibran's *The Prophet*. Continue your search for literary excellence – society needs your intellectual relief!

– Ronald Lee Nichols, M.D.

William Henderson Professor of Surgery

Professor of Microbiology and Immunology

Tulane University School of Medicine

New Orleans, Louisiana

Table of Contents

INTRODUCTION

Congratulations on your graduation from medical school! Once the jubilation subsides, here are a few things that you should know in order to be a successful and happy physician while you adjust to your new role.

Practice humility. All your life you've been taught to be aggressive and forceful – now it's time to be humble and non-threatening. Ask for help if you need it.

Be prepared to get yelled at, on occasion, by a disgruntled patient or family member, as you will not be able to please everybody. I use the Bruce Lee defense: "Be like water making its way through cracks. Do not be assertive, but adjust to the object, and you shall find a way around or through it."

With your medical school graduation, your divorce rate, suicide rate, and addiction rate has now doubled. Set aside time every day to spend with your family. Develop a hobby or some activity outside of medicine. Skip illegal drugs and limit alcohol intake.

Learn to accept defeat. All your life, you've been taught to fight for victory and never accept defeat. You must now learn at times to accept defeat, for death ultimately wins.

Don't get angry at yourself if your patient dies and you've done everything possible. Don't blame others and use them as a scapegoat if your patient dies.

Don't let your patient know that you're in a hurry, with one foot always outside the door. If discussing a serious issue, grab a chair and sit down. Learn the art of listening to your patients, for they can often give you the diagnosis.

All your life, you've been taught to be a "Type A" person – always pushing your way to the top. It's time to be a "Type B" person – it's OK for others to pass you!

You will eventually be sued or threatened with a lawsuit. Practice dealing with lawsuits by thinking up questions and then answering them to the best of your ability before your deposition.

Learn to respect the nurses and all other health care workers in the hospital. Learn the names of the housekeepers and say hello to them- thank them for keeping the rooms clean!

Learn to look inward- practice meditation and self-reflection, for in treating others you can learn to heal yourself! Try to "live and forgive" – that way you carry less baggage into the afterlife!

Finally, and most important, this is a book about people – that's really what medicine is all about We must learn to recognize our potential, but also our limitations. And, despite the increasing regulations and interference, we must above all maintain our compassion for our fellow human beings.

Life After Medical School provides valuable insight, not just for graduating physicians, but for anyone with a career or occupation that threatens to be all-consuming!

In these articles and poems, I have sought to portray my experiences as a practicing physician for the past 50 years. Read and enjoy!

Bill Truels, M.D.

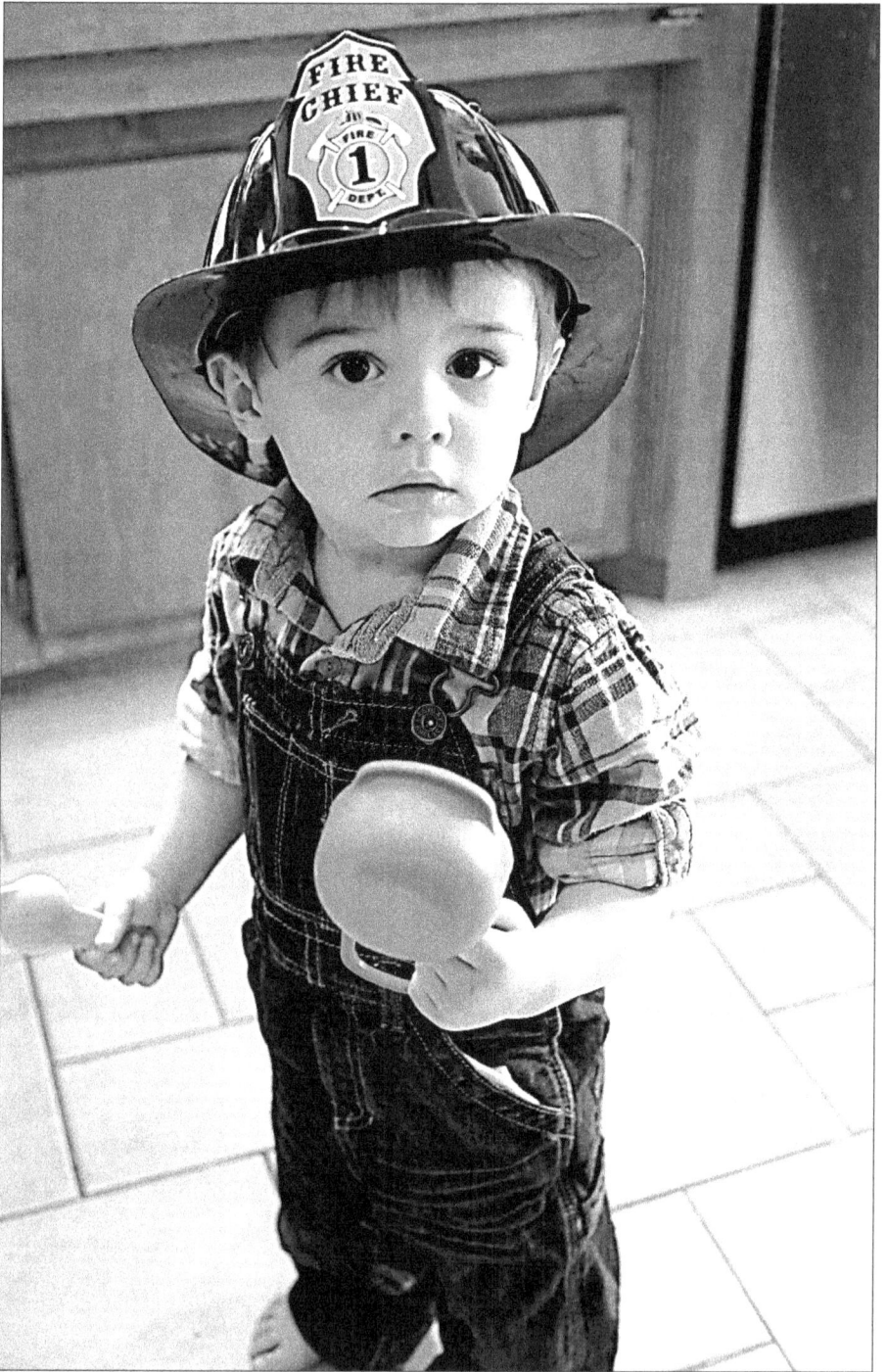

Emmett the FIRE CHIEF – Where's the fly?

THE FLY

You wouldn't think that a harmless little housefly could cause much trouble at a hospital the size of Holy Christian Sinai. But such is not the case. Turf Hopper, the general surgeon, was preparing a patient for gallbladder surgery when, out of the corner of his eye, he noticed a fly in the operating room. A futile attempt was made to kill the little bugger, but, alas, he disappeared under one of the instrument tables. Turf finished the case without incident, but would not let the matter of the fly go unresolved.

At the Operating Room subcommittee, the next day, Turf decided to speak his mind.

"I would like to bring up a very serious matter that until this day has never been discussed," Turf began in a deep, somber tone. "You see, Holy Christian Sinai Hospital has a fly in the operating room."

The room became so quiet you could have heard a pin drop. Flies carry millions of bacteria on their body, the very thing that an operating room abhors.

"I was getting ready to start my gallbladder case, when I saw the little monster out of the corner of my eye," Turf continued. "Now, I want to tell you I've been operating at Holy Christian Sinai for ten years, and I've never before seen a fly in the operating room."

"That's because we've never had a fly in the operating room," Jim Atmoth replied. Jim was the chairman of the Operating Room Subcommittee, and was visibly upset at the prospect of a contaminated insect ruining the sterility of Holy Christian Sinai, which boasted the cleanest operating rooms in town.

"We've got to keep a lid on this thing, Sandy Monarch, the infectious disease nurse responded. "This isn't the kind of thing we want our competition to hear."

"How do you think the little bugger got in?" Turf asked.

"It could have slipped in with the patient," Jim answered.

"Let's be logical," Mo Quito, the urologist, replied. Urologists were fixated on ducts and tubes and secret channels.

"They're renovating the medical records room across from Operating Room One. There's a ventilation duct between the two rooms, and while the duct may be closed, it needs to be sealed to prevent dust and small insects from getting through."

Needless to say, it didn't take long after the meeting ended for news of the insect to fly throughout Holy Christian Sinai Hospital. When the Quality Assurance Committee met two days later, the fly had already been given a name, Alvin, after the chipmunk that always caused trouble.

"As Chairman of the Quality Assurance Committee," Rolyn Poly began, "I'm alarmed that a simple housefly could have so easily slipped past our defenses. We've got contracts with ten HMOs, and the last thing we need is to lose our 'Triple A' rating. This could cost us millions of dollars."

"Alvin must be exterminated before things get out of hand," Dan Raid, the infection control coordinator, replied. A special subdivision of the Safety Control committee was formed. It was decided to look for Alvin on Sunday morning, since the operating rooms were empty that day, as most people were in church, and this would cause the least commotion.

It was quite a motley crew that assembled that morning to hunt down Alvin the fly. Armed with "Mr. Terminator" fly swatters were two urologists, a general surgeon, a scrub tech working overtime, and an infectious disease coordinator to document everything.

Poor Alvin never had a chance. He was spotted sitting on the "A" of the Argon laser control panel when a fly swatter terminated his existence. Just which member of the infection control committee performed the dastardly deed is a mystery to this day.

By the next week, Alvin had become a legend, much to the embarrassment of those involved. The Peer Review Committee even reviewed the case, and determined that the physicians involved had rendered their care in an appropriate and timely fashion.

Poor Alvin even underwent an autopsy and a Covid test. You see, Holy Christian Sinai Hospital has a rule that anyone dying in an operating room within twenty-four hours after admission is a medical examiner's case. The final report stated, "cardiac arrest secondary to massive blunt trauma" as the cause of death, but the hospital intervened and called it a Covid death when the test came back positive.

As I drove home that night, I couldn't help think about Alvin the fly. By the time the incident was over, four committees involving seventeen physicians, three nurses, one infectious disease coordinator, one scrub tech, and one hospital fire safety officer spent a total of twelve man-hours to kill one fly. In the process, they generated thirty-six pages of paperwork and instituted a procedural policy on "The Treatment of Flying Insects in the Operating Room Environment."

The total cost for exterminating Alvin, including lab fees, was $10,500 dollars. Now, who ever said hospitals aren't cost effective?

MY OLD COUNTRY ROAD

When I was a child
I walked off to school
Down a long, winding road
Where the weather was cool.

I'd carry my books
In a bag on my back
I'd carry my lunch
In a brown paper sack.

I'd walk with my sis'
Down that old country road
The wind from the north
Would be blustery and cold!

But then in the Spring
All the fields turned green
With flowers and birds
'Twas a beautiful scene!

The water would rush
Past the old wooden bridge
We'd see the fish jump
As we rounded the ridge!

I still walk this path
As I think about life
How we hustle and run
And fill it with strife!

For though we are many
We travel alone –
We all have to make
That long journey home!

THE GREAT MASQUERADER

As a pre-med student in college at Northwestern, I was working as a busboy on campus at a local sorority on Sheridan Road in Evanston, Illinois to make ends meet. Needless to say, as a full-blown Nerd, I was wet behind the ears.

My job during the first part of the lunch hour was to fill all the water glasses with ice water, as each girl arrived and sat down for her lunch.

Suddenly, I heard one of the girls scream from behind a partition near the lunchroom. The girls at the lunch table simply ignored her and continued with their meal. I poured some more ice water, and then this poor girl screamed again.

"Don't worry about it," one of the girls told me, as I spilled some ice water during one of the screams. "She'll be fine."

But the screaming continued, and finally, my curiosity got the best of me. I calmly put down my pitcher of ice water and quietly walked over to this partition when another scream bellowed out. This poor girl was doubled over in pain, with tears rolling off her cheeks.

I took off my white busboy coat and wrapped it over her shoulders. I noticed that both hands were pressing her right lower abdomen, and that every time she coughed, the pain would get worse.

I decided it was time to take action. I hurried back to the lunch table, put on my white busboy coat, and announced to the girls, "My name is Bill Truewater. I'm a first-year pre-med student and just finished dissecting a frog in anatomy lab, so I know what I'm talking about. I've done a lot of reading, but I worked as an orderly last summer at Lutheran General Hospital in Park Ridge. I have a lot of real-world experience," I boasted.

"This young lady is tender right over McBurney's point in the right lower quadrant," I continued. "She has rebound tenderness and voluntary guarding!"

"The most likely diagnosis is appendicitis, possibly ruptured, causing peritonitis and exquisite pain. Her face is red, and she's breathing fast- she's febrile with tachycardia and tachypnea – I'm afraid she's septic!" I declared.

"Appendicitis is known as The Great Masquerader, but I got this figured out!" I proclaimed. "This is a classic presentation, a slam dunk!"

"She needs emergency surgery and IV antibiotics. We need to get her to the Searle Hall Infirmary right away and get a differential white blood cell count to confirm the diagnosis!" I exclaimed.

None of the girls even looked up – one of them even giggled. Most of them just kept on eating their lunch. I was infuriated.

Finally, one of the girls looked up sympathetically and said, "That's Mary Anne – she does this every month. She's having her period."

Words cannot express how stupid I felt. If there was a hole to crawl into, I would have done so. My face turned a deep shade of red.

But I learned an important lesson. Don't just look at the symptoms. Had I simply asked Mary Anne what was wrong, she would have told me!

I poured some more ice water and resolved to keep my mouth shut for the rest of the lunch hour. Part of making a differential diagnosis is talking to the patient and getting a good history!

One of the girls then said, "You'll make a good doctor someday."

"How's that?" I asked.

"You show compassion," she said.

But there was a bigger lesson here. Among the girls, I detected a quiet support for Mary Anne. They were allowing her to share her pain. But at the same time, the message was to go on with our lives. We must learn to live with our pain, be it Mittelschmerz or Weltschmerz!

In one sense, we are all Masqueraders – putting on a smile despite the frowns!

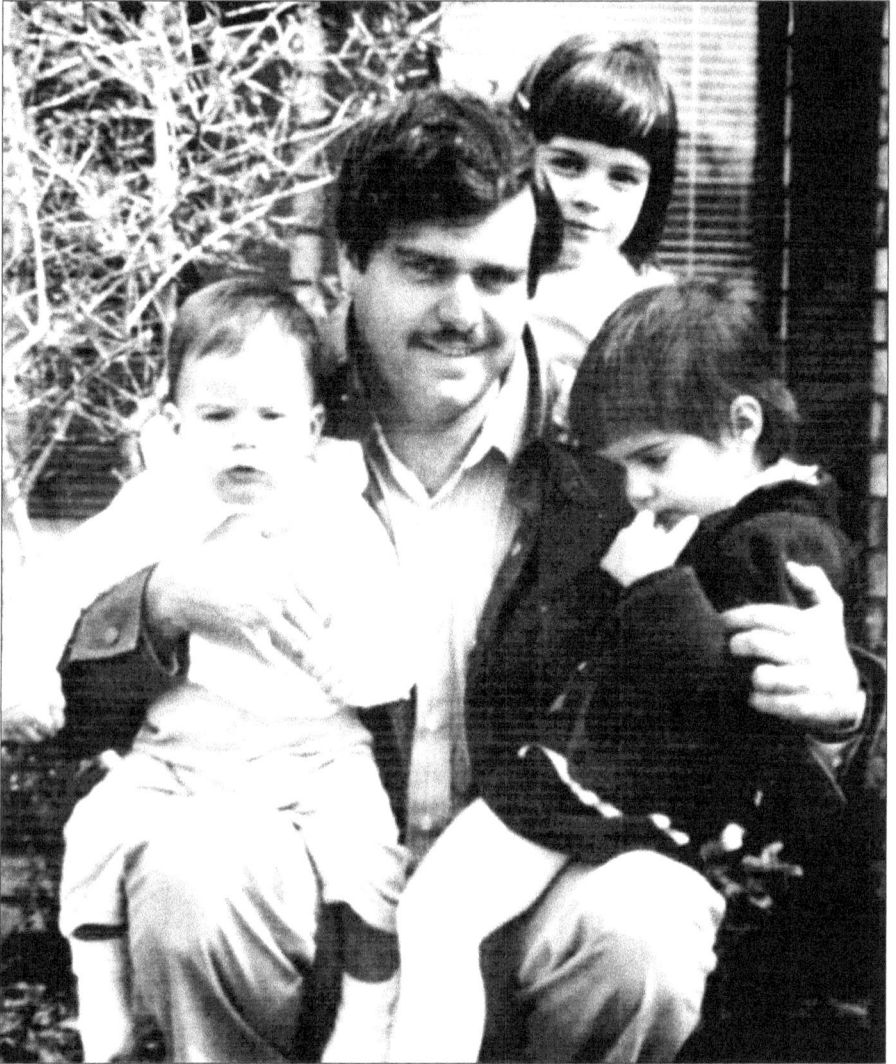

Dr. Truels with his children: Michael, Lisa, and Tracy.

MY DREAM

I made it to a world
That no one else has seen
It's just the kind of place
You'd find in someone's dream!

The world is at peace
There is no need for war
There is no use for weapons
To settle any score.

There are no starving children
There's food for everyone
The children run and laugh and sing
And frolic in the sun.

The air is clean and fresh and pure –
It smells of flowers and spring
It really does my heart some good
To hear the robin sing!

The water flowing in the brook
Plays against the stones
The fish are jumping at my hook –
It's nice to be back home!

MY FIRST CODE BLUE

Probably the one thing I dreaded most as a third-year medical student was the Code Blue. "Code Blue" is a term used by most hospitals indicating that a patient needs emergency resuscitation. I was never exactly sure why they used the term "Code Blue", other than the fact that when someone stops breathing, they turn blue. Some hospitals used the term "Doctor Blue", and I've even heard the term, "Dr. Cardiac". At any rate, the idea was not to alarm other patients and visitors that somebody was about to die (it's bad for business).

I'm sure, however, that not a few visitors wondered why they were asked to avoid using the elevators every time "Dr. Blue" was paged. Perhaps Dr. Blue was so big that no one else could fit in the elevator! Or why interns and medical students would go running through the halls and up and down the stairs every time someone paged "Dr. Blue". They probably thought that "Dr. Blue" was one mean dude!

And if they did figure out what "Dr. Blue" stood for (most of the patients had cracked the code by the second day), what did it mean when the hospital loudspeaker announced, "Cancel the Code Blue"? Had the patient been saved? Were they just going to let him die? Or had he started breathing on his own?

But I'm digressing. As a third-year medical student, the one thing I feared most was being the first one to answer a "Code Blue" – I figured the power of life and death rested in my hands. What if I did the wrong thing? I could kill someone if I gave the wrong drug, or couldn't intubate the patient in an emergency.

To help conquer my fears, I would practice intubating the plastic dummy we called, "George" that was given to our medical school by the Heritage Foundation. I practiced intubating "George" until I could do it blindfolded. Then I took the ACLS life support course and memorized the correct sequence of drugs to use during resuscitation. I gained experience starting IVs and central lines every chance I could get. My group of medical students even had Code Blue practice drills – we'd time ourselves to see how long it would take to get the Crash Cart and start the resuscitation. The "Crash Cart" was the nickname given to the cart that held all the emergency medicine as well as the shock paddles and endotracheal tubes.

Then one night my worst fears came true. I was half-way through my medical rotation at the University. It was two o'clock in the morning. I had just answered a call from Nurse Robinson to start an IV in room 220. This was the first room to the right as you entered the ward. I pulled back the curtain to tell the patient that I would be starting an IV and that I hoped I wouldn't be keeping her up too much longer.

The patient never responded. On closer examination, I noticed that the patient must have just stopped breathing. At that moment, Nurse Robinson came into the room. I bellowed out, "Nurse Robinson, call a Code Blue. We've got a real emergency here. This is no drill!"

"But, Dr. Truewater, the nurse began.

"Don't argue with me!" I interrupted angrily. "There's no time for conversation! Get the crash cart!"

Nurse Robinson looked at the patient and exclaimed, "Dr. Truewater, this patient's dead!"

"Not if I can help it!" I snapped.

Shortly after, some of the other medical students arrived, bringing the crash cart. I had already begun my external cardiac massage, while another student was ventilating the patient with a face mask. When the crash cart arrived, I pulled out an endotracheal tube and, even though she was a little rigid, I managed to pry open the mouth and intubate the patient on the first try. Another of my colleagues had started an IV and given bicarbonate. I was still unable to feel a good pulse, and, in fact, the extremities now felt somewhat cool to touch.

"She's peripherally vasoconstricted," I explained. "I suspect she's going into cardiogenic shock. Pass me the intracardiac epinephrine!"

"But Dr. Truewater," Nurse Robinson began again.

"You'll have to talk to Dr. Lowe outside," I requested. "Pass me the cardiac paddles!" I exclaimed, having had no success with the intracardiac epinephrine.

"Everyone step back from the bed!" I demanded, as I prepared to cardiovert the patient.

In my haste, I had inadvertently spilled some electrode jelly on my scrub pants and failed to stand completely clear of the bed. The only embarrassing moment of the whole resuscitation occurred when I fired the electrode paddles, sending 200 joules of electricity down my left leg. I let out a howl as I fell helplessly to the floor.

Nurse Robinson left the room as I had requested and talked to Dr.

Lowe, my attending physician. I mentally went through my life support check list. We had done everything possible, and yet still the patient showed a straight line on the electrocardiogram.

Dr. Lowe came back into the room and motioned to me. "Dr. Truewater, would you come into the hall for a moment, please?"

I stepped into the hall and recounted my attempted resuscitation procedure to Dr. Lowe. "I did everything I could, Dr. Lowe," I explained, my eyes somewhat watery. "It just wasn't enough!"

Dr. Lowe looked at me sympathetically, sensing my disappointment over not being able to successfully resuscitate my first patient.

He paused for a moment, then said very deliberately, "Don't feel too bad, Dr. Truewater. Jesus Christ himself would have had trouble resuscitating this patient. You see, she was already dead!"

Nurse Robinson finally got her chance to speak. "You see, Dr. Truewater, the patient was terminally ill. She died about thirty minutes ago – that's when Dr. Lowe signed her out. We were just waiting for the family to come for final dispensation."

Just then I remembered that the hospital, for the first time in fifteen years, had just changed room numbers to accommodate their new computer. Room 220 was now at the other end of the hall. I had gone to the wrong room!

Words could not describe my embarrassment. I turned three shades of red. My left leg was still numb from the electric shock. My mouth hung open. I was unable to speak. Besides, what could I say? How do you explain to your attending physician that you just tried to resuscitate a dead patient?

Fortunately for me, Dr. Lowe was in one of his philosophical moods. Twenty years later, I can still remember his advice as clearly as the day he spoke.

"Dr. Truewater," Dr. Lowe began, "There's more to be learned here than the importance of checking the patient chart during a resuscitation and listening to the nurse."

"What you must also remember," Dr. Lowe explained, "Is that we as physicians do not prevent death. We can only hope to delay death and improve the quality of life. The most important role of the physician has not changed in a thousand years – help the family to deal with the loss of their loved one, and never forget the value of compassion. That's what medicine is all about!"

CHANGE OF STATE

I want time to stop –
I'm in a pretty spot –
Things don't have to change –
No need to re-arrange!

I've worked hard to get where I am
I've gotten out of every jam!
Anything now that's new
May put me in a stew!

I suppose I'm getting old –
I'm not quite so bold!
I think and meditate
Upon my present state!

If life stayed the same
I always would remain!
I'd never have to pass
And turn myself to grass!

Such is nature's way
The young will rule the day!
But in all honesty –
That's how I came to be!

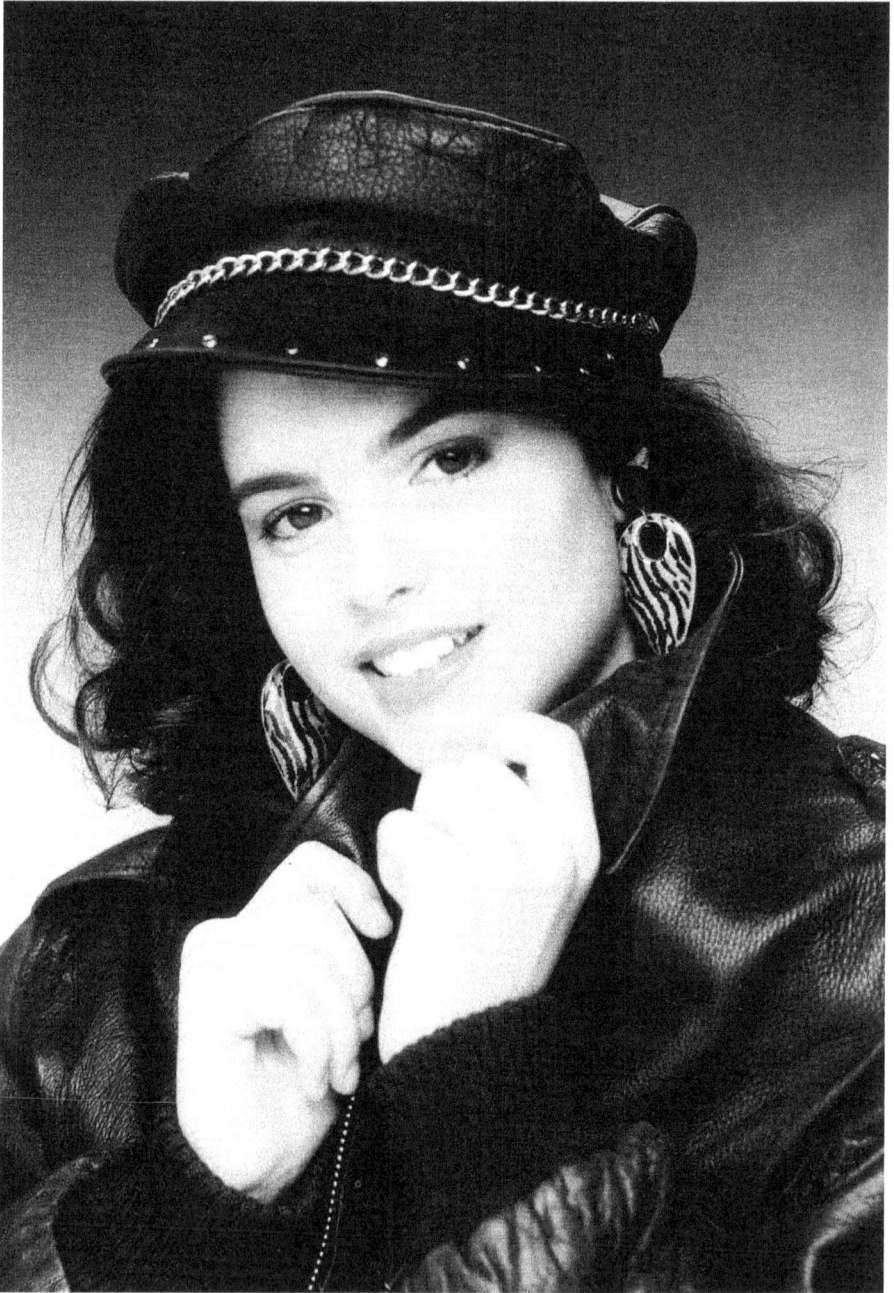

Lisa Truels

MY BEAUTY QUEEN

My teen age girl comes up to me
With a look from off afar
"I had a dream the other night
That I would be a star!"

"Photographers surround me –
I am the beauty queen
My picture's on the cover
Of every magazine!'

"Oh, Father can you tell me
What does this vision mean?
Will I be a famous star
Or is it just a dream?"

I gaze at her a moment
And think about my youth
I dreamed that I could change the world
And make it search for Truth.

"I know not what the future holds,"
I turned to her and smiled,
"But always hold on to your dreams
And go that extra mile!"

"Dreams don't always happen
Just the way we'd like
But they do give us a purpose –
A goal for which to fight!"

"I hope your dreams will all come true
This I'll always pray
Though some may have to change a bit
Upon the light of day."

"But one thing to remember
If times get tough or lean
You'll always be my idol –
You are my beauty queen!"

ON LOOKING YOUNG

My father always used to complain about looking young.

"Whenever I go looking for a job, people always tell me they're looking for someone older!" he would complain.

Little did I realize that when I got older, the same problems would haunt me in the medical profession. While many of my colleagues suffered the ignominious fate of a receding hairline or even premature baldness, I was cursed with a full head of thick, black hair and oily skin that made me look about ten years younger.

At times, this worked to my advantage. One night as a chief resident, I was working late in the Emergency Room sewing up a laceration. About halfway through the closure, my new intern, who was nowhere to be found, suddenly appeared. He was five years my junior, but with his premature baldness, he looked about ten years older.

"Dr. Truewater, may I finish closing the incision?" he asked.

As a courtesy to the patient, I was about to say no, since the closure was somewhat complicated and I was already halfway through the procedure.

To my surprise, the patient, who had been dozing, suddenly spoke up.

"I would prefer, Dr. Truewater, if the intern finished closing the incision," the patient replied. "He looks to be more experienced."

As I prepared to leave, the intern whispered, "What kind of suture should I use to close the skin, Dr. Truewater?"

I whispered back, "Just use your experience!"

With great fanfare, I turned the case over to my intern, handed him the correct suture, and went to sleep for the rest of the night!

At other times, though, looking young can be a distinct disadvantage, especially if you're a surgeon explaining the need for an operation to a nervous patient. More than once I have heard patients whisper as I leave the room, "How old is that doctor?"

Accordingly, during the course of discussing surgery with a patient, I always try to work some reference to my advanced age into the conversation. One time, I had a middle-aged patient from Brooklyn, New York who seemed uneasy about my fixing his hernia.

I casually looked at the chart and said, "I see you're from Brooklyn. Sure was a shame when the Dodgers had to leave Brooklyn!" I complained. Needless to say, I fixed his hernia the same week!

My stepfather was a World War II. veteran and has told me countless stories about his experiences in the South Pacific. One time I had an older patient who was apprehensive about having his gallbladder removed, and I asked him if he was a veteran.

"I sure am a veteran, Doctor," he replied. "I spent four years in the South Pacific and fought in the battle of Okinawa."

"Those kamikazes were lethal," I replied matter-of-factly.

"We knocked three of them down with our six-inch guns," he replied, visibly more at ease. The next day, I removed his markedly inflamed gallbladder.

Another tactic for younger surgeons is to refer to their vast experience. One week, I had removed three gallbladders and was seeing a patient that Friday morning.

"How many of these gallbladders have you removed, Doctor?" the patient asked skeptically, looking at the acne on my face.

"You're the fourth one this week," I replied matter-of-factly. I did his surgery the following Monday.

For a while, I tried wearing my father's bifocal reading glasses. I developed the unique ability of reading out of the top part of the bifocal lenses, which were clear. This added about ten years to my perceived age. After about a month, though, I was getting tired of the headaches and double vision at the end of the day, and reluctantly gave them back to my bemused father!

Lately, my full head of hair has developed some silver streaks, which I initially interpreted as a sign of relief. No longer would I have to convince people of my vast surgical experience or expertise. But, alas, even this development has not solved all my problems.

One day, I was getting ready to schedule my patient for a hernia repair when I detected some apprehension on his part.

"Is there a problem?" I asked.

"Yes, doctor," he replied. "How long have you been in practice?"

"Sixteen years," I confidently responded.

"You probably graduated before they started using lasers," he replied. "I saw an advertisement on TV from the University Hospital. It seems the young surgeons there are using lasers for everything," he added. "Looks to me like lasers are the wave of the future, what with Star Wars and all."

"I've taken two post-graduate courses in laser surgery," I responded defensively. "Lasers have proven themselves in gallbladder surgery, but haven't yet been practical for hernias. In addition, there's a $500 charge for using the laser," I added.

My patient agreed to his outpatient hernia surgery, but I began to wonder if there was ever an ideal age for surgeons. It all came down to one of those good news-bad news stories. I no longer looked too young – I was now beginning to look too old!

THE FALLEN ANGEL

A mallard duck got in the way
Of a busy driver who could not sway!
A dead bird by the side of the road –
A sad site to behold!

The next day I drove by –
A second duck I did spy –
Standing next to his brown mate –
Hoping that she might awake!

The third day that I drove by
He laid down by her side –
How long would he still wait –
And what thoughts did he contemplate?

The fourth day that I drove by –
Two dead ducks I now did spy!
No longer would his heart still ache –
Was it accident or heartbreak?

I parked my car and went inside –
Was this an omen I should bide?
I told my wife, should I die first –
Carry on – for better or worse!

PIRATES AND PRESIDENTS

"It just seemed like once people fell into a system,
they could never find their way out."

The morning air was crisp as I jogged along Canal Street in New Orleans before the last day of my Cardiovascular Horizons annual meeting. Canal Street led to the Riverwalk, where I ran along the boardwalk at the Mississippi River Canal.

I jogged up to an itinerant saxophone player, stopped for a few minutes along the breakwater boulders to listen to this improvising jazz artist, and dropped a few dollars into his basket before resuming my health run.

I had to wind my way past a crowd of tourists, who were boarding the Natchez Steamboat paddle-wheeler for a ride along the Mississippi riverfront, next to the barges and ferries that were busy hauling cargo upstream.

I passed the Jax Brewery, turned down Bienville Avenue toward Jackson Square, then back up Decatur Street toward my hotel. By now, I was a little winded, so I stopped at a park bench at the Jean Lafitte National Preserve.

As I caught my breath, I noticed that I was sitting across from a homeless man. Next to him was a large plastic bag, which most likely contained all his worldly possessions. He was unshaven, wore old ragged clothes, and was holding his head in his hands.

The man lifted up his head, and looked at me for a second or two. I was wearing my jogging outfit with my running shoes, and hanging from my neck was my meeting badge, which served as an I.D. card to get into the lecture halls.

By now, I had caught my breath and thought about getting up.

But the transient quickly eyed my meeting badge and proclaimed, "Dr. Bill Truewater, nice to meet you. My name's Turner Round, but my friends call me Turney."

"Nice to meet you, Turney," I politely replied.

As he caught my eye, I stared down at the empty basket which lay at his feet. I resolved that I would be polite, though I had no intention of dropping him any money.

"Nice morning for a jog," Turney began.

"Yes, it is," I replied. "It's peaceful out here in the morning, before the city wakes up."

"I see lots of people out here every day jogging along the boardwalk, Bill," Turney replied, as he cast his eyes along the waterfront.

"Lots of very busy people, career people for the most part. I see a new batch coming every week – nurses, doctors, lawyers, businessmen and women – all very busy people."

"Why do you think they jog, Dr. Truewater?" Turney asked.

"Well, because it's healthy," I said. "Helps me feel better, too."

"I suppose so," Turney replied. "But, why else do they jog, Doc?"

I really didn't like being put on the spot by a street transient, but I decided to play along.

"Well, I'm a physician," I began, "and I can tell you that jogging will lengthen your life – it keeps your heart in shape. These joggers you see here, they all want to stay in shape and live longer."

"Do you make a good salary, Doc?" Turney asked me.

"Why, yes," I replied. "But I went to four years of medical school after college, and five more years to become a surgeon."

"That's very good, Bill," Turney replied. "You've got me beat by seventeen years of schooling, since I quit after the eighth grade."

"Why did you quit?" I interrupted. "You seem like a pretty savvy person."

"I never liked organized education," Turney replied. "I like to learn things on my own, without a system."

"Did you get a job?" I asked.

"I worked odd jobs for a while," Turney responded, "but I never took to any of the jobs I had."

"It just seemed like, once people fell into a system, they could never find their way out."

"You see, what I really enjoy doing," he continued, "is just sitting here and talking to people – career people like yourself. And, when I'm done, they usually turn around, drop ten or twenty dollars in my basket, and go on."

I laughed. "I mean no disrespect," I quickly added.

"And I don't mean to be rude, Turney, but what could you possibly tell a highly motivated career person like myself that could be so valuable?"

"You know, Doctor, I watch these motivated people, with their cell phones, and their beepers, and their meeting tags jog by me every day, as I sit here in Jean Lafitte Park, and I just have to ask myself, 'Where are they going?'"

"Why, they're going up in the world," I responded. "These are busy people, with goals and ambitions."

"Don't get me wrong," Turney replied. "I admire the work that you doctors do – healing the afflicted, and the disadvantaged. I admire that."

"But tell me about your kids, Doctor."

"My kids?" I asked. "Why, how do you mean?"

"What do your kids think of you, Doctor Truewater?" Turney asked.

"Well, that's getting a little personal," I responded. "But, alright, Turney, I'll play along."

I paused for a moment and reflected, as I watched the Bienville trolley leave Station #5, and the next batch of tourists board the Natchez paddle-wheeler.

"My kids are doing just fine," I responded. "You know, considering they're teenagers and all that."

"They're doing just fine?" Turney asked.

"Well, alright, we've had a few problems," I confessed.

"You know, it's not easy being a doctor's kid – the children try to match their parents' accomplishments, which is hard to do. And if they don't succeed, they feel like they've fallen short of the mark."

"Our family's had problems with drugs and divorce and depression," I admitted. "But we're back on track – we're doing just fine now. There are lots of issues in our modern society today – everybody knows that."

Turney held his head in his hands again.

"You alright?" I asked, as a middle-aged couple in jogging suits strolled by, their meeting badges swinging from their necks like the pendulum of a grandfather clock.

"I'm doing just fine, Bill," Turney mumbled.

"I appreciate your honesty," he continued. "Everybody's so busy these days. It's just that we don't take enough time out to enjoy things, to appreciate life, to spend time with our family and friends," Turney added.

"It's like everyone's on a treadmill, you know, and then they fall off. And then someone else takes their place. Last year, two people dropped dead on this very boardwalk – healthy people, you know, just like yourself. I tried to save them, but it was too late."

"How many hours a week do you work, Dr. Truewater?"

"It depends," I replied, "but it varies between 70 and 100 hours a week."

"That means 70 to 100 hours a week that you're away from your family," Turney said.

"That's true," I replied. "But I play an important role at the hospital. Some people say I'm irreplaceable."

Turney laughed.

"What's so funny?" I asked angrily. "I mean, if you disappeared off this bench tomorrow, how many people would remember you?"

"Not very many," Turney mused. "I mean no disrespect, Dr. Truewater. But how many people really get noticed anyway? You try to make a name for yourself in this world, and what happens?"

"The only people they ever remember are pirates and Presidents," Turney continued, as he cast his gaze along the boardwalk.

"Like Jackson Square over there. Or this national park, named after Jean Lafitte – he was a pirate, you know."

As I stared at Turney, I realized that this sidewalk philosopher taught me more about life in three minutes than I had learned in three days at my cardiology meeting. No one is irreplaceable. Life is short and unpredictable. And the time we spend with our family and friends is the most important time of all.

"Thanks, Turney," I said quietly, as I dropped a twenty dollar bill in his basket. "I hope you get to feeling better."

I decided to skip the last day of my meeting, turned around, and took the next plane home.

I spent the rest of Sunday with my family, talked to my wife and each of my three kids for an hour apiece, and enjoyed the best day of my life. I didn't necessarily solve any of their problems, but I let them know I was on their side, and that I was always available to help them.

That evening, we walked along the Lake Hefner waterfront, then sat down to watch the sailboats and the kites.

"It's funny," I told my kids, as we sat on the park bench and looked out over the sailboats as they skimmed along the lake.

"Enjoy the time you spend with your family. Careers are important. But nobody's irreplaceable."

"And the only ones they ever remember are pirates and Presidents."

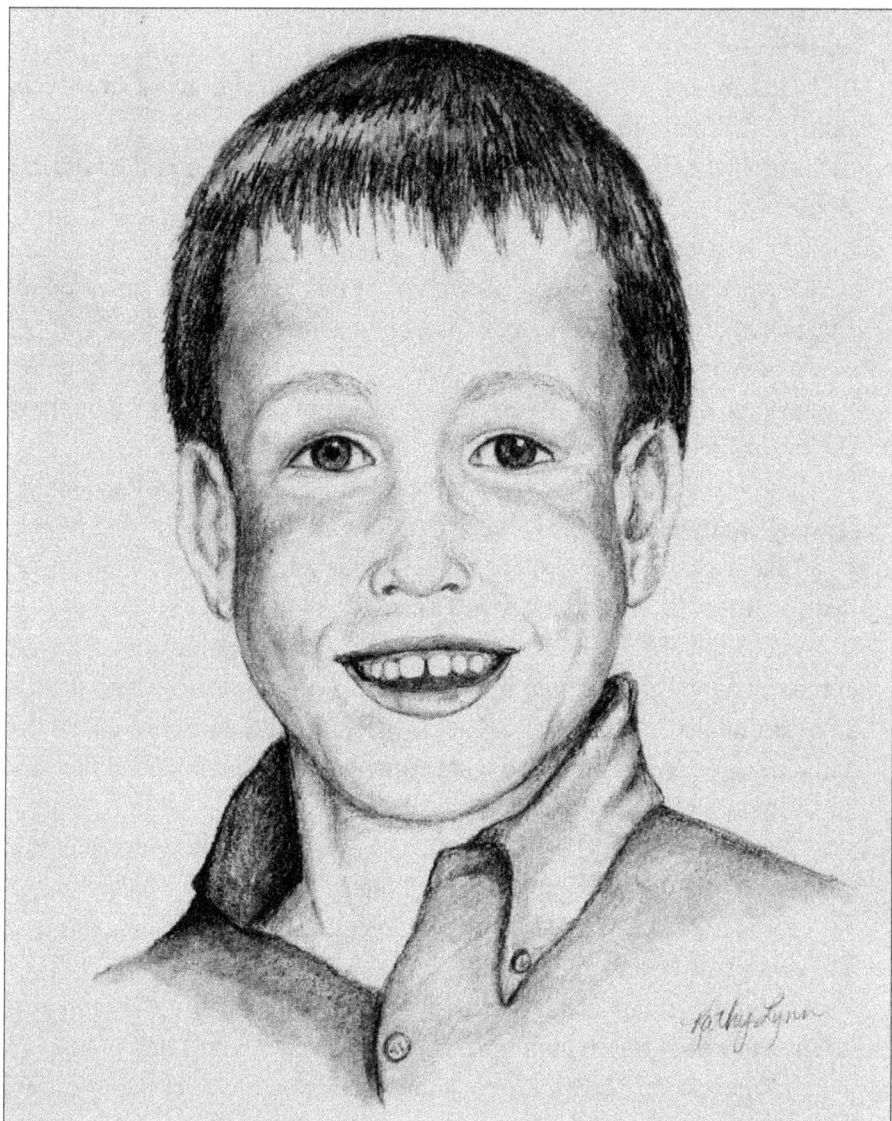

Blake Martin lives in Cedar Valley, Oklahoma, with his two brothers, Bo and Nash, and his parents, Jeanne and Jeff Martin. Blake is an excellent student and avid golfer.

BLAKE

My name is Blake
I cannot hear
But I'm really
Quite a dear!

I'm seven years old
Yet I can read
I'm the smartest kid
You've ever seen!

I catch things
That others miss –
The slightest smile
The softest kiss.

Sometimes the lips
That shape the words
Can tell you more
Than if you heard!

The way you let
Your fingers play
Can tell me more
Than words could say.

Sometimes I wish
I wasn't deaf
But make the most
Of what you get!

When people come
I'm first to greet
I feel the wood
Shake 'neath my feet.

I like to golf
And putt the greens
My dad's the best
You've ever seen.

My two brothers
Treat me right
But my mom
Is really nice!

My name is Blake –
I'm pretty proud
You need not say
My name too loud!

MY FIRST STETHOSCOPE

Most doctors remember their first stethoscope, almost as fondly as their first car or their first date. The stethoscope is the first instrument a medical student buys. It symbolizes one's future role as a physician, and marks a rite of passage into a world of life and death decisions.

The purchase of the proper stethoscope is thus an extremely important matter, not to be taken lightly if the correct diagnosis is to be made.

"Which stethoscope is the best one?" I asked Bradley Chastain, my dormitory roommate. Brad was at the top of the class and always had the best answer, no matter what you asked him.

"Some of them have single tubes and some of them have double tubes," Brad began. "In my opinion the double tube model is better because you can hear twice as much sound. You could miss a subtle heart murmur or diagnostic "click" with the single tube model," Brad explained.

Accordingly, our group of five all got on the Chicago elevated train to go downtown and purchase our double-lumen stethoscopes. We always traveled in our group of five – that was how we were assigned alphabetically to the cadavers. Trefzger, Truels, Truewater, Turner, and Tylkowski – we all shared cadaver number fourteen. We studied together, played basketball together, and on Friday nights we'd all go out and eat pizza together.

None of us knew each other before medical school and we rarely saw each other again, after our training was completed. But in those days, we all shared one common bond – the desire to complete medical school and get on with our lives.

When we arrived at the medical supply store, we looked at all the stethoscopes. The length of the tubing, the size of the bell and diaphragm portions of the stethoscope, even the type of earpiece were all vitally important considerations. The hottest selling stethoscope was the Lumiscope, a Japanese copy of the highly-touted Rappaport-Sprague, for about half the price. We each bought one and carved our initials and the date, 1-7-69, on the bell.

Needless to say, we were all so excited about our new purchase that we decided to wear our stethoscopes on the way home. We tried to act casual, as the people on the subway train wondered why we were wearing stethoscopes around our necks. Certainly, we were too young to be doctors! I even fantasized someone on the subway suddenly developing a heart attack, forcing my stethoscope into active duty to save the day!

My stethoscope would serve me well until I decided to become a surgeon. I would proudly wear the stethoscope around my neck during rounds or when seeing a new patient. I always felt that it lent a sort of professional credibility that overcame my otherwise youthful demeanor. However, the first day on surgery, my junior resident, Alvin Delaney, read me the riot act.

"Dr. Truewater, do you wish to become a surgeon?" Alvin asked in a rather crude tone of voice.

"Most certainly," I replied.

"Then you need to know something about stethoscopes," Alvin replied brusquely.

"I know quite a bit about stethoscopes," I said. "I studied them quite thoroughly as a first-year medical student. The double lumen types give the best audio resolution," I declared.

"That's not what I mean, Truewater," Alvin replied. "The first thing you need to know is that surgeons don't use double lumen stethoscopes. They use single lumen stethoscopes. And they don't wear them around their necks – they stick them in their back pockets!"

"No problem," I replied. "Single lumen stethoscopes are almost as good, anyway."

"You're missing the point, Truewater," Alvin rebutted, grasping my stethoscope and throwing it fifty feet down the old marble floor of the Cook County surgery ward.

"You see, Dr. Truewater," Alvin continued, as I watched my beloved double lumen stethoscope go bouncing down the hallway. "Stethoscopes are used for making diagnoses – internists make diagnoses. Surgeons act!"

"But I don't understand," I replied. "Don't you have to make the diagnosis before you can act?"

"Not in every instance," Alvin responded. "Sometimes you have to take the bull by the horns and operate, even if you don't know the exact diagnosis!"

"And you certainly don't need a cardiologist's stethoscope to listen to bowel sounds!" Alvin continued.

Thirty years later, my wife and I were cleaning the attic. This is always a painful experience for me, as I'm sort of a pack rat and try to hold on to everything I've ever owned. My wife, Margaret, on the other hand, believes in getting rid of unnecessary items that do nothing but gather dust in the attic.

"Do you need this old, broken stethoscope?" Margaret asked, as she held up my beloved Lumiscope.

I looked at my stethoscope, with the old, fractured bell. The double lumen tubing was cracked with age in several places, and the special earpieces had long since disappeared. I wiped off the bell with a rag and saw my initials inscribed, along with the date, 1-7-69.

"That thing looks like it's been through the war!" Margaret added.

"It has!" I replied, as I carefully placed my beloved stethoscope back in its original box. "It's been through the school of Hard Knox. You know, it's hard to believe, but this stethoscope is over thirty years old!"

I've since had my stethoscope restored and mounted on the wall in my office.

"That looks like your original stethoscope!" a patient commented one day during her post-operative visit. I'll bet that means a lot to you!"

"It does," I replied. "I can still remember the day I bought it."

"Do surgeons need stethoscopes?" my patient asked innocently.

"Certainly," I replied. "But surgeons carry stethoscopes in their back pocket, so they won't be confused with internists. You know, it always helps to make the correct diagnosis before you operate!"

PEEPER

We watched through our back window
As the storm blew through the trees
A little nest fell to the ground
Covered by some leaves.

"Those baby doves are really cute,"
My Father turned and said,
"But with their Mom and Daddy gone
They surely will be dead."

I took them both into the house
And made some stew with meat
I fed them with a little stick
To open up their beaks.

Next morning I went to the cage
And I began to cry
One little bird was wide awake
The other one had died.

I picked the little birdie up
He turned to me and peeped
Peeper got his name that day
His brother went to sleep.

Peeper found some feathered friends
They flew up high above
He'd show them he was strong and brave
Just like other doves!

One day Peeper chirped away
Do little birdies cry?
He looked at me and flapped his wings
As if to say good-by!

Peeper never did come back
He flew off in the blue
But every time I see a dove
I always think of you!

THE EYES HAVE IT

My most valuable lesson in patient relations came from an ophthalmologist shortly after I entered private practice. Now, you may wonder how an ophthalmologist could help a general surgeon build his practice. Let me explain.

I was sipping coffee in the Holy Christian Sinai Hospital surgery lounge bemoaning the fact that I had lost a surgical referral to one of my colleagues.

"I just don't understand it," I complained. "I maintained a friendly, professional demeanor, explained the operation in detail to the patient, and I was courteous and polite throughout the interview."

"What happened next?" Seymore Clearly the busy ophthalmologist asked.

"The patient had her gallbladder out two days later by one of my competitors," I complained.

"I guess I just look too young," I added.

"That's not the problem, Truewater," Seymore replied.

"How would you know?" I snapped back. "All you do is look at eyes all day."

"The eyes have it, Dr. Truewater," Seymore replied, with a broad smile.

"Seymore, what could you possibly know about talking a patient into a gallbladder operation, which they obviously need, but don't' want?" I asked.

"Your entire physical exam is limited to two square inches of the patient's body," I added sarcastically.

"But that's an important two inches, Dr. Truewater," Seymore replied. "You see, patients know that they need surgery, but they still have to be convinced."

"But what do the eyes have to do with it?" I asked.

"When you first meet a patient, Dr. Truewater, look them directly in the eyes. Be honest, open, and direct. And always sit down when you're talking to the patient, preferably with your eyes at the same level. Let them know you've got the time to sit and talk with them."

"Sounds reasonable," I replied. "But, I'm doing that already."

"That's just the first step, Truewater," Seymore replied. "Next, you take them back to the exam room, and take their blood pressure."

"But I already know their blood pressure," I answered. "It's on the chart from the referring doctor."

"Then you have them lay down on the exam table and check their gallbladder," Seymour continued.

"But I already know the gallbladder's abnormal," I replied. "Remember? That's the reason they were sent to me – they have symptomatic gallbladder disease, and need to have gallbladder surgery."

"It's easier to skip the exam, and set them up on the surgery schedule," I continued. "Remember, a lot of these patients are still hurting – having them lie down on the exam table may cause even more pain."

"Truewater, Truewater," Seymore replied sympathetically. "How can I put this politely?"

"Let me just say that if you can't get the patient to lay down on the exam table in your office, you're not going to get them to lay down on the operating table for surgery."

"Why not?" I asked.

"Because, Truewater," Seymore replied, "what do people think of when they think of surgery?"

"Why, I always remind them of all the modern advances, technological miracles, lasers, new laparoscopic techniques, and opportunities for feeling better," I answered.

"True enough," Seymore replied. "But what do people worry about when you mention surgery, Dr. Truewater?"

"Death, Truewater," Seymore replied before I could answer. "People are worried that they're going to have surgery and die."

"But, what does that have to do with examining them in the office?" I asked.

"Two things, Truewater," Seymore replied. "First, you're telling them that you care enough to take the time and trouble to examine them."

"Secondly, when you examine somebody, your eyes are temporarily above them – that means that they're trusting you to take care of them. Examine them – gently, of course, and let them know you're willing to take charge, and they can trust you."

"When you get right down to it, Truewater," Seymore continued, "your entire surgical interview has only one purpose – build trust with the patient."

"Of course, you're doing all the things that are medico-legally correct – explaining the operation and its' potential complications. But what you're really doing, Truewater, is building trust with the patient."

"You're absolutely right, Seymore," I replied. "I thought I knew it all when I finished my residency. You know, you spend six years learning the technical aspects of being a surgeon, but you've still got to convince the patient that you're the surgeon they want."

"One other thing I like to do that they don't mention in the textbooks," Seymore continued. "Ask a personal question such as their occupation, or maybe a hobby, or how the family is doing. It's a personal touch, but it means a lot – it shows you care about them as a human being."

"I feel like I have to be a salesman, a preacher, and a surgeon all rolled into one," I added.

"You'll learn with experience, Dr. Truewater," Seymore smiled, as he headed into surgery.

"Remember, look directly into the patient's eyes, be honest, treat them as human beings with understandable fears and anxieties, develop their trust, and watch your practice grow!"

TIPS FOR MEDICAL STUDENTS

I remember my medical student days when some outspoken intern, resident, or even attending would ask some question which would leave me completely flabbergasted and embarrassed in the presence of my peers. But, alas, there is hope! As a practicing surgeon who has worked with medical students, here are a few tips which can be extremely helpful.

The first thing a medical student needs to cultivate is what I call the "disheveled look". The hair must be slightly messed, the collar or tie slightly askew, and the skirt or pants must be ever so slightly wrinkled. In the case of women, pale make-up is in order. When outdoors, both male and female students must always wear sun block to prevent the development of a tan during the summer months.

The disheveled look gives your attending physician the appearance that you have been up all night taking care of patients. The pale look suggests that you have been spending your time at home reading medical books instead of enjoying the summer sun.

Next, you must develop what I call the "enlightening nod". While you need not listen to what your attending is saying, learn to smile and nod whenever he pauses, as if suddenly receiving some pearl of wisdom that will forever change your life. If you have a note pad handy, pretend to furiously scribble for a few seconds, as if preserving his words for posterity.

Now comes the hard part. Your attending physician singles you out during rounds, and asks some obscure question that nobody is able to answer.

For example, your attending may say, "Tell me, Dr. Truewater, what is your recommended treatment for decubitus ulcers in light of the work by Ramrod and colleagues at the Brigham using white mice with wet pressure patches?"

Now, rather than stammering and stuttering for the first few seconds, the first thing you must do is force yourself not to speak. You must learn what I call the "meditative pause."

For five long seconds, you say and do absolutely nothing as you look your attending straight in the eye. A deep, introspective sigh may also be employed to add drama to the moment. This gives the impression that you are mentally reviewing a vast amount of information about decubitus ulcers and white mice stored in your memory banks. Looking your attending physician straight in the eye convinces him that you are not afraid or insecure (which, of course, you are).

Regardless of the question, the first sentence of your answer must always be the same. You must know that surgeons pride themselves on being hard-driving, industrious, and capable of curing all medical and social problems. Surgeons would much rather make an error of commission than omission.

Your first statement should be uttered with almost religious conviction: "I think it's important to be aggressive in treating this problem."

Of course, feel free to expand on the above idea. For example, you might add, "I hate treating decubitus ulcers conservatively. Too often, the conservative approach does nothing more than waste time and money. You still end up taking these people to surgery."

Oftentimes, the above explanation is sufficient. However, your examiner may want you to be more specific. In this case, tell him or her what you know about the subject, but use what I call "battlefield terminology".

In the above example, you might say, "Aggressive local debridement would be my first plan of attack. If that fails, then I'd pull out the big guns and rotate a skin flap. Of course, I'd have to protect my rear with triple antibiotic therapy to combat the very real risk of infection."

If you are in oil-drilling states like Oklahoma or Texas, you might say that you'd have to do a "deep dive" on the subject and review the latest literature.

If your attending physician presses you for more information, you'll have to pull out your ace in the hole. Every prospective medical student should read a book about some famous deceased surgeon, such as Warren Cole or William Halsted. Whenever surgeons get together, they always share some tidbit that their professor taught them in residency thirty years before, no matter how trivial or unimportant it might seem to the uninitiated. Whenever they speak of this man or woman, there is a warm glow on their face as if revering the very teachings of Christ or Mohammed.

Thus, when your attending presses you for more information, simply roll your eyes upward, as if looking to heaven, and say, "William Halsted believed in the principles of meticulous hemostasis and close approximation of skin edges for proper wound healing. Those principles are just as important today as they were one hundred years ago!"

Your attending may press you on Halsted's principles of wound healing, but these you've already committed to memory. You've now successfully switched the subject from white mice with decubitus ulcers to something more familiar and easy to recall. Your friends are dazzled and amazed at your vast knowledge, and your attending is convinced that he's recruited another outstanding surgical candidate!

Author's disclaimer to medical students: the above article was written in jest. Please do not try this with your own attending physician!

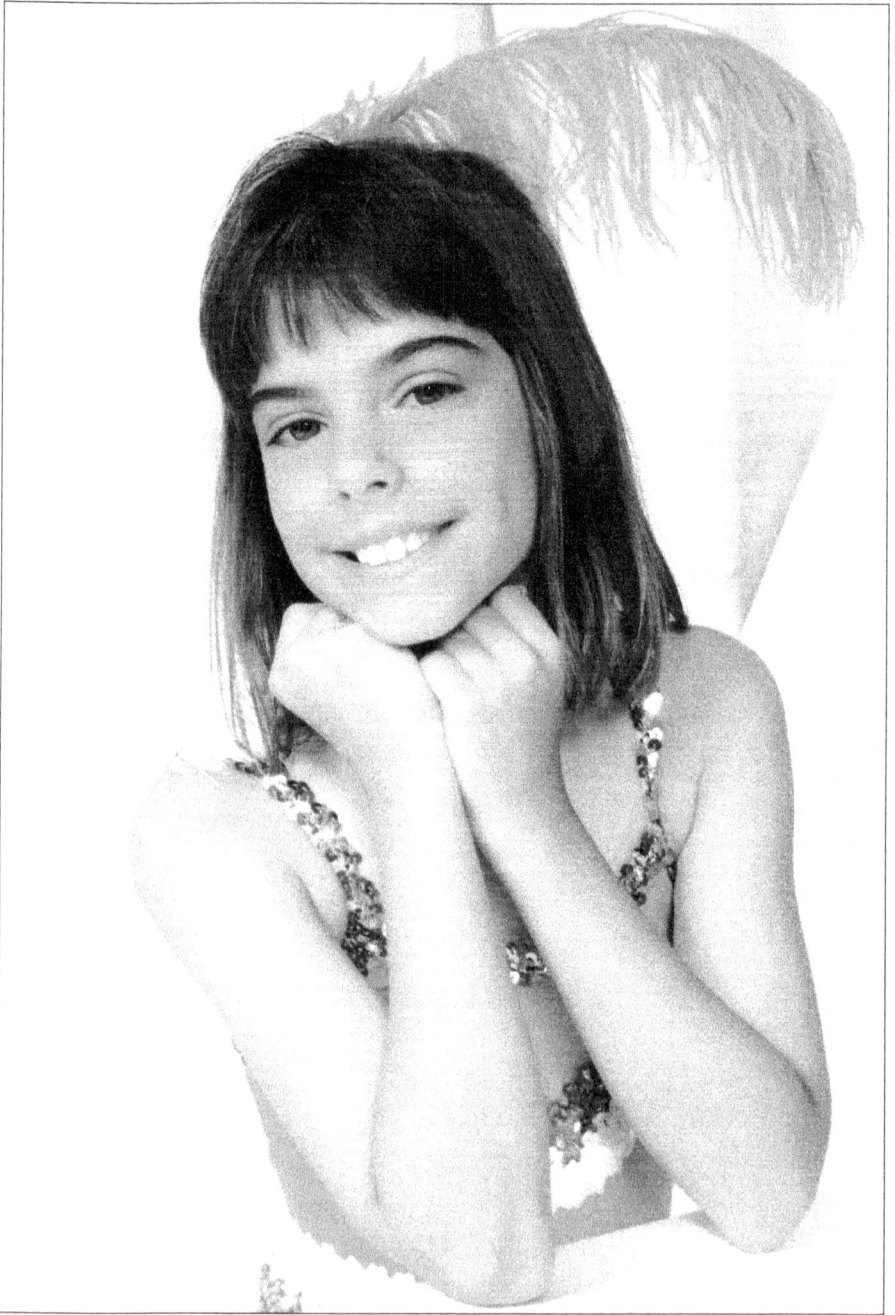

Tracy Truels, the ballerina.

AM I PRETTY?

My little girl sits on my knee
She's almost eight years old
"Am I pretty? Am I smart?
This I'd like to know."

"I see the boys in second grade
Grin and wink their eyes
Am I really all that cute
Or do they fib and lie?"

"I don't know what the others see,"
I turn to her and smile,
"But I think you're the cutest girl
I've seen in quite a while."

"But beauty is a funny thing
Like flowers in the field
You must learn to appreciate
You're as pretty as you feel!"

MAKING CONTACT

My teen-age daughter and I were suffering from a failure to communicate. I attended a CONTAK session at our church, in hopes of finding a solution (the letters stood for COuNseling for parents of Teen-Age Kids.) The speaker, Harry Petersen, was a drug rehabilitation counselor for teen-age children.

"The only way to understand today's generation of kids is to make contact," Harry began. "Talk turkey with them. Take time to learn their language. It shows them that you care, and that you're willing to communicate! Remember, everything's cool!" Harry concluded.

When I got home that evening, I couldn't wait to call my daughter, Lisa, into the living room for a friendly father-to-daughter chat.

"Lisa," I said, "teach me some of your vocabulary words."

"Dad, some of the words I know, you don't want to hear!" Lisa responded.

"No, no," I replied. "That's not what I meant. Let me give you an example. A long time ago, believe it or not, I was in high school, just like you! There were two groups of kids, greasers and snobs."

"The greasers earned their name because they liked to put oil in their hair and make it shiny. Greasers liked to work on cars and were planning to go to a trade school," I continued. "Some of them were quite talented."

"They usually wore leatherjackets, smoked cigarettes in the washroom, wore patent leather shoes and never opened a book."

"My Dad was actually kicked out of Lane High School in 1937 in Chicago for smoking. Then, when he got drafted in 1942, the government gave him a gun and handed out free Lucky Strike cigarettes!"

"Today, we call them skaters," Lisa interrupted.

"Skaters?" I asked.

"Yes," Lisa responded. "They own a skateboard and practice at school during recess. They usually wear baggy pants, multi-colored tennis shoes, and T-shirts to school."

"The other group we had when I was in high school were called the snobs," I continued. "The snobs wore dress slacks or Levi jeans, penny loafers, and usually shirts with button-down collars. The snobs prided themselves on studying, cheerleading, and student counsel activities."

"We call them preppies," Lisa replied. "Preppies are wearing penny loafers again, like the dorks they are. They wear designer jeans, leather jackets, and Polo shirts, or some other logo."

"You mean," I asked, "that Beverly Hills Polo Club shirt we waited in line for over an hour at that restaurant in Chicago is now gathering dust in the closet?"

"I never wear it!" Lisa replied firmly, as she got up with her skateboard and walked toward the door.

"Where are you going?" I asked.

"Skateboarding," she replied. "I don't want people to think I'm a poser."

"What's a poser?" I asked.

"A poser is somebody who claims to be a skater or a preppie, but really isn't," Lisa replied.

"Did we leave anybody out?" I asked.

"No," Lisa replied, "except for the geeks and nerds."

"I'm afraid to ask!" I exclaimed.

"Geeks and nerds – you know – those kids that are real smart, wear adhesive tape on their glasses, usually button their shirts wrong, wear butterfly collars, and carry books home from school," Lisa explained.

I looked down at my open butterfly collar. Only last week the dog had broken my eyeglasses, and I had repaired them with adhesive tape. There was no doubt as to which group I belonged.

"Well, gotta be going, Dad," Lisa added impatiently, as she walked toward the front door with her skateboard tucked under her arm. "I'm really glad we had this heart-to-heart talk!"

"Me too," I added. "Everything's cool!"

That night I had the strangest dream. I dreamed my future son-in-law was coming to meet me, and ask for my daughter's hand in marriage. He was standing on a skateboard, had black, shiny hair, wore patent leather shoes, and offered to tune up my car every spring, if I let him marry my daughter.

"I woke up screaming, lunging for his throat, and yelling, "You're just a poser!" before my wife managed to wake me up.

"Wake up, Bill! It's only a nightmare!" Margaret yelled. "By the way," she asked, "what were you dreaming about?"

I paused for a moment's reflection.

"Everything's cool!" I finally responded, when my pulse returned to normal. "I just made contact with my future son-in-law!"

THE OPEN CHART

Holy Christian Sinai Hospital has an "open chart policy", which it prides itself on maintaining. At any time they wish, patients are free to "browse" through their hospital chart to see how their progress is coming. Oftentimes, however, patients misinterpret what they read, as medical jargon can be misleading.

I was making rounds one night on Jenny Ulster, a middle-aged woman who had recently undergone a hemorrhoidectomy.

"Hello, Mrs. Ulster!" I began. "How are you doing today?"

"Not very well, Dr. Truewater. I'd like to check out," Jenny answered abruptly.

"It's a little early," I replied. "You just had your hemorrhoid surgery yesterday. Anything wrong?"

"I read the nurse's notes, and I decided those nurses don't like me. One of the nurses described me as 'a middle-aged woman who appears her stated age.' Now, Dr Truewater, most of my friends tell me that I look younger than my stated age!"

"Oh, that's just medical jargon," I replied sympathetically. "Sometimes we say a patient looks older than her stated age if we suspect some undiagnosed problem or stress."

"Then another nurse wrote that I had a 'good noc'," Jenny continued. "I don't remember anybody knocking into me last night!"

"That's Latin," I replied. "The word 'noc' in Latin means night – it just means you slept well, Jenny."

"And what about the nurse who described me as a 'well-developed, well-nourished female'?" Jenny asked. "Was that a polite way of saying I'm overweight?"

"No, no Jenny," I answered. "That's just medical jargon for a healthy-looking patient."

"And what does this mean: 'Patient denies illegal drug usage'? Of course I deny illegal drug usage. I've never taken anything illegal in my entire life!"

"I know that, Jenny," I replied. "Nobody's accusing you of taking drugs. That's just more medical slang."

Jenny looked at me rather suspiciously, like she wasn't sure if I was telling the truth, or just trying to dig my way out of a difficult and embarrassing situation – I was actually doing both.

"That's all well and good, Dr. Truewater," Jenny finally rebutted.

"But I'd still like to check out. You see, after I read the nurse's notes, I went on to read the doctor's notes."

"I can explain everything," I began.

"First of all," Jenny interjected, "I'd like to know why they call them 'progress notes'. Most of the patients around here don't look like they're making too much progress!"

"I'm not sure," I answered. "I guess it's because we doctors always like to emphasize the positive."

"Then, why did you describe me as a 'rectal spazz?'" Jenny asked indignantly, as she re-adjusted her hemorrhoidal heating pad. "That doesn't sound very positive to me!"

"No, no," I explained. "I wrote that you're suffering from 'rectal spasm' as a result of your hemorrhoidal disease. That's why we did the surgery. Your rectal muscles were in a state of spasm."

"Well, the handwriting wasn't the clearest I've ever seen," Jenny responded. "It took my ex-husband and sister two hours to decipher four progress notes!"

"Well, I admit to not writing very clearly," I answered. "But you should know you're one of my star patients, Mrs. Ulster," I reassured her.

"Perhaps so," Jenny responded. "But why did you describe me as a chronic smoker and an S.O.B.!" Jenny complained, as she fought back the tears. "I've been trying for years to quit smoking! And now you think I'm an S.O.B.!" Jenny sobbed.

"And what's this about 'morbid obesity'? I'm a little overweight, that's all. What's morbid about that?"

I now realized that reading the patient chart had become a traumatic experience for Jenny, and I sat down next to her to try to assuage her feelings.

"Jenny, 'morbid obesity' is just a term we use for people who need to lose weight," I explained. "It's not meant to be derogatory."

"And 'S.O.B.' just stands for 'shortness of breath' – I wasn't trying to cast any aspersions on your character. You've had some shortness of breath as a result of your cigarette smoking. That's all. It's medical jargon. We use medical abbreviations as a form of shorthand all the time."

As I left the room, I vowed that I would write more legibly, and never use medical abbreviations again. They were simply too confusing for patients – and probably other medical personnel – to understand.

"Thanks for spending the time to explain those medical terms and abbreviations, Dr. Truewater," Jenny replied. "I realize you've had a long day, and it's getting late."

"No problem," I answered.

"Oh, and one more thing," Jenny smiled.

"What's that?" I asked.

"Have a good 'noc', Doc!"

THE VALUE OF HONESTY

Dear Jesse,

I am honored by your selection of me to discuss the value of honesty as a practicing physician. As I look back, I view honesty as an inborn trait. The young baby or child, with wide open eyes and undeveloped bias, looks at the world with a purity and openness that we adults can only envy. In the words of the romanticist, William Wordsworth, "the child is the father of the man."

As we mature, our perceptions become clouded by our experiences. We call this the learning process. We learn to judge the world around us. And we develop barriers between ourselves and other human beings. We become competitive and learn to place ourselves first.

The "survival of the fittest" becomes the basis for a "me first" philosophy, not only in business, but in our personal lives. Dishonesty thus arises as an attempt to place ourselves first. We deny some part of the truth for what we perceive as a greater gain.

What, then, is the value of honesty? As a practicing physician, I can say that honesty builds trust. This is far more important than any transient gain from lying or dishonesty. With trust, one builds permanent friendships, and with friends, we are never alone.

Good luck, Jesse, with your future career!

Your friend,

– *Bill Truels, M.D.*

Author's Note: the above letter was written in response to a request by Jesse White, a student at McGuiness High School in Oklahoma City, to discuss the value of honesty.

PUT MORLEY IN THE BRINE!

"Do you want to go on a deep-sea fishing trip for physicians, Dr. Truewater?" Phil asked me, as I sat in the doctor's lounge waiting for my case to start.

Phil was my scrub tech, but had a 100-ton Master Pilot's license. He had organized several deep-sea Pacific fishing trips that traveled over 1,000 miles out of San Diego in his 122-foot boat, past Guadalupe Island.

"What do you fish for?" I asked.

"Tuna," Phil replied. "It's quite a challenge."

"Tuna?" I asked. "Aren't those the little fish that come in the tiny cans?"

"Those are sardines," Phil laughed. "No, tuna come in all sizes. Why, on the last trip, Dr. Atkinson from Okarche caught a 200-pound cow."

"I didn't think cows could swim," I quipped.

"No, a cow is a large female tuna," Phil laughed again. "I can see you're in dire need of some deep-sea fishing experience."

"The trip sounds interesting" I answered. "How'd your last trip go?"

"It was very successful," Phil replied. "Each doctor caught at least one tuna as well as dorado and wahoo. We had fifteen doctors on a sixteen-day excursion."

"We left out of San Diego, and each doctor said it was the trip of a lifetime."

"Sounds fantastic," I replied.

"Well, except for one doctor," Phil added.

"One doctor?" I asked.

"Dr. Morley Oaks," Phil replied. "He didn't have such a good time."

"Well, let me qualify that," Phil added.

"For the first eight days, Dr. Oaks – he told us to just call him Morley--had a great time – the time of his life, he kept telling me."

"Then what happened?" I asked.

"Well, Morley was about 60 years old. He worked for 30 years as a cardiologist in Kingfisher. Never got to spend his money. But that's what kids are for."

"Anyway, Morley had been out in the sun and the salt breeze for sixteen hours a day for the previous eight days, and he got all excited – he managed to hook a big tuna cow. I guess you could call it a heart stopping experience."

"You see, tuna herd their prey, forcing smaller fish such as anchovy and herring to the surface in an ever-smaller circle. We were in the middle of this circle, and all the docs were getting some action."

"Sounds exciting," I replied.

"That's when I noticed Morley – he'd hooked into a yellowfin cow tuna and was getting spooled. Then he sort-of slumped against the side rail and dropped his fishing reel."

"What'd the other docs do?" I asked.

"Well, one of the other docs quick grabbed his reel as it went skittering across the deck – they knew Morley had hooked a big one."

"No, I mean what did they do for Morley?"

"Well, there was really nothing they could do. I mean, his buddies tried to resuscitate him – they pounded on his chest and all that, but it was no use. Besides, we were four days – 850 miles – from the nearest civilized land, and we didn't have a satellite phone."

"So then what happened?" I asked.

"Well, we left Morley on the deck so we could reel in his cow. Then, after the tuna left, we all gathered in a circle. One of the doctors – his name was Grule – had spent two years in seminary school before going to medical school, and he said a small prayer for Morley."

"That was very considerate," I said. "It must have been a solemn occasion."

"Dr. Grule said that Morley had been a good doctor, and that the same God that watched over the tuna watched over Morley."

"He said that just as Morley had reeled in the tuna, God had chosen to reel in Morley. It was very touching. There wasn't a dry eye on the boat."

"I imagine you must have cut the trip short, and headed back," I said. "It must have been a somber return home."

"Well, not quite," Phil replied. "The fourteen remaining doctors took a vote – we had two more days of fishing left, so we decided to continue the excursion."

"You kept on fishing after Morley died?" I asked.

"What was the vote?"

"Thirteen to one," Phil replied. "One of the doctors – I think he was a plastic surgeon – got seasick."

"Well, life must go on," I answered. "But what'd you do with Morley?"

"We wrapped him in his fishing gear and threw him in the brine, next to his cow tuna."

"You threw Morley in the brine?" I asked.

"Sure, I mean, what else could we do? He was dead, after all. We put him on top, and face up, to show respect. We even left on his fishing cap. He floated there for eight days before we got back."

"Well, what did Morley's wife say when you got back to shore?" I asked.

"I called her on the phone and gave her the bad news. She cried for a few minutes, then she said that's what Morley would have wanted."

"Why would Morley have wanted that?" I asked.

"Well, you know, to die while you're doing what you love most – no ventilators, no electric shock, just go in peace."

"Let's face it," Phil added. "Life – sometimes just staying alive – is a battle – one that we will all eventually lose. The idea is to make the most of it while you can – that's what Morley was doing."

"True enough," I said, as I slipped on my mask and headed back to surgery.

"I guess you could say Morley got to sleep with the fishes!"

SHADOWS

Each one of us lives in a cave –
'Tis our lot in life
We see our shadows on the wall
But cannot see the light.

I live inside my little world
Spinning out my days
I think I see another life
Hidden by the haze.

There is a land beyond my view
Ready to unfold
Where all the riddles man has asked
Are waiting to be told.

The Earth's a funny place to live
For every now and then
We pass from light to shadow
And back to light again.

Just when we think that all is right –
The answers finally found –
Another problem comes along
And knocks us to the ground!

But for now it shall suffice
To live without the sun
How oft' the greatest thoughts are made
Before the night is done!

And one day when the Angels call
In the stillness of the night
I'll step out of my shadow
And back into the Light!

MY BIOPSY

For a number of years, I had noticed a slow-growing lump on my right shoulder. As a surgeon, I knew that this was most likely a benign lipoma, or fatty tumor. One day, I finally decided to go ahead and have it removed. I made a point of not telling anybody, and asked my surgery crew not to broadcast my name.

I decided to have the surgery at Holy Christian Hospital, because that's where I work, and that's where I felt most comfortable. But, I hated the thought of my closest co-workers viewing my naked, bony, unconscious body as I lay asleep from the anesthesia. So the hospital agreed to schedule me as Bill Trueblood instead of Bill Truewater – to help keep things confidential.

The surgery went so well that I only missed one day of work – I was back making rounds at 7 o'clock the next morning. The pathology report came back as "benign lipoma", and so I figured things had pretty much returned to normal.

Or so I thought. I ran into Jim Fetters, one of the regular surgery scrub techs, who had a big smile on his face.

"What's so funny, Jim," I naively asked.

"Nothing," Jim responded.

"No," I said. "Tell me what's so funny. Were you at my surgery yesterday?"

"All I'll say, Dr. Truewater, is that you're one bony dude."

"Thanks, Jim," I replied. "At least I'm not overweight," I added, as I looked at Jim's rather ample features.

But it didn't stop there. In fact, things got worse – much worse. When I arrived at my morning clinic, everybody was in a somber mood.

"Are you alright, Dr. Truewater?" my head nurse, Karen Boulder asked.

"I'm just fine," I replied.

"Well, I don't mean to pry into your personal affairs, Doctor Truewater, but the word's gotten out that you had a lump removed yesterday from your back. We're all pretty concerned."

"Oh, it's nothing to worry about, Karen," I reassured her. "It was just a benign lump."

"I'm sure it was," Nurse Boulder replied. "But you sure kept it quiet, like you didn't want anybody to know. You didn't even use your real name on the surgery schedule."

"Look, I'm just fine," I replied. "I was just a little embarrassed, you know, what with my naked, bony body and all, I wanted to keep things on the QT."

"I can understand that," Nurse Bolder replied.

"You do look a little skinny, Doctor," my lab tech, Jim Murphy chimed in. "Have you lost weight?"

"I haven't lost any weight," I replied defensively. "I'm just fine."

"And I noticed your hair's falling out," Nurse Chatwick added. "You're not on chemotherapy, are you?"

"It's called a receding hairline," I answered. "It's what happens to men when they get older."

"Look, I appreciate everybody's concern. But reports of my cancer have been grossly exaggerated – the pathology report was benign. I'm not dying of some terminal disease."

At this point, Cindy Morrow, the ward clerk, started waving her hands. "Dr. Truewater, personal call on line two!"

It was my preacher, Norman Snow. Now, I must confess I haven't been to church in two months. What with the summer break, and my kids preparing to go off to college and playing sports, I had skipped my usual church activities.

"Look, Norman," I began defensively, "I'm sorry I haven't been to church lately – I've been busy with the kids and all."

"That's O.K., Bill," Norman began. "I just want you to know that you've been one of my best parishioners over the years, and I really appreciate you."

"Well, thanks, Norman," I responded.

"I just want you to know that we're all praying for you, Bill. Why, every hour around the clock, one of your Bible partners from your Wednesday morning men's group is sending up a prayer. We know you're going to pull through this just fine."

"Really?" I said. "Pull through what?"

"Your back tumor, Bill. We're all with you on this – why you're even on the prayer list on this Sunday's bulletin – 1,400 Christians will be praying for you!"

"Remember, God never gives us more than we can handle."

"Norman, I want to thank you and the parishioners," I replied, still in a state of shock. "It's nice to know that people can all pull together in a crisis. But, you know, this is a benign lump – nothing bad here."

"I know, I know," Pastor Snow replied. "And we all respect your desire for confidentiality. It's between you and God, and that's all."

I no sooner hung up the phone with Pastor Snow that my first patient, Gene Rose, decided to offer a few well-intentioned words of advice.

"Dr. Truewater, may I say something?" Gene began.

"Sure, Gene," I replied.

I had taken care of Gene's diabetic leg problems for a number of years. I figured I could count on Gene for a few words of reassurance.

"I had a dog once – an Irish setter named Mackey," Gene began.

"I sure loved that dog," Gene added, as he wiped a tear from his eye.

"Well, Mackey had a lump on his back – the veterinarian took it off, and told us everything was just fine."

"I've been trying to tell people, Gene, that these things happen all the time," I said. "It's nothing to worry about."

"I'm not finished yet, Doctor Truewater," Gene added.

"It wasn't six months later that Mackey died. You know, I think that lump was cancer all along, and the vet just didn't have the heart to tell us. You've got to watch out for these things, you know. People don't always tell you."

"That's how things were decades ago, Gene," I responded. "Doctors – and sometimes families – wouldn't tell their loved one they had cancer. But times have changed – we've got treatments, now, for cancer that can result in cures. And people are a lot more open now than they used to be about these things."

As I drove home that night, I had a moment of inspiration. People thought that I was dying. What was the result? Instead of just walking by, individuals who hadn't said hello to me in months stopped to say hello. When my relatives heard about my biopsy, I got post cards from aunts, uncles, nieces, and nephews who hadn't written to me in years, telling me how much they appreciated me, and the good times we had together.

I decided to quit trying to tell people that my biopsy was benign. I reveled in the attention that I was now getting, no matter how ill-founded. Besides, maybe I've got cancer somewhere else, and just don't know it. Or maybe I'll get clobbered by a giant beer truck while driving to the hospital tomorrow, and that'll be the end of things.

I must admit, I changed as well. I started saying hello to people, instead of just walking busily by on my way to rounds or to the clinic. I wrote post cards to my relatives, telling them that I was doing fine.

Sure, I was busy. But we should never be too busy to stop and talk to our friends and acquaintances. Regardless of the results of my biopsy, or anybody's biopsy, for that matter, we are all in this realm for only the shortest of times. Take time to smell the roses.

Take time to stop and say hello.

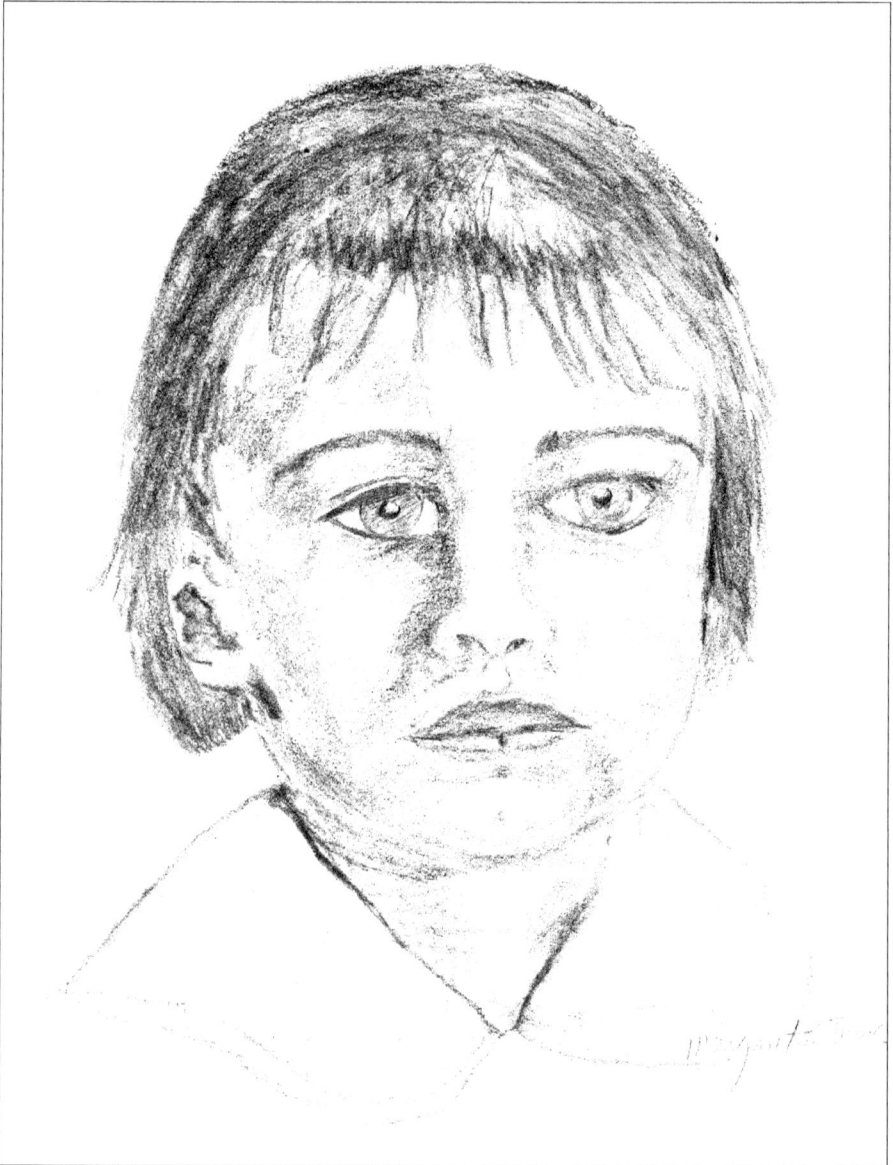

Stephanie Marie

STEPHANIE MARIE

Tell me, who was Stephanie Marie?
A child that never came to be
Eight months she spent with her brother
God picked one but not the other.

Little twins they were to be
Until Fate changed their destiny
Robert Stevenson was born that day
But Stephanie Marie would never stay.

Like colored pictures in the sand
Life weaves its forms upon the land
Some will stay their marks to make
Others God will choose to take.

Tell me, who was Stephanie Marie?
A little bit like you and me –
For even though we live to die
We never know the reason why.

TAKING LIFE TOO SERIOUSLY

I was informed of a surgery resident yesterday who took her own life. The final precipitating event involved one of her patients not doing well. She apparently blamed herself for the patient's death, although this was not at all the case.

My first reaction was sorrow. My second reaction was that we physicians sometimes take our roles, and probably ourselves, too seriously. True, we are involved in life and death decisions.

But one thing I learned after leaving medical school was that doctors don't prevent death – they at least can hope to delay death. While we must bear responsibility for our actions, we must also realize that much greater forces are at work than a doctor can hope to control. Our role through the centuries as healer is partly technical but more importantly emotional.

People look to physicians for a cure to their problems, but much of that cure involves the patient's belief in his physician – a belief grounded just as deeply in folklore as in science. If a patient does not believe in his physician, then no cure is possible.

The physician must realize, as have healers and high priests throughout the centuries, that there will be shortcomings – there will even be failures. Such failures are an inevitable part of our transient existence on this earth. To hold oneself responsible for those failures is at best self-deception and, at worst, a painful form of self-destruction.

But this is a burden that all physicians must carry. Did I do enough? Should I have done more? One thing that separates us from mere technicians is that we are dealing with people, and we must carry the burden of our own conscience. At times, this is good, for it can stimulate us to do better. At other times, when we dwell too heavily on our mistakes, it can impair our performance, and even our sense of well-being.

And do not fear death. Look it straight in the eye. Talk to your patients who are dying. Talk to their families. Death is not a failure – only a transition from one world to another. Help your patients across the threshold. By doing so, you will help yourself to understand the world around you. Not that you will find all the answers. Hopefully, you will find enough answers to keep you searching. And to keep you living.

My only suggestion to young physicians, who I have found to be terribly conscientious, is don't take yourself or your role so seriously that you blame yourself every time a patient fails to do well. It is the unfortunate lot of the human race that we don't do well – we will all die! That is a fact we cannot escape. The best we can hope for is to improve the quality and perhaps the length of our patient's lives by a few years!

Those who live in the quiet suffering of a grievous loss

Carry a burden which can never be lost –

You toil in the present and smile at the last –

As flashes of memory break through from the past!

FAMILY PICS

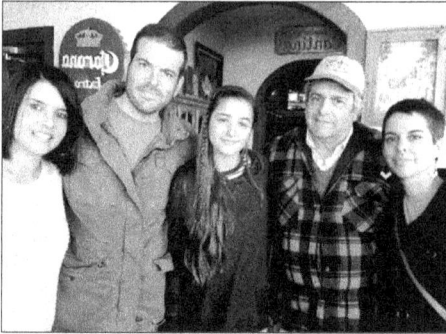

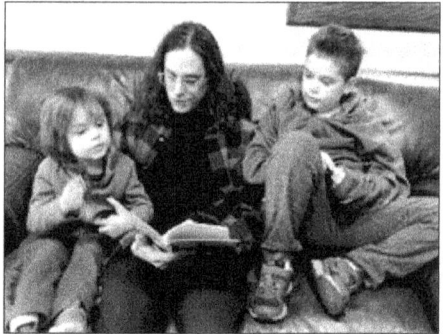

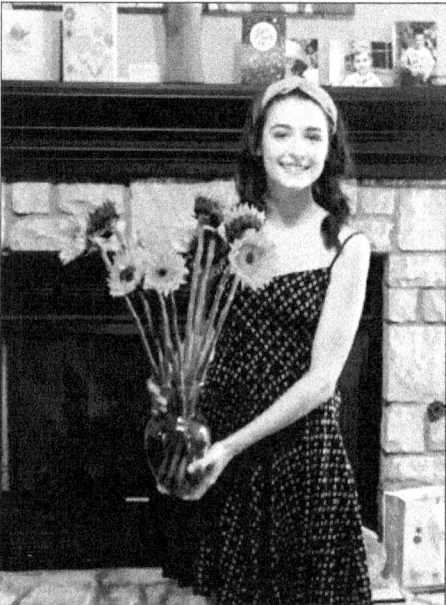

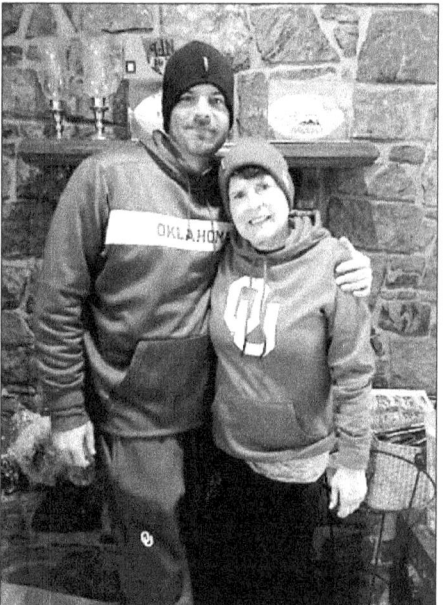

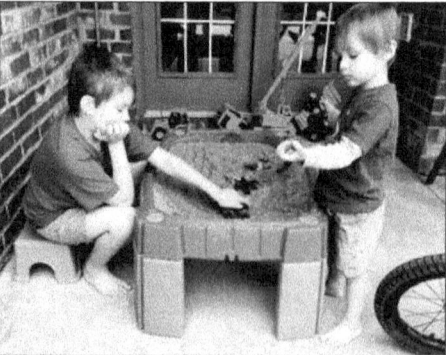

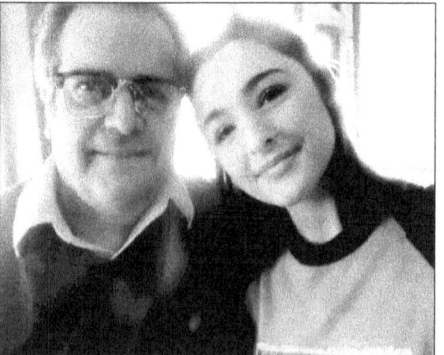

TIME PASSAGES

I regret the passing
Of each and every day
My children growing up
And moving far away.

I wish I had a camera
I'd freeze each day in time
We never would grow old and gray
We'd never say goodbye.

But life is always changing –
Will nothing ever last?
The flowers of each newborn spring
Are but echoes of the past.

So treasure every moment
Heed the children's pleas
Take time each and every day
To count your memories!

A SHOCK OF GRAY

I brushed back a shock of hair in front of the twelve-inch mirror that Holy Christian allows in the surgery lounge, while waiting for my case to start.

Herb Minder, the plastic surgeon, happened to notice me.

"I notice you've got a shock of gray, there, Dr. Truewater," Herb quipped.

"It's premature gray," I replied.

"At your age, Truewater, I wouldn't call it premature."

"Very funny, Herb. Besides," I added, "I don't really mind gray hair. It makes me look more distinguished when I go out to talk to the family after surgery."

"You know what they say."

"No, what do they say, Herb?" I asked, already getting irritated.

"Gray today, gone tomorrow! You need to start thinking about retirement, Dr. Truewater," Herb chided me.

"I'm not about to retire," I grumbled. "I've still got three dysfunctional kids to support, who are only in their thirties. My dear wife wants to re-do the kitchen again – this time with granite countertops. And my grandkids are approaching college age. College is a lot more expensive now than it used to be."

"You've got to start thinking about yourself, Truewater," Herb replied.

"I am thinking about myself, Herb. You see, I enjoy being a surgeon. I don't plan to quit before my time," I answered.

"And when is your time, Dr. Truewater?" Herb asked.

"I haven't decided yet," I replied.

"Maybe it's not your decision, Bill."

"How do you mean, Herb?"

"Let's face it. Nobody knows how long they've got on this green planet. Look at that new general surgeon, Mary Chalmers – after twelve years of college, medical school, and surgery residency, she gets diagnosed with multiple sclerosis. Why, you could have pancreatic cancer right now, Truewater, and not know it. Only God knows that – God decides how long you've got."

"Of course," I replied. "But I feel just fine."

"Surgeons are workaholics," Herb continued. "They don't know when to quit. Then they drop dead in their surgery scrubs."

"I don't plan to drop dead in my surgery scrubs, Herb," I answered.

"Nobody does," he replied. "It just happens, that's all. And it all starts with gray hair – that's a warning, you know."

"I don't think God is warning me," I replied. "I think God wants me to keep doing surgery. He just wants me to look a little older, a little more distinguished, that's all."

"Besides," I added, "with this shock of gray hair, patients no longer wonder if I'm too young."

"Wait a few more years, Truewater," Herb quipped. "With a little more gray, you'll look too old, and they'll start wondering again."

"At least I've got hair," I replied angrily, as I looked at Herb's balding head. "You're just jealous 'cause I've got hair on my head, no matter if it's brown or gray."

"I've been bald since I was forty."

"Anyway, being bald is kind of sexy these days," Herb added, as he rubbed the shiny orb that once represented a full head of dark hair back in medical school at the University of Chicago.

"Besides," Herb added wistfully, "I'm a victim of my genetics – male pattern baldness, and all that."

"That's 'cause you've got too much DHT – you've always had too much testosterone, Herb," I joked.

"That's better than not having enough, Truewater," Herb replied. "Besides, I've never had patients think I was too young to be a plastic surgeon."

"The only thing I don't like about this gray hair," I replied, as I again tried to brush it back, "is that it's too stiff. It's won't lay down like it's supposed to."

"That's because it doesn't have the natural oils," Herb explained. "You see, as you get older, Truewater, things kind of dry up."

"So I've noticed," I replied. "I remember back in the fifties my dad used to use Vitalis – the greaseless grooming discovery."

"Never heard of it," Herb replied. "Do you mean the 1950's? You're not that old, Truewater."

"I'm afraid I am, Herb. Why, I remember when the Chicago Cubs played the Brooklyn Dodgers. Bob Rush pitched for the Cubs. His wind-up was so slow that Jackie Robinson stole home!"

"Brooklyn doesn't have a team anymore," Herb answered. "They moved to Los Angeles – what a pity."

"I thought you weren't that old," I said.

"Some things I choose not to remember," Herb replied. "I don't want to give away my age, you know."

"There's nothing wrong with getting older, the way I see it, Herb."

"This gray hair is just part of Nature's process. Besides, older people are more respected in our society – they're looked upon as opinion leaders and judges."

"Then, why do older people dye their gray hair black?" Herb asked.

"Some people just want to look younger, that's all," I replied.

"Look at all the senior physicians on our staff," I added. "With gray hair comes respect and honor."

"And senility," Herb added. "I remember when you memorized all your patients' names and hospital room numbers. Now, I see, you carry a list."

"That's because I've got more patients, now," I said. "I'm not getting senile, just because I've got a shock of gray hair."

"Nevertheless, Dr. Truewater, that gray hair is a harbinger of things to come."

"Good things to come," I replied. "I choose to look at the positive."

"Okay, then some day you're positively going to die."

"Sure, everybody knows that. I'm not afraid of death. After all, I'm a doctor."

"And?" Herb asked.

"And doctors aren't afraid of death," I answered. "That's why they became doctors. They deal with death all the time. They take courses on it in medical school. They read books about it. Doctors are trained to deal with death. Why, they dissect cadavers in medical school. Next to preachers, doctors understand death better than anybody. They counsel the dying patient. Death is a natural part of the life process. We're born, we live, we get a shock or two of gray hair, then we die."

"It's all very simple," I added, as I brushed my hair in the mirror.

"Say, what have you got in that brush?" Herb asked suspiciously.

"Nothing," I replied.

"Then, why does your hair keep getting darker each time you brush it?"

"It's just a little hair color, that's all," I said. "My wife started me on it, and she says I look ten years younger. Once a day takes out the gray – you've seen the commercial, where the man brushes out the gray and becomes more attractive and self-confident."

"So, you're living a lie – telling me you don't mind the gray hair, then brushing it out."

"I don't mind this shock of gray hair," I replied defensively. "I just don't want it quite so soon – that's all. And I'm not quite ready to assume the mantle of elderly physician."

"Of course not," Herb replied. "I understand completely."

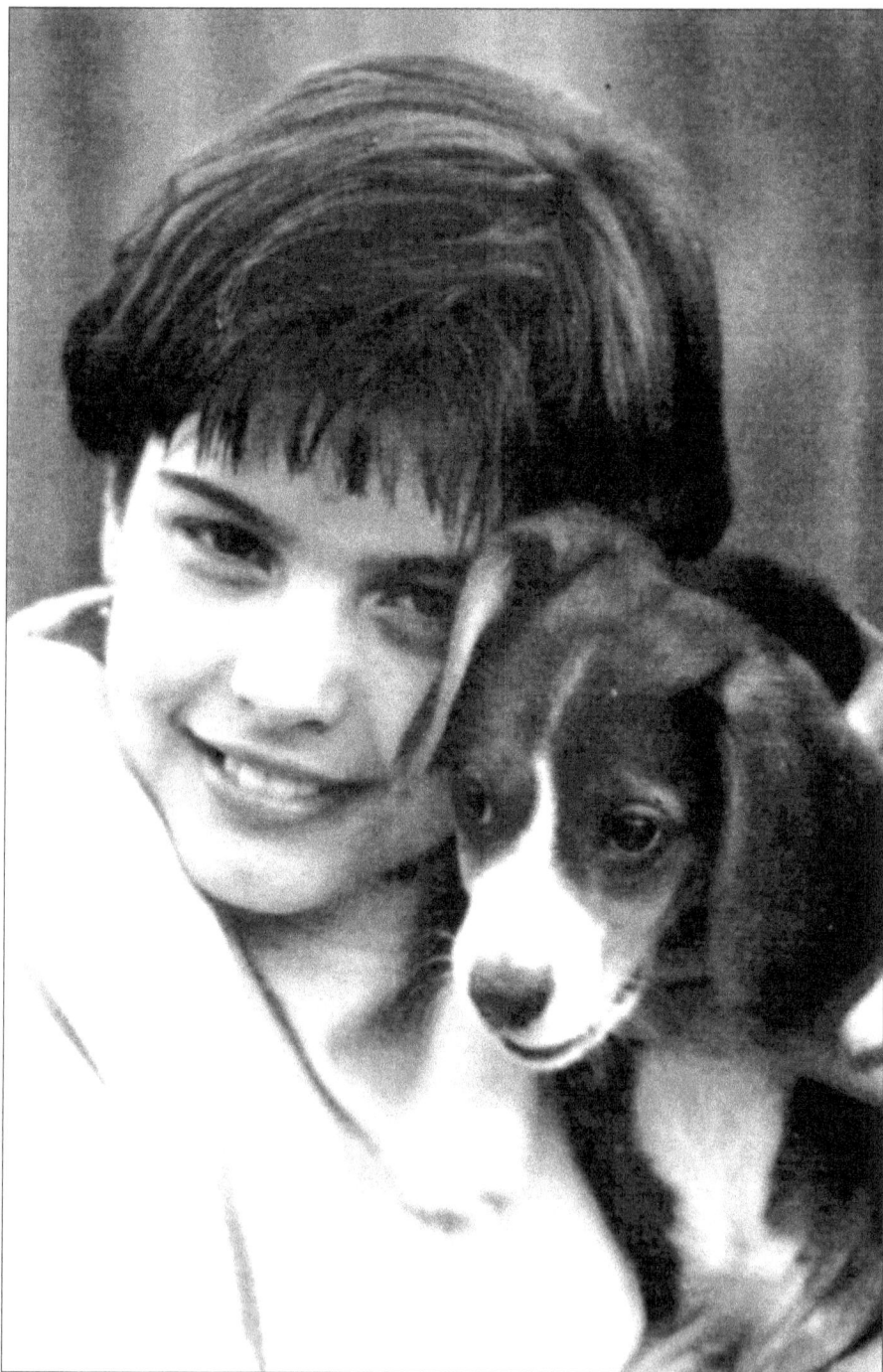

Lisa Truels with furry friend

BUTTERCUP

I want a dog
Oh, yes I do!
I'd like a friend
To see me through

A little puppy –
What a surprise!
With short, thick hair
And big brown eyes!

I'll make a home
For him to stay
It'll be a place
For him to play!

I'll feed him once
Each day and night
And train him so
He wouldn't bite!

I'll wash him well –
My Mom to please
So that he won't
Come down with fleas!

I'll walk him
Morning, noon, and night,
To keep the carpet
Clean and bright!

I'll warm a spot
Down at my feet
Each night that I
Retire to sleep!

I'll train him well
To do his job
And guard the house
From those who rob.

He'll be a gift
From God above
And I will give him
All my love!

I think I'll call him
Buttercup!
Oh, won't you please
Get me a pup?

GRANNY'S ON A HIGH

"Have you got your marijuana license yet, Doctor Truewater?" Herb asked me, as we ate corned beef sandwiches for lunch in the doctor's lounge.

The sandwiches were provided gratis by a pharmaceutical company – only after we signed a federally mandated statement that we wouldn't let corned beef sandwiches influence our decision over which antibiotics to use.

"I beg your pardon?" I said, as I munched on my sandwich and guzzled down a Diet Coke.

"I don't use drugs – illegal ones, that is, and that includes marijuana."

"Of course not, Truewater," Herb replied. "But the great city of San Francisco wants to legalize marijuana for medicinal use, and at the same time provide funding for a San Francisco garden to grow medical marijuana for the use of its citizens."

"I thought most San Francisco gardens already grew marijuana," I replied.

"This would be legal," Herb responded. "San Francisco wants to avoid the Canada Debacle."

"What's the Canada Debacle?" I asked.

"Well, Canada legalized marijuana for medicinal use – you know, for seriously ill cancer patients as a pain killer, for example. The only problem – there were no legal suppliers of marijuana, so these cancer patients were buying marijuana off the street – at $300 per ounce!"

"Well, we can't have that," I replied.

"Sounds to me like you don't believe in the medicinal uses of marijuana," Herb responded.

"I remember back in my medical school days at the University of Illinois," I reminisced. "The pot smokers back then were in a constant state of euphoria – and they demanded an end to the Vietnam War, free sex, and legalized drugs. I always thought they smoked one mushroom too many, but they all became fine doctors – at least most of them."

"Marijuana is not a mushroom, Truewater," Herb replied. "It's an herb."

"I know it's an herb. And you're a Herb whose had too many mushrooms," I joked.

"Marijuana has serious medicinal uses," Herb ignored me.

"Like what?" I asked.

"Marijuana has been approved in Canada for the terminally ill, those with multiple sclerosis, spinal cord injury or disease, AIDS/HIV infection, severe arthritis, and epileptic seizures."

"In addition, those with serious medical conditions like hepatitis C, in which conventional treatments have failed, are also eligible, with decisions from two medical specialists."

"Marijuana helps control pain as well as nausea. It increases the appetite. And it provides a feeling of euphoria, and well-being."

"Most recently, some have pushed to get those with serious depression approved for cannabis use."

"Cannabis?" I asked.

"Marijuana, for the uneducated," Herb quipped.

"Well, the symptoms you just described, including depression, would cover about half the adult population. That's a lot of marijuana."

"I can see it now," I added. "Soon cancer wards, rife with the acrid odor of marijuana, will smell like the Sigma Alpha Epsilon fraternity house on Masquerade night! Pass the water pipe, Nurse Riley!"

"I wouldn't jump to conclusions, Truewater," Herb responded. "This is a serious issue, and you're not taking it seriously!"

"I'm taking it seriously," I replied. "I'm just trying to be realistic."

"You can't have the Little Old Lady from Pasadena driving up and down Colorado Boulevard smoking a water pipe to relieve the pain of osteoarthritis! You just can't have that."

"Would you pass the mustard, please?" I added. "This corned beef sandwich is a little dry."

"People smoking marijuana would be prohibited from driving," Herb replied.

"Of course," I said. "And people drinking alcohol are prohibited from driving, too – but they do it anyway. That's what keeps us trauma surgeons busy on Saturday nights."

"That's a problem for law enforcement," Herb answered.

"Now there's a solution," I replied. "Juice up the public with marijuana as well as alcohol, let them crash their cars into each other to the tune of 50,000 traffic fatalities and one million injuries per year, and then let the peace officers issue traffic tickets! And that's ignoring another 40,000 suicides per year, many due to drug usage."

"If you ask me," I continued, "smoking marijuana isn't going to solve our problems. It will only increase them, as people try to tune out the world and ignore the search for solutions."

"Now you're taking things too seriously, Truewater," Herb answered. "I've always thought you were kind of a straight arrow. We're only on this earth a short period of time. What's wrong with a little enjoyment? Besides, sometimes, if you're facing the pain of cancer, or a chronic, debilitating illness for which there's no cure, or even nuclear annihilation, a little euphoria isn't such a bad solution. Lighten up! You know, certain Greeks championed hedonism – the pursuit of pleasure."

"Now we're talking nuclear annihilation?" I asked.

"I just thought I'd throw that in – for a little perspective," Herb said.

"The Greeks also used to say, 'Nothing to excess'," I replied.

"I suppose an appropriate solution would be to approve the use of medicinal marijuana in selected instances," Herb proposed.

"I'm just afraid that's going to open up Pandora's box," I answered, "and everybody from A to Z – from arthritis to herpes zoster – will be demanding medical marijuana before long."

"Relax and enjoy!" Herb responded. "Have another corned beef sandwich – you'll like it!"

"Thanks," I replied, as I took another sandwich.

I concluded that some problems were just too complicated to solve over lunch.

A CHANCE ENCOUNTER

Have I met you before
In a world long ago?
Tell me the answer –
Don't torture me so!

Was there a world
Where dreams never die?
Or was it a place
Of hello and goodbye?

Was there a time
When love conquered all?
Or was it a place
Where flowers must fall?

My hands touch your hair
As it blows in the wind
Your skin touches mine
As we meet once again.

Sometimes I think
When I look in your eyes
Was it good that we met?
Does God really cry?

You look so familiar
With that same pretty smile
I'd like to take pause
And linger a while.

But though our paths cross
As we stand by the sea--
I must suffer the loss
Of what cannot be!

TRANSITIONS

I wish you well in your retirement, Tom. I know that retiring is a very difficult decision after your long and distinguished career as a surgeon. Retirement represents one of life's most difficult transitions.

But you have made other transitions that were equally difficult. Going from civilian life as a medical student to becoming a B-24 bomber navigator in World War II. was no easy chore. One minute you're in school, the next minute you're navigating a bomber with eleven brave souls over enemy territory, watching the flack burst around you.

It took courage to do that, and to live with the fact that some of your buddies didn't make it – something that only a war veteran can understand. I know, Tom, that you had difficulty being a member of a bomber crew, as any caring young man would. I am very proud of your distinguished military service to advance the cause of freedom and defeat the enemy.

You were ready now for life's next transition – from navigator to surgeon. Now you were in the business of saving individual lives. Besides being an excellent surgeon, you took a personal interest in your patients.

In this impersonal world, where insurance companies and the federal government refer to patients as clients, and discourage personal involvement with a single physician, you insisted on treating your patients as human beings with real thoughts and feelings. You cared about your patients, just as you cared for your own children.

You were a great father and family man, Tom. You once said that you would do anything to help your children, and I believe you. Because that's the kind of person you are. Unlike some physicians who mistakenly placed their career ahead of their families, Tom, you placed your family first. You cared about your children, and you were there to help them with their own transitions – the recitals, the birthday parties, and the fatherly advice to help them navigate life's difficult passages.

And you cared deeply about God. As the Bible says, "Your faith shall sustain you." I have no doubt, Tom that your faith in the Almighty, and your faith in the Goodness of Man, carried you through those difficult times.

But perhaps your most endearing quality, Tom, is your sincerity. The open, honest way you deal with people is something I will always remember. In our complicated, modern world, riddled with competition and false fronts, we sometimes lose sight of the beauty of simplicity, honesty, and sincerity in dealing with our fellow man. Perhaps our memory of you will show us the way.

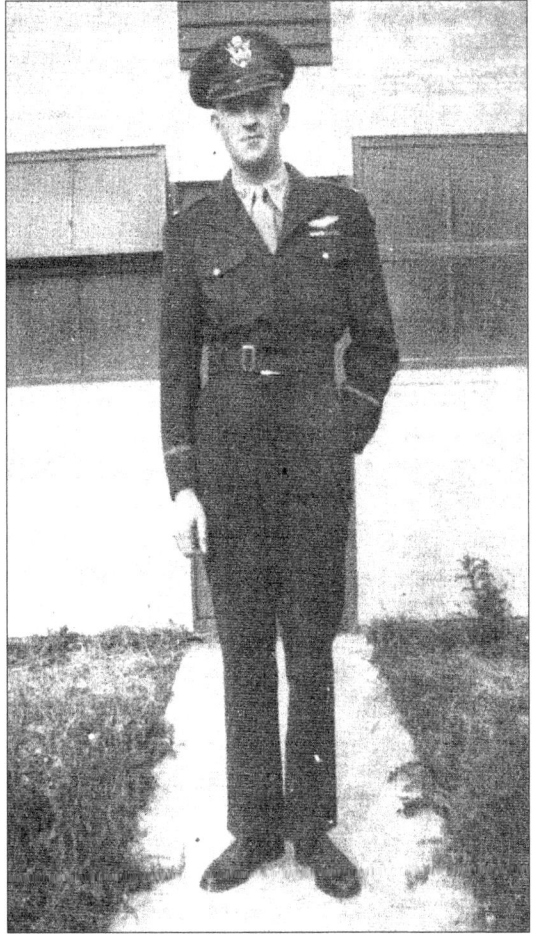

Now you are ready for the next transition, Tom, that of retirement. I know it won't be easy giving up the career you love. But I know you'll make it. You love to garden and work on the farm.

And I know you'll be back to visit us from time to time. As your friends, we will be here to help you. And, hopefully, Tom, you will be here to help us!

Tom Henley practiced general surgery at Mercy Hospital in Oklahoma City from 1962-1992. He is pictured above in April, 1944, at the Tibenham Air Force Base in England.

SPEAKING FRANKLY

I sat in the doctor's lounge with a concerned look on my face. One of my patients, Jeb Armstrong, was dying of cancer and didn't have long to go.

"You seem a little down today, Dr. Truewater," Herb replied, as he sipped on some Java juice contributed to the surgery lounge by one of the pharmaceutical reps.

"Let's just call it a look of consternation," I replied.

"Well, okay, Dr. Truewater, why the look of consternation?"

"I've got a patient who's dying," I answered without looking up over my Java juice.

"Join the club," Herb replied. "I've got a few myself. It happens. Get over it."

"I'm over it," I replied. "It's just that it's not a very nice thing to say to someone."

"What's that?" Herb asked.

"What you tell your very sick patients," I answered.

"What do you say?" Herb asked.

"I told Mr. Armstrong, 'You're probably not going to make it.' That's not exactly a cheer-you-up kind of thing to say to your patient."

"I mean, patients just don't go to their doctor to hear that kind of prognosis. Why, in the old days, the English king would kill his doctor if he made that kind of prognosis. In Egyptian days, the priest, who also acted as a physician and healer, would be entombed with the Pharaoh in the pyramid."

"Don't worry, Truewater," Herb replied. "No one's going to bury you alive if your patient dies. Families are more understanding these days."

"Sometimes I'm not so sure," I interjected.

"But let me get this straight, Truewater," Herb continued. "You actually tell your patients they might die? I mean, people don't want to hear that."

"People only want to hear good news," Herb added. "It's human nature."

"Sometimes it's better to say, 'You've got a chance of pulling through this thing.' I mean it's true. There's always a chance that your patient might pull through. You don't want to be too pessimistic here."

"Sometimes what you don't say can be more important."

"But being realistic isn't so bad either," I responded. "And you're less likely to be misunderstood if you speak frankly with your patient and his family."

"I mean, most of our lives we live in a state of denial. We live our lives like we're going to live forever. We go to work – sometimes 60 or more hours a week – we rush our kids to baseball or soccer practice, we pack them off to school, and then we let little things upset us, like whether someone has a new car or a new house, or who likes us or who doesn't like us."

"Those are important things," Herb quipped. "But, what's your point, Truewater?"

"My point is that we lose sight of the big picture. We lose sight of our transient existence on this planet. Oh, to be sure, we get jolted to reality when a close friend or relative dies. But, after a few days, we're back on the trivia track – you know, getting preoccupied with the daily details of life."

"Well, what's the alternative, Dr. Truewater?" Herb replied.

"Are we supposed to sit in a circle all day, smoke mushrooms or drink moonshine, and contemplate the meaning of life or the reality of God?"

"I mean, as doctors, we've got to get caught in what you call the 'trivia track' – our patients' lives depend upon our daily attention to detail and our work ethic."

"True enough," I answered. "But, as doctors, we must not get so caught up in the details of our patient's care – you know, checking the electrolytes, the blood gases, the X-rays, and so on, that we forget to tell the family the painful truth – that death is imminent, or that the chances of survival are very slim."

"Well, let's face it," Herb replied. "You don't go through four years of college, four years of medical school, and then four or more years of residency in a sub-specialty, just to have your patient die."

"I mean, the whole point of all that education is to enable you, as a doctor, to save that patient's life. When a patient dies, there's a tendency for the doctor to view himself as a failure."

"Sometimes the hardest thing for a doctor to accept is that his patient is dying."

"Just then, Nurse Havisham announced over the intercom in the doctor's lounge that my patient was ready for surgery."

"Doctor Truewater – ready in room nine!"

"I've got to get back on track, Herb," I replied, as I put down my cup of Java juice.

"I've got to fix this inguinal hernia, and then I've got another patient for a lap gallbladder."

"See you later, Dr. Truewater," Herb answered. "It's always nice to philosophize a bit before getting back on the trivia track!"

"Just don't forget to keep track of the big picture!" I added, as I laced up my mask and headed back to the operating room.

STAY CLOSE

Stay close
Put your arms around me tight
Save me
From the gremlins of the night.

Take me
To your lovely home
Keep me
From being all alone.

Tell me
The words I want to hear
Spare me
From all the things I fear!

Kiss me
And show me that you care
Teach me
All the things you dare!

RELAX AND ENJOY!

"I hate standing in line," I told Herb, as we waited for the grand opening of the latest "*Fast and Furious*" movie sequel.

"You'll like the movie," Herb said, trying to distract me.

"It's got lots of action – cars zooming around, even dropping out of airplanes with a parachute. It's one those IMAX giant screen extravaganzas in three dimensions and Dolby stereo with surround sound."

"I still don't like standing in line," I said.

"Relax, Dr. Truewater," Herb replied.

"You're retired now. We've got all day. There's nothing else we have to do today."

"I just don't like standing in one place without moving," I answered.

"You don't have to be a 'Type A' anymore," Herb answered.

"I'm not a 'Type A", Herb," I replied angrily.

"I mean, I got 'A' grades in school because I went out and tried harder. There's nothing wrong with that."

"In fact, that's how I got to be a doctor," I added. "I had to push myself to get ahead."

"That's what I mean," Herb answered. "You've been pushing yourself all your life. Now it's time to learn how to relax."

"Well, we had to work hard, Herb, in order to make the grade. Why, in residency, I put in a hundred hours a week – I was on call in the hospital every other night – that was part of the surgery training."

"Why, at Cook County in Chicago, we'd operate from Saturday afternoon to Sunday morning during the summer, when the Knife and Gun club was in action. You had to be able to take the stress."

"And what good did it do?" Herb asked. "How many doctors do you know that are divorced or alcoholic or even committed suicide because of the stress?"

"Well, if you can't take the heat, then get out of the kitchen – that's what Harry Truman said," I replied.

"You know, this line hasn't moved an inch," I added angrily. I hate spinning my wheels and not getting anywhere."

"Then quit spinning the wheels," Herb answered. "Learn to take your foot off the gas!"

"Then, you're never going to get anywhere, Herb," I answered.

"Why, I drove to Houston last week to see my wife's family – now there's a dysfunctional family – and they're not even doctors!"

"Anyway, I tried doing the speed limit of 75 miles per hour on the Texas Interstate. And you know what happened?"

"No, what happened, Dr. Truewater?" Herb asked.

"I got passed by all these pick-up trucks and cars going 85 miles per hour. I even got passed by a semitrailer truck!" I replied.

"So, let them pass, Truewater," Herb answered. "You know, John Lenin said that life is what happens when you're making plans."

"Take your foot off the gas. Slow down and enjoy the view!"

"I suppose you're right, Herb," I answered. "I should just relax and enjoy the movie."

"But, take a look at that teenager making popcorn at the concession counter," I continued. "He's taking all day to make the popcorn and serve the hot dogs – he'll never make it in the real world."

"You remember the race between the turtle and the hare?" Herb asked.

"Sure – the turtle won," I replied. "The hare was so fast that he got distracted, didn't keep his eye on the goal."

"That's right," Herb answered. "Slow down and finish first – and enjoy life along the way."

"Learn to spend time with your family and friends, get a fun hobby, and take time to appreciate each day!"

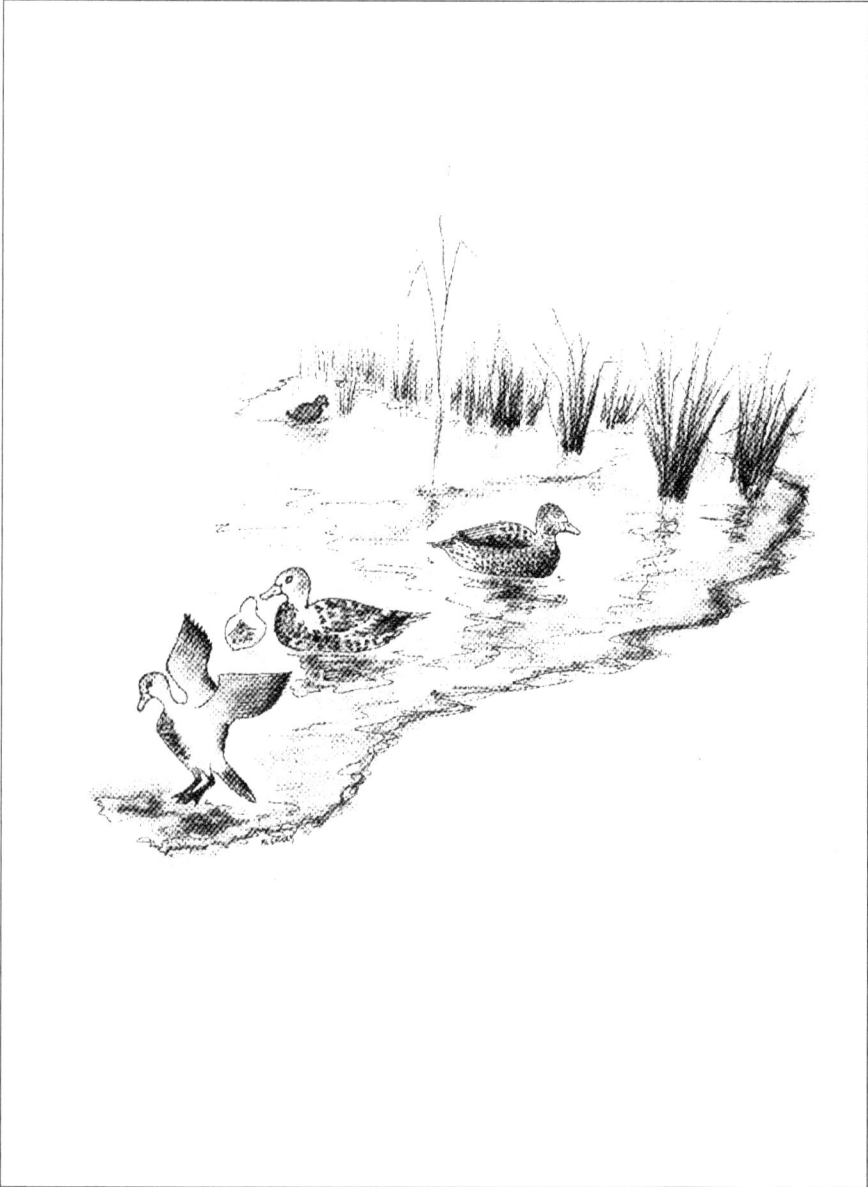

Lake Hefner Duck Pond

MY DUCK POND

When I wish to clear my mind
I think of something very fine.
A duck pond with pretty trees
Helps to put my mind at ease.

I just lean back and close my eyes
And what a scene I then surmise!
Beautiful birds with colored feathers
Swim around in sunny weather.

The water laps upon the shore
Where little children there explore.
Seagulls sail in the cool breeze
As the wind blows through the trees.

I walk upon the fertile land
And feed the ducks with open hands.
The quacking ducks sing their refrain
And fight each other for the grain.

I often come to linger here
My peace with nature gives me cheer
The children ask if I can play
And wonder when I'll come to stay.

The telephone rings and spoils my view
I've got lots of work to do!
I've had my time to meditate
My duck pond was a nice escape.

CUDDLE TIME

"Cuddle Time" was developed so the hospital could allow compassion between seriously ill patients and their spouses, and not be seen as some cold, uncaring institution.

I walked into the Holy Christian Hospital surgery lounge with a flustered look on my face.

"Cat got your tongue?" Herb asked with a smile.

"I guess so," I replied. "I sure didn't know what to say when I walked into my patient's room this morning!"

"What happened?" Herb asked.

"Well, I did a laparoscopic gallbladder surgery on young Miss Susie yesterday. She was nauseated after the surgery, so I decided to keep her overnight."

"Sounds reasonable so far," Herb responded.

"Usually, I knock before entering, but this morning I walked into the room without looking and simply said 'Hello.' I sat down in the chair, opened the chart, and started to write some discharge orders. When I looked up, I had the shock of my life."

"She had her street clothes on and ready to go?" Herb asked.

"No, just the opposite," I countered. "Miss Susie was lying in bed with her boyfriend, or significant other, or whatever he's called."

"That's not good," Herb replied. "What'd you do?"

"Well, at first I pretended like he wasn't there," I answered.

"I asked Miss Susie how she was doing, and she said just fine. Her nausea had resolved, and she had eaten most of her breakfast."

"Then what happened?" Herb asked.

"Then her boyfriend introduced himself, so I was forced to confront the issue. 'I'm Joe Atwater, Miss Susie's significant other,' he said."

"Don't get up," I replied, as I stood to shake his hand. "I never met a 'significant other' before. Nice to meet you."

I had a pleasant but brief conversation with the two of them and then left.

"You should have reported them," Herb replied.

"For what?" I asked.

"For conduct unbecoming a patient, and a lack of moral turpitude," Herb said.

"Sounds like the military," I answered.

"Holy Christian hospital has rules about these things," Herb replied. "There's such a thing as maintaining moral turpitude in a hospital setting."

"What's 'turpitude' mean?" I asked.

"I'm not exactly sure," Herb replied, "but there're rules against it. We can't let Holy Christian hospital turn into a brothel."

"Of course not," I answered. "But what's the hospital policy on this?"

"It's called 'Cuddle Time Protocol'," Herb replied pontifically.

"It was developed so the hospital could allow compassion between patients and their spouses, and not be seen as some cold, uncaring institution."

"Sounds reasonable," I said.

"It was developed for cancer patients," Herb continued.

"Most of my cancer patients are Medicare age," I replied. "They've long since quite cuddling."

"Nevertheless," Herb continued, "the significant other is allowed to cuddle with his or her mate for a prescribed time period. It's believed that this touching, compassionate bond can actually help promote healing, or at least allow the two partners to express themselves by physically touching and caressing their mate."

"Of course, a 'Cuddle Time' sign in large letters is placed on the door to ward off visitors, nurses, doctors, medical students, nurses' aides, nursing students, housekeeping, or maintenance engineers who might inadvertently enter a patient's room during this period of mutual appreciation."

"It's become quite popular," Herb continued.

"We've actually had some patients make their own sign and hang it on the door, so they could get a few hours sleep while they were in the hospital!"

"Let me get this straight," I interrupted Herb's pontificating. "You've got to have cancer before you're allowed to cuddle?"

"Not just cancer," Herb replied. "You're also allowed to cuddle if you have multiple sclerosis, lupus, diabetes, or Lou Gehrig's disease."

"Sounds perfectly reasonable," I replied.

"I suppose they also have a definition for 'cuddle'," I said.

"Of course," Herb replied. "I was on the Compassionate Care Committee with the Sisters of St. Gregory Hospital, and we helped set up the definitions and guidelines."

"The verb 'cuddle' is defined as the touching or coddling of a significant other, without the transfer of bodily fluids."

"Sounds very proper," I said. "The transfer of bodily fluids is the kind of thing that should never occur in a hospital setting."

"But no set of rules is complete," I continued, "without a means of enforcement. In the case of my patient, Miss Susie, for example, what happens if a patient violates the Cuddle Time Protocol and commits an act of moral turpitude?"

"Very simple," Herb replied. "Hospital security is called, and the significant other is escorted out of the hospital."

"I'm not opposed to intimacy," Herb continued. "It's just that there's a time and place for everything, and we at Holy Christian Hospital are trying to maintain the high ground, while at the same time showing a compassionate face to the seriously ill patient."

"I couldn't have said it better," I told Herb, as I left to make rounds on my next patient.

Next time, when I approach my patient's room, I'll be sure to knock before entering!

THE TUMOR BOARD

I attended the Holy Christian Sinai Tumor Board Conference today. Now, you've got to understand that once you put a bunch of doctors in one room, it's hard to get them to agree on anything. But today's Tumor Board Conference was particularly exciting. The patient being presented was a 75 year-old man with a very rare cancer, called a transitional cell carcinoma of the prostate.

Fleck McWaters, the urologist was summing up the case.

"In conclusion, we have an otherwise healthy 75 year old man with "Stage A" (early) cancer. It's a tough choice between surgery, chemotherapy, or radiation therapy," Fleck concluded, knowing full well that, as a surgeon, he felt surgery was best. Whenever a surgeon says that someone is "otherwise healthy", that means he wants to operate.

Harold Curtain, another urologist, rose to speak. The other doctors all render their opinions while seated, but Harold is very deliberate and prefers to stand before he speaks, in order to lend emphasis to what he has to say.

"Dr. McWaters," Harold begins, "as a surgeon, I have to say the only way to completely remove a cancer is with an operation. This man needs a standard cancer operation to give him the best chance of survival."

Having spoken his piece, Harold sits down and Jim Garden, the other urologist takes his turn.

"I totally agree with Dr. Curtain," Jim begins. "God only knows that there may be other nodules within the prostate that the needle biopsy missed. Without surgery, these people die of their disease. With surgery, I could keep him alive long enough so that he would die of his cardiac or pulmonary problems before his cancer could finish him off."

Now, all this time, Jo Trendelenberg, the radiation therapist, was doing a slow burn. Jo likes to eat bananas for breakfast, and, with banana in hand, he began waving frantically for recognition.

"I've had it!" Jo exclaims, waving his banana at Harold Curtain. "You surgeons think that the only way to cure cancer is with the knife! Those cancer cells are just as dead when I hit them with my cobalt rays or electron beams, and with a lot fewer complications!"

Dr. Curtain rises to speak, but Jo isn't finished.

"Sit down, Harold!" Jo exclaims. "I'm not finished speaking! All my life, whenever I get patients, they come to me with this hopeless look in their eyes. The surgeon has told them that surgery is useless and sends them for radiation or chemotherapy. I'm tired of being second banana!"

Dr. Curtain rises to speak again, but this time the chemotherapist, Fred Korker, chimes in.

"In my opinion," Fred begins, "chemotherapy is the best treatment for cancer, because it is so selective – it only kills rapidly dividing cells – and it can be done as an outpatient. In some cases, chemotherapy should be done first, before the surgery, in order to assure the best chance for disease free survival."

Dr. Curtain rises one more time to speak and is recognized. He obviously wants to make peace with his fellow comrades.

"This is a very rare case," Harold states, "and there is not enough information in the literature to state dogmatically which treatment is best. There's more than one way to skin a cat."

"We're not skinning cats! We're treating cancer, Dr. Curtain!" Jo Trendelenberg responds angrily. "Look at the Queen Elizabeth Hospital experience."

The group fell silent. Now, whenever Jo Trendelenberg wishes to make a point, he always pulls out his ace in the hole – the Queen Elizabeth Hospital experience in Canada. No one else is familiar with the Queen Elizabeth Hospital experience. Jo spent two years at Queen Elizabeth in Toronto, a hospital that treats everything with radiation therapy, including warts on your nose and even acne.

"The Queen Elizabeth experience treated seven patients with "stage A" transitional cell cancer of the prostate in the last twenty years and reports a 30% five year survival."

"I can do that well with surgery!" Jim Garden retaliates.

"Or chemotherapy," Fred Korker interjects before Jim Garden can quote his statistics. "There's a new study out of the Petersen (referring to C.D. Petersen Clinic in Waco, Texas) using the "LAF" protocol (leucovorin, adriamycin and 5-FU). This might be a good patient to put on the Baylor protocol."

The radiologist, Rod Bean, had not yet voiced his opinion. Radiologists always seem to be requesting more information and establishing baselines for future testing.

"I think a CAT scan would be helpful, along with a bone scan and liver scan to further stage the patient. You might even consider an ultrasound to rule out a cystic lesion and a PET scan to be definitive. Even if they're negative, they'll provide a good baseline for future tumor staging."

"There's also a study at the University using interferon," Dave Hayes, another chemotherapist, argues. Dave Hayes trained at the University at a time when beta interferon was thought to be the new miracle drug for the eighties.

"We might consider sending this man to the University for the new interferon protocol," Dave adds.

By now, things are threatening to degenerate into total confusion. Jo Trendelenberg is waving his banana again. Harold Curtain is standing to speak, and four more doctors are requesting recognition. My beeper goes off, and it's time for me to head off to surgery.

As I walk to the operating room, I think about how great it is to be in a scientific profession, where decisions are made not on opinion, but on fact, and where you can start your day off right with a peaceful morning breakfast!

Author's note to patients and medical students: Most tumor board decisions are not this controversial, and are well-grounded in scientific analysis.

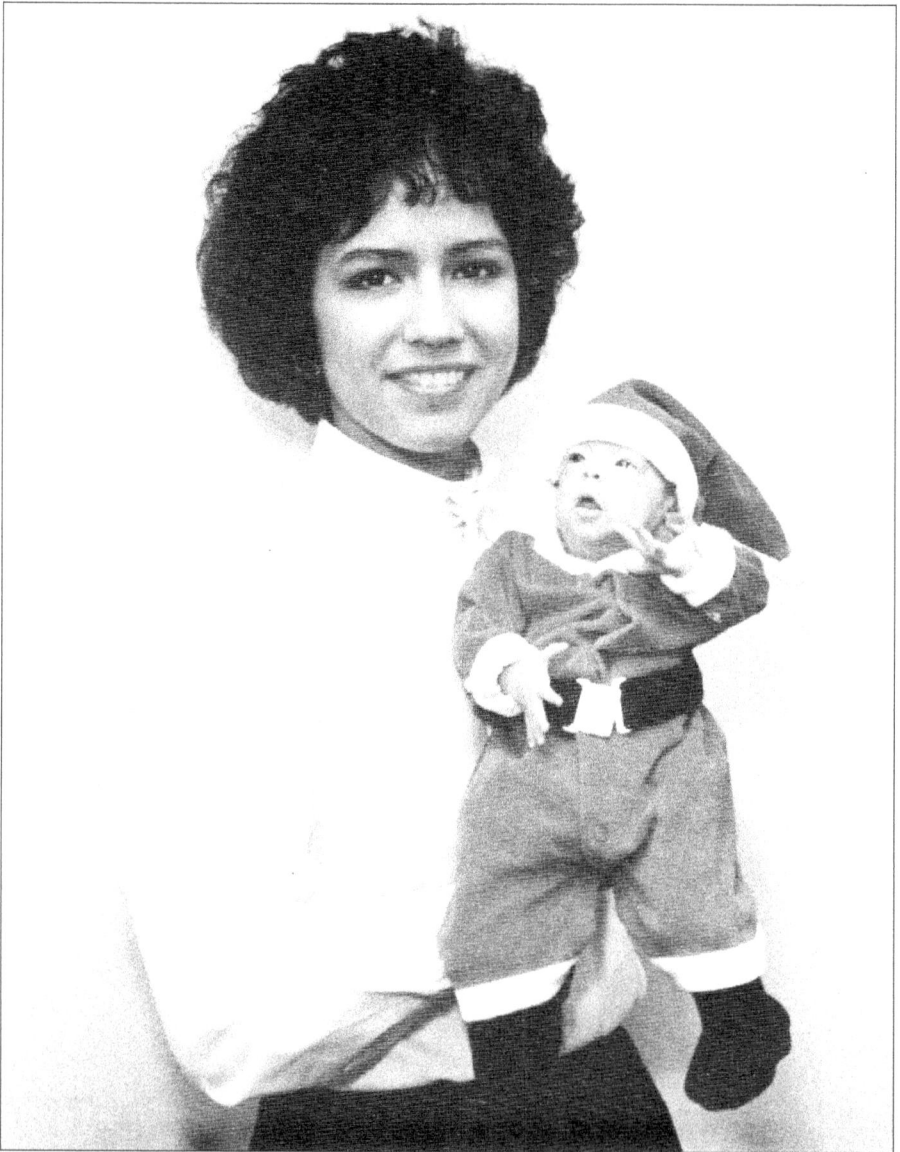

Neonatologist Sylvia Lopez, M.D., holds an infant in the Neonatal Intensive Care Unit at Presbyterian Hospital, Oklahoma City. The baby, Elora Lopez, from Oklahoma City, is the daughter of Marcelino and Veronica Lopez. She weighed 2 lbs. 12 oz. at birth.

THE KEEPER

I am the keeper of lost souls
A refuge in the night
A shelter for the homeless
A haven from the fight.

I am a healer for the wounded
A provider for the lame
A warm and present comfort
For those who suffer pain.

My door is always open
For the tired and the poor
One day we'll have an answer
Someday we'll find a cure.

Enter little children –
The road is hard and long
We'll share the bread and water
And fill each day with song!

But when your soul has rested
And your journey must restart
Always reason with your head
But never lose your heart!

THE DOCTOR'S DIVORCE

When they graduate, a lot of doctors think their
medical practice is more important than their family.

Herb walked into the doctor's lounge with a tired look on his face.

"What's wrong, Herb?" I asked. "Were you up all night operating or something?"

"Not exactly," Herb replied. "It's personal," he added.

"Martha wants to divorce me."

"I'm sorry to hear that, Herb," I answered. "You two seemed like such a good couple."

"We were a good couple," Herb replied. "It seemed like we had everything."

"I mean, think about it," he continued. "You're married to a doctor. What more could you want? I mean, isn't that supposed to be a part of the American dream – grow up and marry a doctor or lawyer and live happily ever after?"

"Not a lawyer," I replied. "Malpractice premiums are going up 40% this year."

"O.K., not a lawyer," Herb answered. "But, marrying a doctor – isn't that what everyone dreams of – to marry a doctor and live happily ever after?"

"More like happily never after," I quipped.

"How do you mean, Dr. Truewater?" Herb asked. "Look, I work hard, I make good money, I pay my bills, we belong to the Country Club, we live in a nice house, we drive two cars, we have two lovely children. What's so bad about that?"

"I didn't say being married to a doctor was bad," I began.

"It's just that it's difficult. It's not all that it's cracked up to be. Think about it. If you're a doctor's spouse, you've got certain expectations you're supposed to live up to."

"Such as?" Herb asked.

"Such as trying to raise your kids, and keeping up with the Jones," I answered. "It's like you're in a competition, or something – you know, the best car, the biggest house, even the nicest golf clubs and clothes."

"I suppose so," Herb answered. "But that's not a whole lot different than our society at large."

"True enough," I replied. "Then there's the stress of being married to someone who works all day in a pressure cooker environment, dealing with life and death matters, and then comes home at night to collapse."

"It can be a little difficult being married to someone who collapses when they get home. It's not easy carrying on a one-way conversation."

"I'll admit I'm a little tired when I get home," Herb replied. "And I haven't communicated as well with my wife as I probably should have. I'll admit to that."

"And then there's the kids," I continued.

"My kids are doing just fine," Herb replied defensively.

"Of course they are," I said. "But how well do you know them?"

"As well as you can know teenagers," Herb answered.

"I think it can be harder to raise doctor's kids, just like it's harder to raise a preacher's kids – there's a certain set of expectations that people place on you, and it's hard to live up to that. Furthermore, the kids often grow up with one or more parents absent most of the time."

"When you're in medical school, there's all this emphasis on how important it is to practice good medicine. You're taught this obsessive-compulsive behavior and the importance of the work ritual. The family takes a back seat."

"When they graduate, a lot of doctors think their medical practice is more important than their family. That makes it harder on the spouse as well."

"Well, is it any easier to be married to a businessman or a hard-working tradesman?" Herb asked.

"I suppose not," I replied. "What's important is that the parents spend time with their kids and that the parents spend quality time with each other."

"As a doctor, it's hard to find quality time," I continued. "Why, when I worked in Hollis, Oklahoma, I would tell people I was out of town for the week-end, and they'd actually drive by my house to make sure I was gone! One man even wheeled grandma up the driveway so I could give her a flu shot!"

"I spend quality time with Martha," Herb replied defensively.

"Why, we go out golfing every Sunday afternoon."

"That's important," I said. "But, what do you talk about?"

"Why, we talk about golf," Herb replied. "You know, making birdies and pars and deciding which way the putt is going to break."

"That's good, Herb," I replied. "But I wouldn't consider that quality time. You need to sit down with Martha and have a heart-to-heart talk about why she's unhappy."

"I've done that," Herb answered.

"And?" I asked.

"I don't want to get too personal, here, Dr. Truewater," Herb replied, as he poured himself another cup of coffee and bit into a donut.

"Maybe that's part of the problem," I volunteered. "Not getting personal enough."

"Oh, alright, I'll tell you," Herb answered. "I mean, we've only known each other since medical school. If I can't tell you, who can I tell?"

"Your wife," I replied smugly.

Herb paused for a moment.

"Alright," Herb began. "I've started noticing other women – you know, looking at them when I'm with Martha. She doesn't like that."

"Well, stop looking," I said. "That's easy enough to fix."

"And I've started thinking about my mortality – I'm sixty now, you know. Patients who are my age and even younger are dying. I'm going to more and more funerals these days. That gets a little depressing, knowing that your mortality is approaching."

"Of course," I replied. "I've noticed the same thing myself."

"Is that all?" I added, knowing that I had heard some things through the grapevine.

"No, that's not all," Herb answered.

"I'm having an affair with a younger woman I met at the Penny Heights Weight Control and Healthy Living Center. We rode exercise bikes next to each other."

"That's not good, Herb," I answered.

"I'm not really in love with her," Herb quickly added. "It's just that she seems to fill a niche in my life that I need right now. Maybe man wasn't meant to have just one partner."

"I've heard that argument before," I responded. "Have you tried counseling?"

"We're going next week," Herb responded. "We're going to see that orthopedic surgeon, John Grunsfield, who quit medicine after fifteen years, and became a Deacon at Holy Christian Heights. I hear he does a lot of personal counseling for doctors."

"I wish you and your wife the best, Herb," I replied, as I headed back to surgery.

One of the more difficult things about being a doctor, or any career person for that matter, is to keep in touch with your family. Just as work is required to maintain a career, so work is required to maintain a marriage and family.

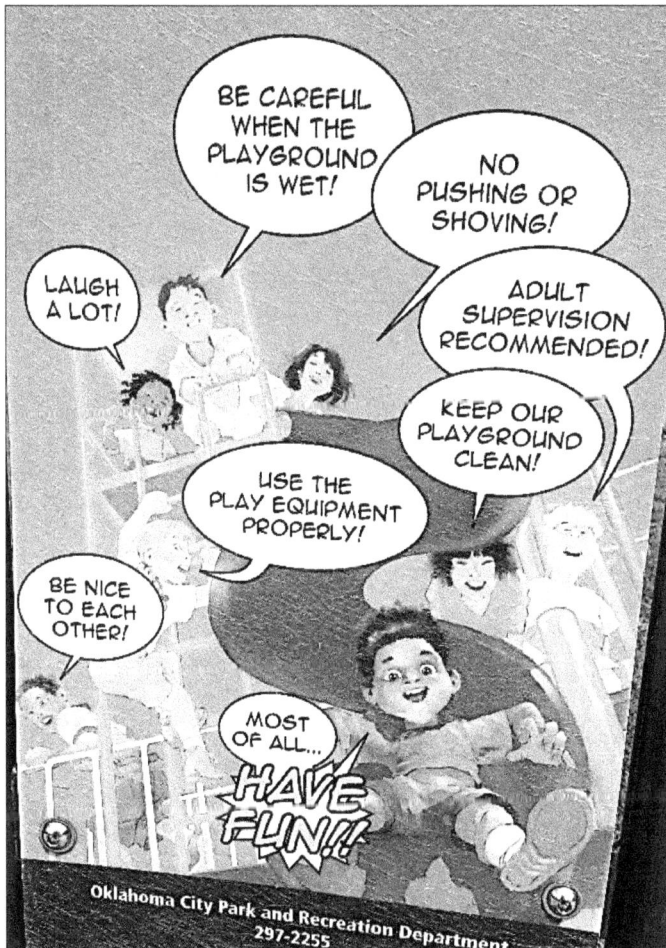

Everything I need to know I learned in Kindergarten!

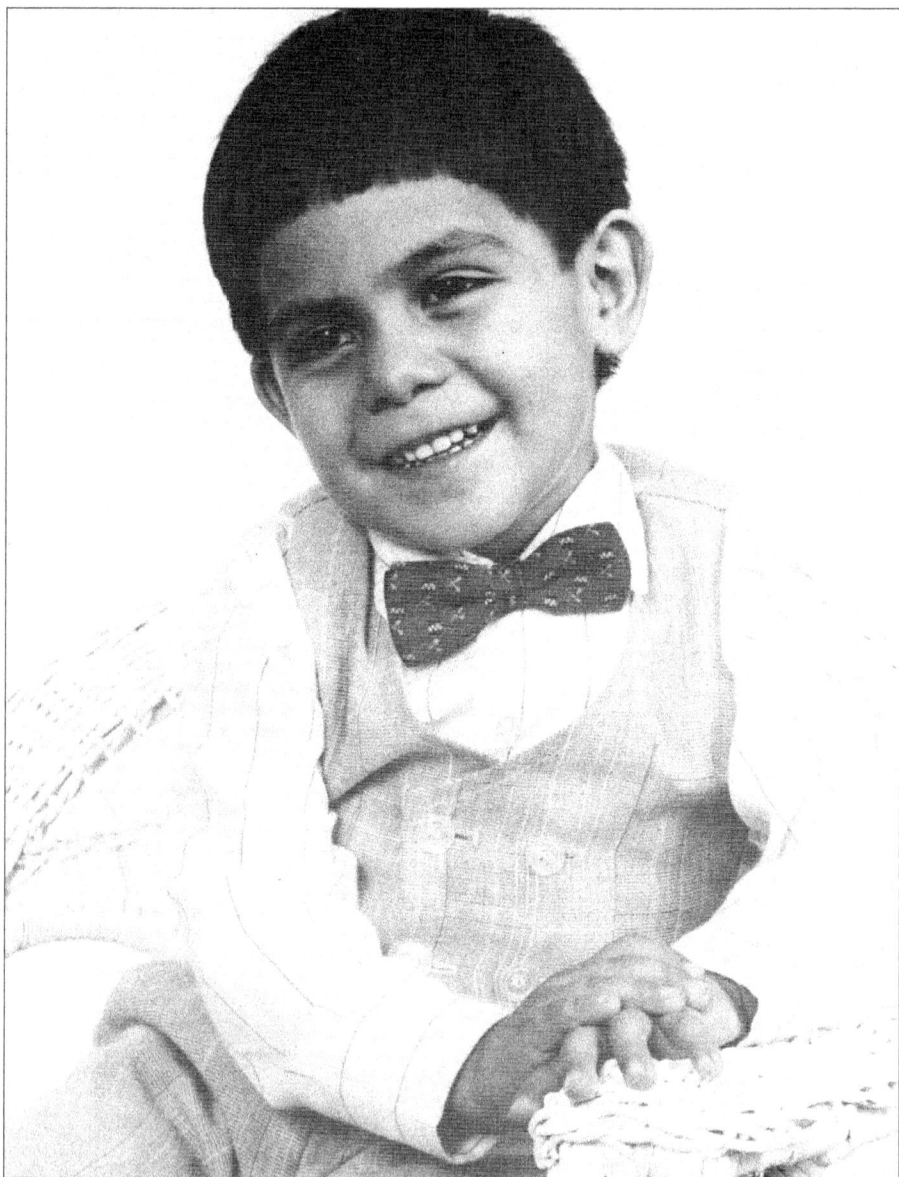

Ricardo Melendez, age 3, is the son of Maximina and Benigno Melendez. Ricardo is a patient at the Baptist Medical Mission Clinic, founded by Dr. William Hale of Oklahoma City.

WE ARE DIFFERENT

No two snowflakes are the same
It's part of Nature's plan
The ice that glistens on the tree
Is unique in all the land.

No two people are the same
It's just that simple too
Each one of us has different traits
And things we like to do.

Some will sing their music
Others play their bow
Some will swim across the seas
Or race upon the snow.

Nature's great variety
Gives each a different view –
Like the colors of the rainbow
Each one's a different hue!

BREASTFEEDING ON THE RISE

*In our culture, it's perfectly acceptable to use breasts to
sell products, but it's not OK to use breasts to breastfeed,
the purpose for which they are biologically intended.*
— La Leche League

"A funny thing happened on the way to the surgery lounge,"
Herb smiled as he sat down for a cup of coffee before starting his
hernia repair."

"What's that?" I asked.

"A woman exposed her breast to me in public," Herb exclaimed.

"You should be honored," I said.

"Let's just say I was surprised, and certainly unprepared," Herb
answered.

"Well, that's been known to happen," I replied. "I'm sure you've
seen some of those spring break videos from Fort Lauderdale."

"No, it's not like that," Herb replied.

"Well, you shouldn't be offended," I replied. "It's all very natural.
You don't want to be a prude about these things."

"What things?"

"Breasts," I replied. "As a physician, you should know that breasts
are just a normal part of the female anatomy."

"Of course I know that," Herb replied. "And I'm not a prude. You
see, this woman was breastfeeding in public."

"Breastfeeding in public is now perfectly acceptable," I told Herb.

"Why, in the old days, women used to breastfeed in the bathroom,
dressing rooms, or even behind closed doors. One La Leche member
states that breastfeeding women have come out of the closet. They're
proud of their breasts, and there's nothing to be ashamed of in today's
new world."

"I just wasn't ready for it, that's all," Herb replied.

"Like many of us, you're just a victim of today's culture," I added.

"Society today equates breasts with sexuality. But breasts are more than just an object of beauty and poetry. They happen to be functional organs, and are intended for a specific purpose."

"I recently read an article about a woman from the La Leche League. She was interviewed in the Daily Oklahoman on December 29, 2003:

"In our culture, it's perfectly acceptable to use breasts to sell products, but it's often not OK to use breasts to breastfeed, the purpose for which they are biologically intended."

"The article went on to describe a waiter at a restaurant where La Leche members were dining. When one woman pulled out her breast and started breastfeeding, he started giggling and held his hand in front of his face and walked away."

"How rude!" Herb quipped.

"They had to get the manager to have a talk with the ill-informed waiter. In fact, the manager sent the waiter back for a second look, in order to apologize to the lactating mother."

"Other breastfeeding women have complained that they have been made to feel nasty or embarrassed when they expose their breasts in public, and have threatened to file lawsuits."

"Lawsuits over public breast feeding? Dr. Truewater, you're putting me on," Herb interjected.

"But that's not all," I continued. "Some pediatricians are designated their waiting rooms and exam rooms as 'Public Breast-Feeding Zones.'"

"And what will the symbol be for designating a Breast-Feeding Zone?" Herb asked maliciously.

"I'm not going there," I replied.

"Let me get this straight," Herb responded. "You can't pull out a cigarette in a doctor's office or a restaurant, but you can pull out a breast and start breast feeding?"

"It's all about health," I replied.

"And, you'll be seeing more breasts in the future – courtesy of the federal government," I added.

"That can't be all bad," Herb interjected.

"You see, the federal government has issued a Healthy People 2010 initiative, which mandates 75% of mothers to initiate breast feeding at the time of birth and to continue breastfeeding until their infants are at least six months old."

"You're making this up, Dr. Truewater," Herb replied angrily. "The government can't do that."

"I'm not making this up, Herb. You can read it for yourself."

"Sounds like Big Brother at work," Herb added.

"Furthermore, the American Academy of Pediatrics says breast milk is an important source of nutrition for babies, and has protective substances that ward off illnesses. In addition, women who breastfeed return more quickly to their pre-pregnancy weight, and have a reduced risk for ovarian and premenopausal breast cancers."

"I'm all for more breast feeding," Herb answered. "I could get used to it."

"Advocacy groups are urging state lawmakers to allow lactating workers flexible time to breastfeed or pump milk. And one state representative wants to exempt breastfeeding mothers from jury duty."

"That would probably increase the birth rate," Herb quipped.

"And thirteen states now exempt breastfeeding mothers from public indecency laws. Nineteen states allow mothers to breastfeed in any public or private location," I added.

"Of course, all this is really nothing new," Herb replied. "I'm Greek, and in the old country, Greek women would publicly breastfeed until the child was five or six years old. It's been that way since ancient times."

"For that matter, Roman men attending sporting events in the Coliseum were forbidden to wear clothes," Herb added. "It was all very natural, you know."

As I headed back to surgery to start my case, I wondered, with modern women baring their breasts like days of old, what might be next. I dreaded to think what forbidden part of their body men might expose as we entered the Brave New World.

And would they be exempt from jury duty?

NO MORE FAT!

The nurse walks in with your first solid meal in a week, lifts off the lid, and leaves you staring at a bowel of dry cereal, low-cholesterol eggs, and dry wheat toast with no butter.

I was sipping on my Cappuccino coffee in the doctor's lounge, waiting for my hernia case to start, when Herb Silverstein, the plastic surgeon, walked in, quietly munching a bacon, sausage, and egg biscuit.

"Good morning, Dr. Truewater," Herb mumbled in a garbled voice, as he continued eating.

"Hello, Herb," I replied.

As I stared at his bacon, sausage and egg biscuit, I couldn't help commenting about the new hospital dietary guidelines.

"I don't mean to be critical, but that's a lot of fat and salt you're ingesting there, Herb," I began.

"You should know that Holy Christian Hospital doesn't approve of what you're eating – you're setting a bad example for your patients," I chided him.

"I've been eating bacon and eggs for breakfast since I was a kid," Herb responded.

"Why, it's part of the Southern tradition – along with biscuits and gravy," Herb added.

"I suppose so," I said. "But Holy Christian Hospital has issued a new set of dietary guidelines. They're hoping to promote healthy heart nutrition by deleting excessive fat and salt from the menu."

"Starting the first of this month, Holy Christian Hospital will no longer serve bacon or sausage to its patients for breakfast," I proclaimed.

"Why, that's preposterous!" Herb exclaimed. "We'll lose all our patients!"

"Nonsense!" I rebutted.

"We've got to stop eating like pigs, and it's time for doctors to set an example," I added, as I stared longingly at the remainder of Herb's sausage and egg biscuit.

"Stop eating like pigs?" Herb rebutted. "You should know, Dr. Truewater, that pigs are vegetarians and eat mostly corn."

"Alright, Herb, you know what I mean," I answered. "I'm referring to all the fat and cholesterol in the American diet. Obesity in this country has become a national epidemic, and heart disease kills over 500,000 people every year."

"I'm all in favor of reducing obesity and lowering cholesterol," Herb said, as he looked at his rounded gut, "but I'm not sure that eliminating sausage and bacon from a patient's breakfast tray is the answer to the problem."

"I mean, think about it. Let's say you're a patient and you haven't eaten in five days, because you're recovering from a ruptured appendix or a ruptured colon. The nurse walks in with your first solid meal in a week, lifts off the lid, and leaves you staring at a bowel of dry cereal, low-cholesterol eggs, and dry wheat toast with no butter. Now, wouldn't that make you start vomiting all over again?"

"It's a matter of re-training you're eating habits, Herb," I replied. "And what better place to educate than in the hospital? People have just got to learn to eat healthy."

"Well, who's to say that eating sausage and bacon isn't healthy, Dr. Truewater? You know, these guidelines aren't exactly written in stone."

"I'm aware that there's a debate about this in the medical literature, Herb," I replied, "but cardiologists that I've talked to recommend the low-fat diet – along with running or some other aerobic exercise three times a week."

"I'll bet any diet would be acceptable if you did aerobic exercises three times a week," Herb quipped. "Why did you see that one cardiologist who runs through Penny Heights every morning at 6 am? I mean, is he obsessive-compulsive or what?"

"Why, if I made as much money as those cardiologists, I'd probably do everything I could to live an extra year or two myself!" Herb added with envy.

"This has nothing to do with money, Herb," I interjected. "It's all about building lean muscle mass. Statistics show that people with lean muscle mass are happier, healthier people, who are less likely to die from heart disease."

"And more likely to die from cancer," Herb chided.

"Well, you've got to die from something," I replied.

"Alright," Herb conceded, as he put down a second sausage biscuit on the chair next to me. "No more sausage and bacon for breakfast. But just let me have my biscuits and gravy. I was raised on biscuits and gravy. That's part of the Southern tradition, too, you know."

"No, Herb, biscuits and gravy are not allowed either," I said. "Well, let me put it like this – you can have the biscuits, but without the gravy."

"Dry biscuits?" Herb whined. "Cholesterol free eggs? Dry cereal? Toast with no butter? I think I'll just have a cup of coffee for breakfast and go directly to lunch."

"Coffee's O.K., Herb," I said – "as long as it's decaffeinated."

Just then, Herb left the doctor's lounge to start his cleft palate repair. I looked surreptitiously around the doctor's lounge, which was now empty. I slowly unwrapped the sausage and bacon biscuit that Herb had given up only moments before. As I munched away on my breakfast, I realized that it was a lot easier to give advice than to take it.

"Forgive me, Herb," I said to myself, as I bit into a juicy morsel of sausage and bacon.

Some habits are just too hard to break.

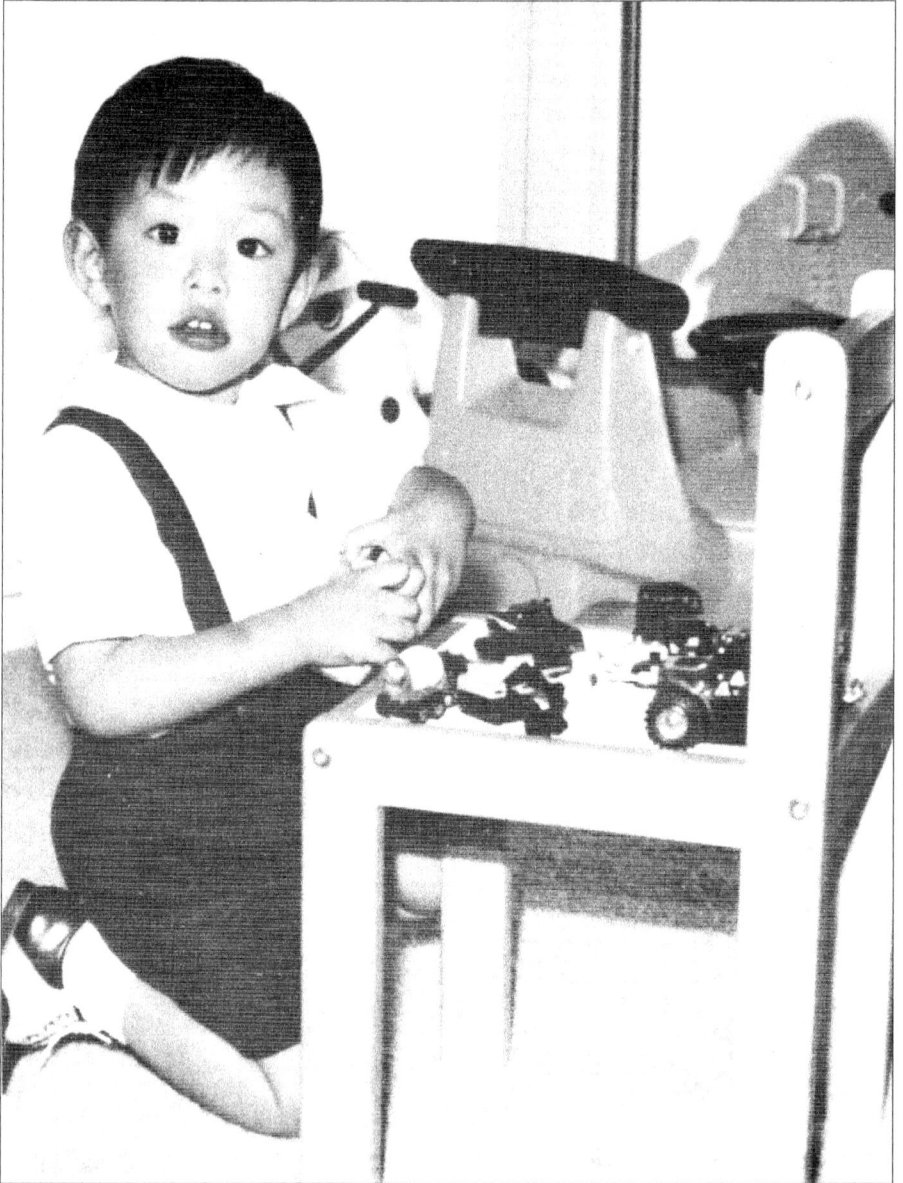

Christopher Huy Cao, age 5, is the son of Hoang and Huong "Thi" Cao, of Oklahoma City.

THE ICE CREAM MAN

Hurry up and get your dime!
The ice cream man is right on time.
The kids are waiting by the street
Anxious for a frozen treat!

The ice cream man gets off his bike
And waves to all the little tykes
He greets each little child by name
And then begins his ice cream game.

"Hello Mary! Hello Jim!
It's really nice to see that grin!"
He reaches down inside his box
And pulls out ice cold cherry pops!

"I used to work hard every day
Before I learned just how to play.
Now I'd rather see a smile
On each and every precious child!"

One day I heard the children cry –
Their little ice cream man had died
He left his bike beside my door
We never saw him anymore.

Now I ring the bells and chimes
That play the little nursery rhymes
How I love to see the smile
On each and every precious child!

GOING TO CHICAGO

I was sitting in the surgery lounge, munching on a custard-filled doughnut when Herb walked in with a rather dejected look on his face.

"What's the trouble, Herb?" I asked.

"You remember Mrs. Lucas, my elderly patient with leukemia that I put a central line in the other day?"

"Sure, Herb," I replied. "You said she was pretty sick, and you weren't sure she would live much longer."

"Well, Mrs. Lucas expired this morning," Herb replied.

"I'm sorry to hear that," I consoled Herb. "Sounds like Mrs. Lucas was a real nice lady, and you worked hard to try to help her."

"Thanks, Dr. Truewater," Herb replied.

"There's just one thing," I added, as I finished my doughnut and sipped on my cappuccino.

"What's that?" Herb asked, as he sat down waiting for his next case to start.

"I don't like it when the nurse tells me my patient just expired."

"Well, no doctor wants to hear their patient just died," Herb replied.

"No, of course not," I answered.

"This may sound kind of picky, but I don't think the word 'expired' should be used when a patient dies."

"Well, why not?" Herb asked.

"To me, the word 'expire' should be used, say, when your parking meter expires, or your driver's license expires, or your library book is overdue. I mean, people don't expire."

"Of course they do," Herb replied. "The word 'expire' comes from the Greek – it means 'to breath out' – in a sense, to take your last breath, or to conclude."

"Well, people don't expire," I insisted. "You're not like some carton of milk with the date stamped on it, where you suddenly turn sour or rancid."

"I think the undertaker might disagree with you on that," Herb quipped.

"Our death isn't pre-determined," I continued. "In fact, that's what doctors are for – to prolong life and improve the quality of life beyond some arbitrary number of years."

"Well, when I was a kid," Herb interjected, "If Grandma died, the parents would simply tell their kids that Grandma went to sleep."

"I know," I added. "I've been afraid to sleep ever since."

"You know, patients are funny," I continued. "They don't want to go to a doctor whose patients die – like they might die if they go to see him. Let's face it--we're a death-denying society. People aren't supposed to die. Like old soldiers – I guess we're just supposed to fade away."

"Well, in our office," Herb replied, "We use a code phrase for death, in case the patients in the waiting room overhear the doctor."

"A code phrase?" I asked.

"You see," Herb continued, "When I ask my nurse why Mr. Smith missed his doctor's appointment, instead of saying that Mr. Smith died, my nurse will say, 'Mr. Smith went to Chicago.'"

"That way, if the patients in the waiting room overhear us, they won't go running out of the building."

"Makes me think twice about traveling to Chicago," I quipped.

"But why pick Chicago? I mean, I grew up in Chicago – Chicago always gets the blame. There were just as many gangsters in New York or Los Angeles, but Chicago gets the wrap for gangsters."

"Okay," Herb answered. "Maybe you'd like it better if the nurse told you your patient just passed."

"Passed?" I asked.

"You know, like someone passes away," Herb added.

"People don't pass away either," I said. "I mean, to me the word 'pass' has always been associated with good things – you pass your board exam, or you get a free pass to get into a ball game, or you pass inspection."

"If you pass, that means you go on to live," I concluded. "People don't pass when they die. If anything, when organ systems fail, patients go on to die."

"Okay, you want the nurse to tell you that your patient just 'failed' when they pass?" Herb queried.

"It would make more sense," I replied.

"Perhaps you're looking at death the wrong way, Dr. Truewater," Herb continued.

"This may be getting into metaphysics and religion, but when your patient passes, he travels from one world to the next – he passes on."

"Ah, yes," I replied. "In Grecian mythology, the souls were ferried by Charon across the river Styx to reach their final abode."

"When you pass on, Dr. Truewater, you'll travel from one world to the next – be it heaven or wherever."

"What do you mean, 'wherever,' Herb?" I asked.

"Well, of course, we don't all go to the same place," Herb continued. "In my religion, if you've been a good doctor, or a good person, you'll go to heaven, and, if not, well, Lord help you."

"Are you suggesting that I'm not a good doctor, Herb?"

"No, I don't mean that at all. It's just that nobody really knows where they'll end up. I've been taught that there's a heaven and a hell and that we all await judgment day."

"For all I know, we may all end up in eternal damnation."

"You're talking fire and brimstone, no doubt."

"No, for you Dr. Truewater, eternal damnation will mean poring endlessly through Webster's dictionary looking for the true meaning of life."

"Surely, you jest, Herb."

"Of course, Dr. Truewater. I'm sure that you and I will both pass through those pearly gates. It's just that I'll be greeted by Moses and you'll be greeted by Jesus, and others by Mohammed or Buddha."

"You mean, after you pass on, you'll be greeted by a representative of your own individual religion?" I asked. "Sounds like a cruise ship or a travel agency."

"I really don't know the answer to that," Herb replied. "How about if the nurse just tells you that your patient crossed over?"

"Crossed over?" I asked. "You mean, like crossing over the Golden Gate Bridge into Sausalito?"

"No, I mean like crossing over into another world," Herb replied. "The Christians talk of a land of milk and honey and streets lined with gold."

"I kind of like the Islamic idea of being greeted by 72 virgins and 80,000 servants in the seventh heaven," I replied. "Actually, I might even settle for one or two virgins. I don't think I could handle 72 virgins, especially at my age."

"You have to die a martyr to get 72 virgins," Herb added.

"As physicians, we're all martyrs," I replied. "Just last year, malpractice lawyers filed over 100,000 lawsuits against physicians. That's one lawsuit for every six doctors annually. For surgeons, the rate is even higher – it works out to one lawsuit every three years. We're like lambs going to the slaughter. It's been predicted that at this rate, we'll run out of paper – and surgeons – in ten years. We'll have to go back to papyrus or rice paper, and start letting the barber do surgery on the kitchen table."

"Why don't we just say that, instead of passing on, or expiring, your patient just up and died?" Herb replied.

"Do you have a problem with that?" he added.

"Of course not," I said, as I finished my cappuccino and headed off to surgery.

"It's all a matter of semantics. Life must go on."

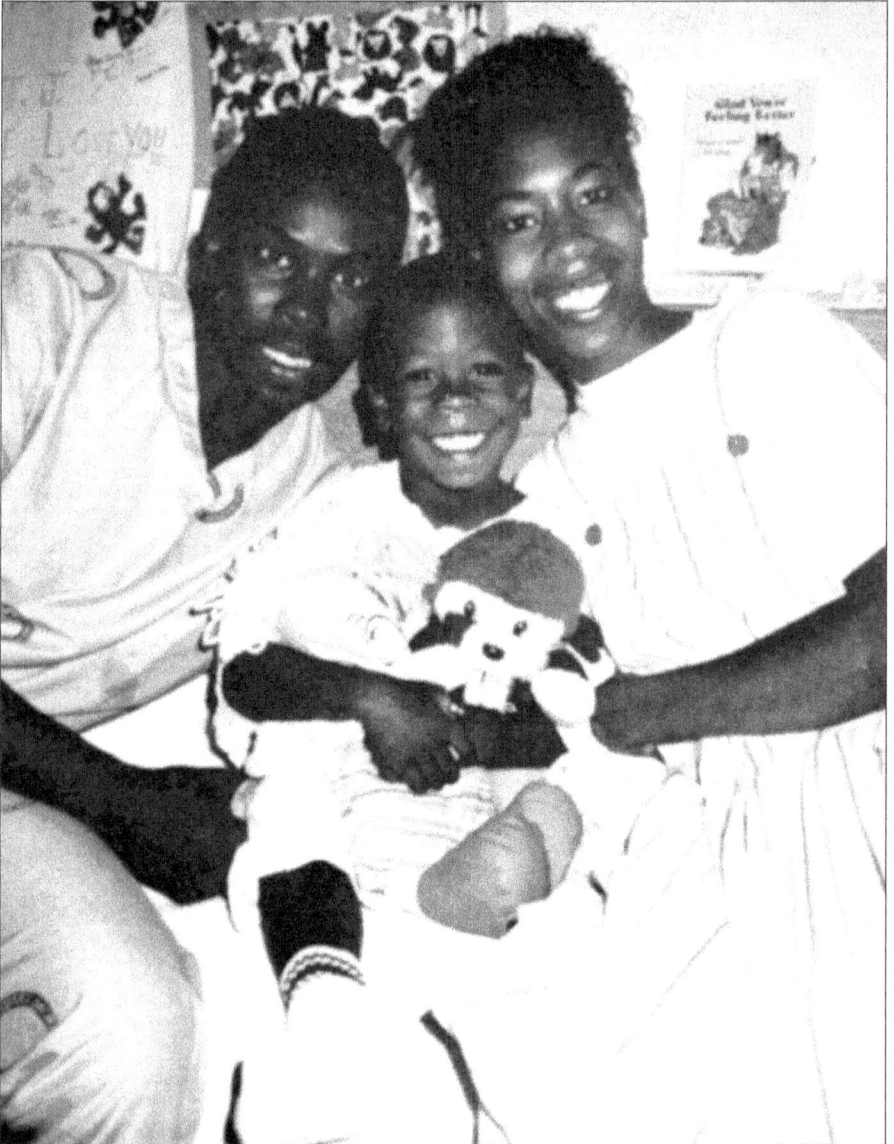

Troy Bowen, Jr., is pictured with his parents, Troy and Carmen Bowen, during a recent hospitalization. Both parents are employed at Baptist Medical Center in Oklahoma City. Troy, Jr., is doing very well, and especially enjoys playing video games.

HURRY AND GET WELL

Hurry and get well, my son
We've got so much to do
We could go down by the pond
And catch a fish or two.

You really gave me quite a scare
The day that you fell down
I tried and tried to wake you up
But you wouldn't come around.

We got you to the hospital
I thought that you were dead
Then you opened up those eyes
And sat up in the bed.

You asked me for your teddy bear
I knew you were alright
But even though you're almost well
I think I'll spend the night!

I think about you day and night
And what I almost lost
If I should ever lose you, son,
I couldn't bear the loss!

CONFESSION TIME

If you ever really want to know about somebody, talk to their anesthesiologist or priest. In the case of the priest, people will tell their most intimate secrets for fear of holding out on the Almighty. But the anesthesiologist is the one who really holds the cards. Let me explain.

Tom Williams was referred to me by Dr. Allan Flowman to fix his hiatus hernia.

"I've got a good case for you," Allan phoned one day. "I've been treating Tom Williams for about six months for peptic esophagitis and regurgitation. He's had all the medications I can think to give him, he's elevated the head of his bed at night, and he still has the same problem. I think he needs surgery," Allan concluded.

"Sounds like a good case," I replied. "He's a real medical failure."

People who don't respond to medical therapy are called "medical failures". Surgeons like to get "medical failures" – the patients have already resigned themselves to surgery, and it's usually just a matter of explaining the operation and putting them on the schedule. Nobody can accuse you being "knife happy" because the patient's already had his medical trial.

Besides, most surgeons feel that medical therapy is only a prelude to the definitive surgical correction – sort of a formality that has to be observed before you can get on with the show.

"You'll like Mr. Williams," Allan continued. "He's an avid skier, and works as a technical support engineer for the telephone company. I've known Tom for over fifteen years – his oldest daughter is dating my son."

"I appreciate the referral, Allan," I replied. "I'll call your office when we get him on the surgery schedule. Thanks again."

When Tom Williams arrived at my office, he was a model patient. Neatly dressed, courteous to the office crew, and with a quick sense of humor. Tom was a star. At the end of my interview, I went through all the usual questions.

"Now, I've got some routine questions to ask you, Tom, that I need to know before we go to surgery," I began somewhat sheepishly.

"Go right ahead, Dr. Truewater. I've nothing to hide," Tom replied matter-of-factly.

"Any allergies to medications?" I began.

"None," Tom replied.

"Alcohol or tobacco usage?" I continued.

"Never," Tom answered.

"Past history of drug abuse, such as narcotics or amphetamines?" I asked.

"Aspirin's the strongest medication I've ever taken," Tom replied.

One week later, Tom was in the holding area of the hospital, waiting for his surgery. The anesthesiologist, Dr. Charles Baxter, was conducting his routine interview. As I reviewed the chart, I overheard Charlie's pre-anesthetic interview. I couldn't believe he was talking to the same Tom Williams who I was getting ready to operate.

"How do you do, Mr. Williams," he began. "I'm Dr. Charles Baxter. I'll be putting you to sleep for your surgery. I need to know everything about you so there won't be any mistakes."

"Mistakes?" Tom asked, with a quiver to his voice.

"Yes," Charlie continued. "As you know, unknown drug interactions can be fatal. Do you smoke?" Charlie asked.

"I'm down to two packs a day," Tom replied.

"Do you drink alcohol?"

"I've been through drug rehab twice," Tom replied. "I haven't had a drink in two days."

By now I couldn't believe my ears. I had to take a quick peek from behind the curtain to see if this was really my patient. Sure enough, there sat Tom laying quietly on the patient cart, handkerchief in hand, spilling his guts like he was on his way to the gallows and Charlie was giving him the Last Rites.

"Anything else I should know?" Charlie continued.

"Yes," Tom confessed. I take a gram of amphetamines a day – I've been doing it for twelve years. I've tried everything I can to break the habit, but Lord knows my weaknesses!"

"That's no problem," Charlie continued. "I see it all the time. Now tell me, have you ever used intravenous drugs? I have to know if there's a risk of AIDS."

"Is it really necessary?" Tom whined.

"This is all strictly confidential," Charlie continued in his most serious voice.

"I've never taken intravenous drugs, but I've had boyfriends – lots of them – but I prefer my wife. I'm really a family man at heart. It's just that, well, Lord knows my weaknesses," Tom sobbed.

"That'll be all," Charlie concluded. "I don't expect any problems with the anesthesia.

At the end of the case, Charlie showed me the history and physical that I had dictated from my office.

"You really need to interview your patients more thoroughly," Charlie chided. "This man is bisexual and has a serious drug and alcohol problem."

"I'm sorry, Charlie," I replied. "When I asked him about drugs in the office, he denied having any problems. In fact, his referring physician didn't know about it either!" I added sheepishly.

I concluded that the priest and anesthesiologist are really the only two people who really know their constituents. Most of us live in a pseudo-world of false fronts and first impressions.

Sitting in the doctor's office chatting with the family physician, or even the surgeon doesn't cut the mustard. Put those same people in the confession box at church or the holding area in surgery, when they are getting ready to face the unknown, and all manner of confessions spring forth!

THE BULL RIDER

The First Baptist Church in Atoka, Oklahoma, will never be quite the same. Over 3,500 cowboys and cowgirls from Colorado, Texas, and Oklahoma, wearing rodeo hats and championship rodeo belt buckles, have come to bid their hero farewell. They fill the sanctuary where their hero rests. They stand on the sidewalk, even the street in front of the church, to hear the Reverend Willard Moody, a former professional calf roper, eulogize their fallen comrade.

"Lane Frost was only 25 years old," Willard tells the gathering. "He rode the giant bull, 'Red Rock', after 308 attempts by others. In Oklahoma, they don't give up – they just keep trying until somebody wins, somebody conquers the insurmountable. And Lane Frost was their winner. He conquered where others failed. He kept on riding until he was the best. He rode 'Red Rock'"!

To the city dweller, it's hard to explain why people ride bulls, or even why people have rodeos. To the Oklahoma cowboy, riding the bull is man's challenge against Nature, man's attempt to order his world, to overcome the forces that would rule him. But these cowboys don't talk their philosophy – they live it. Men of action in a world of inaction, men who take chances in a world that is overly cautious – that's what the pioneer spirit is all about.

Lane Frost was the champion. But he was not proud or vain. He loved to teach kids as much as he loved the rodeo. He taught little Jakus White, at the age often, to ride small calves.

He built self-confidence in Jakus by teaching him to rodeo. And he would talk to Jakus about his problems – any problems – at any time of the day or night. Lane loved people. And Lane loved children.

"Good-bye, Lane," little Jakus sobbed, as he laid a red rose on his hero's chest. "I will always remember you!"

They buried Lane Frost next to Warren "Freckles" Brown of Soper, another world champion bull rider, at 2 p.m. in Hugo, Oklahoma. Warren "Freckles" Brown had ridden "Tornado" in 1967 after 211 previous tries. The cowboys removed their giant hats and watched with reddened eyes as Lane was placed next to "Freckles".

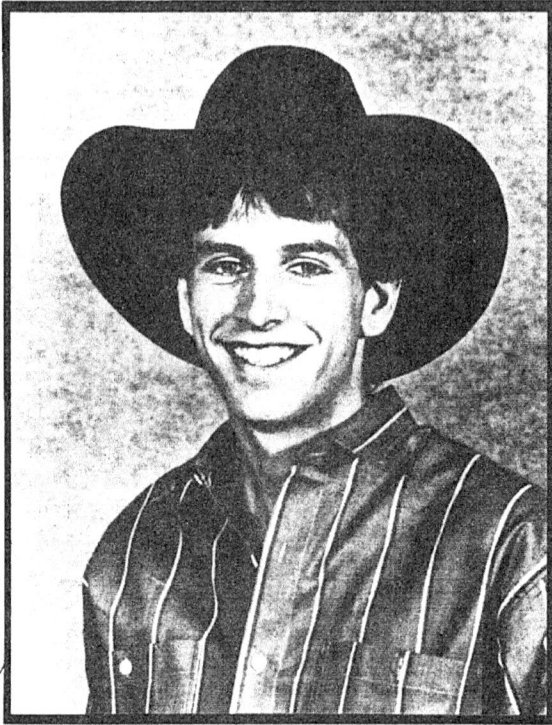

LANE FROST
LANE, OKLAHOMA
1987 WORLD
BULL RIDING CHAMPION
$105,698

PROFESSIONAL RODEO COWBOYS ASSOCIATION
101 PRO RODEO DRIVE
COLORADO SPRINGS, COLO 80919
303 593-8840

Photo of Lane Frost in 1989 bull riding competition in San Angelo, Texas.
The author thanks Clyde and Elsie Frost of Lane, Oklahoma.

Afterwards, the people talked about Lane. "He was the finest person you'd ever meet. He didn't have no enemies. Why did he have to die?"

Lane had successfully ridden "Takin' Care of Business", scoring an 83 at the Cheyenne Frontier Days, when the bull suddenly turned, and rammed him from behind. Lane died several minutes later.

"He didn't have to die," the people said. "It wasn't his time."

But any cowboy can tell you that you can't pick your time. You fight the odds and hope to win. But you can't win forever.

Eventually, the forces of Nature, be they chance or evil, will take their toll and claim their victory.

And who's to say that living and dying sensibly, from diseases of the aged, is a better way to conduct one's life? Not that we should be foolhardy, just that occasionally we ought to take chances, challenging the forces that would control or limit our potential. We may not always win, but we will always learn. "Lane was like the catcher in the rye," one cowboy observed after the funeral. "He was always watching after the little kids, afraid that one of them might fall over the edge, and he'd have to go catch him."

"Trouble is," the cowboy continued, "There was nobody to catch Lane Frost."

No national newspaper carried the story that day. But the people of Oklahoma will always remember. Lane Frost was the best bull rider ever!

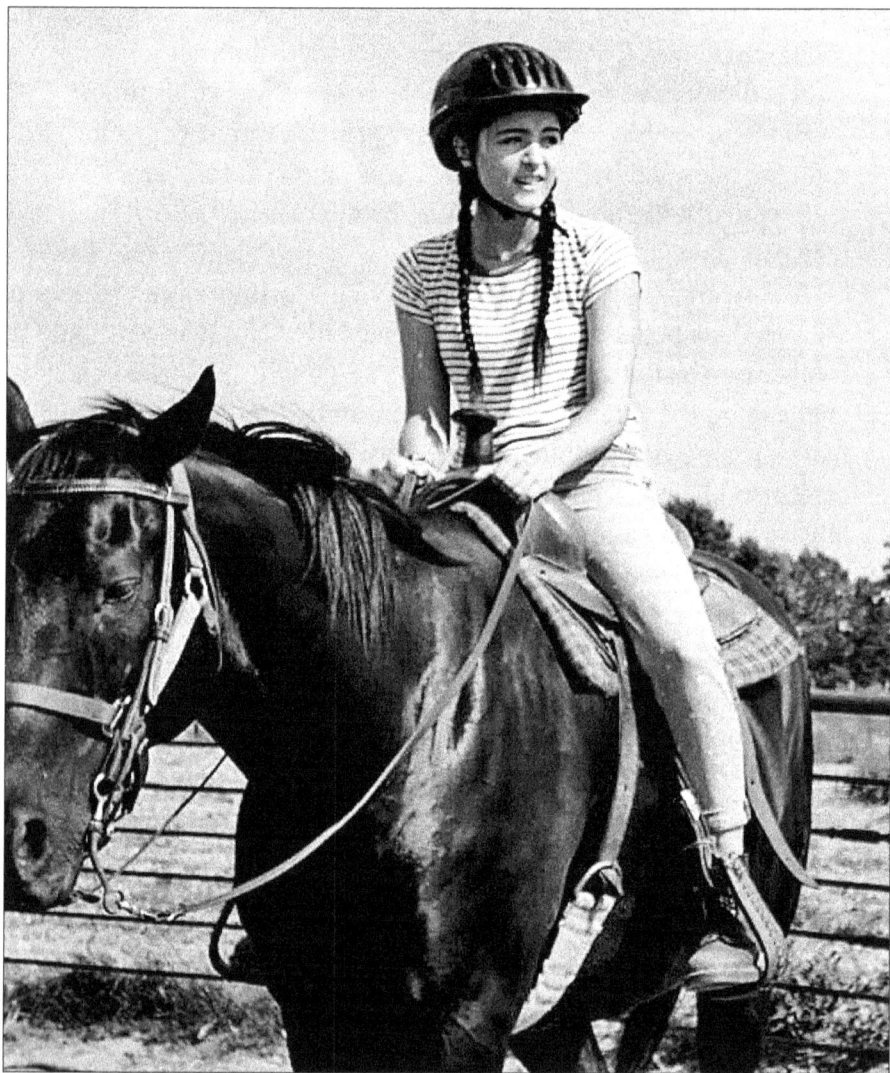

Jaedn Moddrell, daughter of Lisa Truels

WHAT IS LOVE?

by Jaedn Moddrell

"Love" is defined by Merriam Webster as:

1. Strong affection for another arising out of kinship or personal ties
2. Affection based on benevolence, admiration, or common interest
3. Warm attachment, enthusiasm, or devotion

In other words, the definition of love in our society involves an emotional attachment to another individual. It is this basis for love that determines who we should marry. But is this a good definition?

For example, many couples marry based on this emotional attachment—we often hear the phrase, "love at first site". But is this genuine love? Love isn't rushed and should go beyond first impressions. Real love involves finding someone who can continue to grow with you.

And if love is based on emotional attachment, why do so many marriages, over 50%, end up in divorce? What happened to the warmth and emotion? Furthermore, the divorce rate for subsequent marriages is even higher, according to the American Psychological Association.

Too often, I see stories of "true lovers" who have formed a strong emotional attachment that rapidly dissolves as the relationship evolves. Love today has become commercialized, based on good looks, proper dress, and traveling to exotic islands. People date each other in a flurry of emotion, then quit dating when the excitement fades—only to look for another round of excitement in a new relationship.

Relationships typically begin with an "infatuation stage", which extends through courtship and the honeymoon. This is followed by an "adjustment stage" where each member sees the "dark side" of the other member. After another six months, or longer, the relationship enters the "compatibility stage", where each member learns to accommodate both the good and bad points of their mutual relationship.

Popular entertainers talk about creating a "stage character" while entertaining—you put on an act in order to entertain the public. People were shocked to find out, for example, that Elvis Presley was very humble, but often moody and angry in private. In the same way, first dates and often first impressions are often totally misleading as each person "puts their best foot forward." One comedian's wife was shocked to find out that her husband wasn't very funny in private—she kept asking him to "say something funny!"

Love involves a grounding in reality that is too often ignored by our popular culture! One song describes love as a "many splendored thing." Love is many splendored—but it involves finding a person who I can live with 24/7, through all the ups and downs that life delivers. At times, love can be hurtful until a mutual compromise can be achieved.

True love, in my mind, goes beyond any emotion, and involves finding a "soul mate" who shares and compliments my needs and desires. In Eastern societies, parents by custom will pick their child's future spouse, based on integrity and compatibility, and these Eastern marriages have a higher success rate than Western societies.

In my opinion, true love arises out of a compatibility with another person that goes beyond a fleeting emotional bond. It is said that the infatuation stage of a marriage lasts about two years. The marriages that last the longest are the ones where people develop a compatibility or friendship with each other that carries them through the inevitable ups and downs of our everyday experiences.

One simple option would be to skip the infatuation and adjustment stages and go directly to the compatibility stage—pick a number of people who you feel most at home with –then marry the one you like the best!

This analysis is not intended to take the romance out of a relationship, or to dwell upon the downside of discovering your partner's weaknesses. But the sooner you can get to the compatibility stage of your relationship, where you feel most comfortable sharing your innermost thoughts, the sooner you will be able to cement a lifelong bond with your significant other!

MOVING OUT

My clothes are in the trailer
Everything is cool
I guess it's time to say goodbye
I'm heading off to school.

Thank you for the times we shared
They were really great
The football games, the marching band
The times we stayed out late.

It doesn't seem that long ago
I started off to school
I used to walk the old dirt path
And think the boys were cruel!

Then we'd go in our back yard
I loved to swing up high
I'd stand up on the monkey bars
And try to touch the sky!

Now I'm off to college
I'm not that little girl
I'd like to be out on my own
And test the real world!

Of course I'll still be coming home
Every chance I get
I'll try and call you every week
You know I won't forget!

Most of all, I thank you, Mom
Through the good times and the bad
You were there to comfort me
And for that I am so glad!

THE LIVING WILL

One of our esteemed Congressional leaders has proposed a new piece of legislation requiring doctors and other health care personnel to inform patients of their Constitutional right to make a living will. I have no doubt that the proposal is well-intended. After all, sometimes patients become incapacitated during their hospitalization, and are unable to make their own life-support decisions.

I decided to inform my very next patient of his right to a living will in order to better prepare me for the upcoming legislation. His name was Harold Outback, and was referred by Dr. Jim Wellston for an inguinal hernia repair.

"Hello, Mr. Outback," I began. "My name is Dr. Bill Truewater. How may I help you?"

"My pleasure, Dr. Truewater," Harold replied, as he knocked some red clay off his cowboy boots. "I've got this hernia, Doc, and every time I rope a steer, my hernia bulges out and hurts."

I examined Mr. Outback after he removed his gun and holster, and confirmed that he indeed had a painful inguinal hernia. After the exam, I explained the procedure of inguinal hernia repair, as well as the risks and complications.

"Now, Mr. Outback," I began, "the malpractice lawyers inform me that you have a right to know all the things that can go wrong with your hernia surgery. Following any surgery, it is your right to know that you could have a stroke, heart attack, paralysis, or even death."

"Forget all that legal stuff, Doc," Harold replied. "I trust my old friend, Dr. Wellston, to send me to a good surgeon. I know that I ain't gonna live forever, and I know that things can go wrong. Now, I've got to get back to roping them steer. The only reason I came to the city was to get this here hernia fixed. How soon can you do it, Doc?" Harold asked.

"We can fix it tomorrow as an outpatient, Harold," I replied. "Now, there's one more thing you need to know."

"What's that Doc?" Harold asked.

"You have a Constitutional right to a living will," I said.

"A what?" Harold asked.

"A living will," I replied. "If anything goes wrong, it directs us about what to do with your estate."

"I don't have an estate, Dr. Truewater," Harold replied. "All's I got is my gun and my horse, Red Rider, and don't nobody want her."

"The living well also tells us if you want to be placed on a life support system, Harold," I added.

"Doc, just how serious is this hernia repair?" Harold asked.

"It's just a precaution," I added. "The federal government wants to make sure nobody gets put on a life support system that doesn't want one—needless pain and suffering, you know, to say nothing of the expense. Why, they're even talking about rationing health care."

"Doc," Harold said, "I can tell you right now, I don't want to be put on no respirator. If I can't sit on Red Rider and rope steer every day, life ain't worth living."

"And I'll tell you somethin' else," Harold added. "I had me an Aunt Clara at a nursing home for twenty years, and that ain't fer me."

Harold reached across the desk, grabbed me by the lapels of my lab coat with his deeply calloused hands, and pulled me closer, as if confiding his deepest, darkest secret.

"Doc," Harold whispered, "I don't want to be no vegetable in no nursing home. If there ain't no hope for me, I want you to take out 'ol Betsy here, and shoot me twice in the head!"

"Oh, come now, Mr. Outback," I replicd, as I reeled in shock from his request. "I couldn't do that—I'm a doctor!"

"Why not?" Harold replied. "That's what I'd do fer my horse, Red Rider, and that's what I'd want done fer me!"

"Well, for one thing, the federal government would never approve it," I replied jokingly. "Furthermore, hearing that gunshot would scare the wits out of the other patients. And it'd give the hospital a bad reputation to boot!"

"And it'd put me out of my misery," Harold added.

"We can't do that, Mr. Outback," I answered firmly. "Besides, there's always a small chance that the patient might make a miraculous recovery. I'm sure you've heard stories of people whose condition was thought to be hopeless, who miraculously survived."

"Doctor Truewater," Harold replied, "I respect you and I respect the medical profession. I don't want to tell you how to run your business. But the last thing this country needs is for the doctors to start reading patients their Constitutional rights every time they come in the hospital!"

I must admit I felt uncomfortable discussing such issues with Mr. Outback the day before his surgery. Fortunately, he underwent his hernia repair without difficulty, and was back roping steer within a few weeks. It never seems like the right time to discuss end-of-life issues, but as physicians, it's important that we discuss these matters ahead of time!

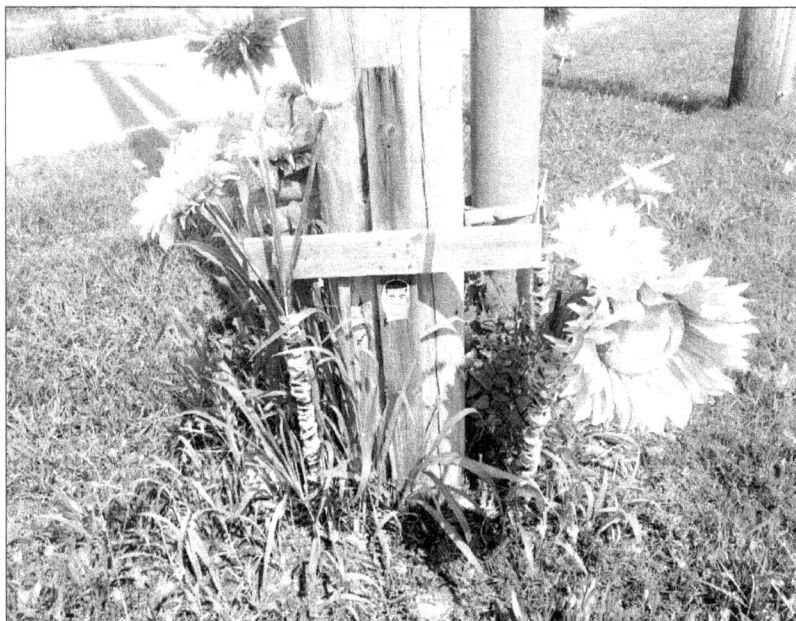

GONE TOO SOON

Gone too soon
While life was young
We played beneath
The rising sun.

I miss the days
Not long ago--
We planted flowers
And watched them grow!

In high school games
You were the star!
I watched you climb
The highest bar!

The accident that claimed your life
Has filled my world with grief and strife!
I'll leave these flowers for all to see
Where fate has ruined our destiny!

THE ACCIDENT

"Looks like you had an accident, Dr. Truewater," H.T. Park, the urologist chided me, as I sat in the Doctor's lounge waiting for my case to start.

"How about that?" I replied, with some embarrassment, as I glanced at the small spot on my scrub pants.

"I guess I was in a hurry," I added. "Could happen to anybody."

"Could happen to anybody," H.T. replies, "but it happened to you, Dr. Truewater."

"What's that, H.T.?" I asked.

"Dribbling, Truewater," H.T. answered. "We call it dribbling."

"Not a very scientific name," I replied. "Sounds more like I'm playing basketball."

"The technical name would be 'post-voiding incontinence', Dr. Truewater, but we rarely use it."

"I'm not incontinent," I snapped indignantly. "You make it sound like I'm ready for the nursing home. No, I just had a small accident. Things like that happen when you're in a hurry."

"And getting older," H.T. added.

"Look, H.T.," I replied indignantly, "Every male over the age of 40 has a little benign prostatic hypertrophy. I'm not going to worry about it."

"I agree, Bill," H.T. answered. "Still, it wouldn't hurt to have a flow study."

"A flow study?" I asked. "What's that?"

"That's where you urinate into a commode, and we measure how long it takes you to empty your bladder."

"How long?" I asked. "And, who's 'we'? I'm a little sensitive about these things."

"The nurses," H.T. replied.

"Male or female nurses?" I asked.

"Look, Dr. Truewater," H.T. responded. "We're all professionals here."

"Of course, no problem," I replied. "What comes after the flow study?"

"A digital rectal exam," H.T. answered. "It's important to make sure there aren't any prostatic nodules."

The thought of urinating into a commode under professional supervision was one thing. But when the urologist discussed a digital rectal exam, my sphincter muscles went into a state of acute spasm.

"A digital rectal exam," I said. "Which digit?"

"Why, the index finger," H.T. answered, as I looked at his rather large hands. "With lubrication, of course."

"I don't think I can handle this," I replied.

"It's not as bad as it seems, Dr. Truewater," H.T. reassured me. "If I feel a nodule, we can do a non-invasive ultrasound study."

"Non-invasive?" I asked.

"Of course, Dr. Truewater," H.T. replied calmly. "The ultrasound probe fits easily into the rectum."

"Sounds pretty invasive to me," I flinched.

"Look, H.T." I added, after a moment's reflection. "I respect your professional judgment in urologic matters, and I appreciate your concern for my welfare. But the rectum is a part of me that not too many people know or share. Maybe I'm overly sensitive, but I consider any procedure that violates one of my body cavities to be invasive."

"Very well," H.T. answered. "Then I would recommend a PSA blood test to help rule out prostatic cancer. Besides, even if there is a prostatic nodule on digital exam or ultrasound, we can easily do a trans-rectal needle biopsy. Doesn't hurt a bit."

"Doesn't hurt you, maybe, but what about the poor sap who gets a six inch needle up his rectum in order to biopsy the prostate?"

"We use local anesthesia, Dr. Truewater," H.T. hastened to add. "Just like having a vasectomy."

By now, another part of my body was beginning to cringe.

"I think it's time for me to be going," I said. As I stood to leave, I noticed that the small spot on my scrub pants had dried.

"Look!" I smiled jubilantly. "The spot's gone, I'm cured!"

As I headed back to surgery, I exclaimed, "It's a miracle! Thank you, Lord! I promise not to ever spot again!"

"Denial!" H.T. muttered to himself as I left. "I see it all the time!"

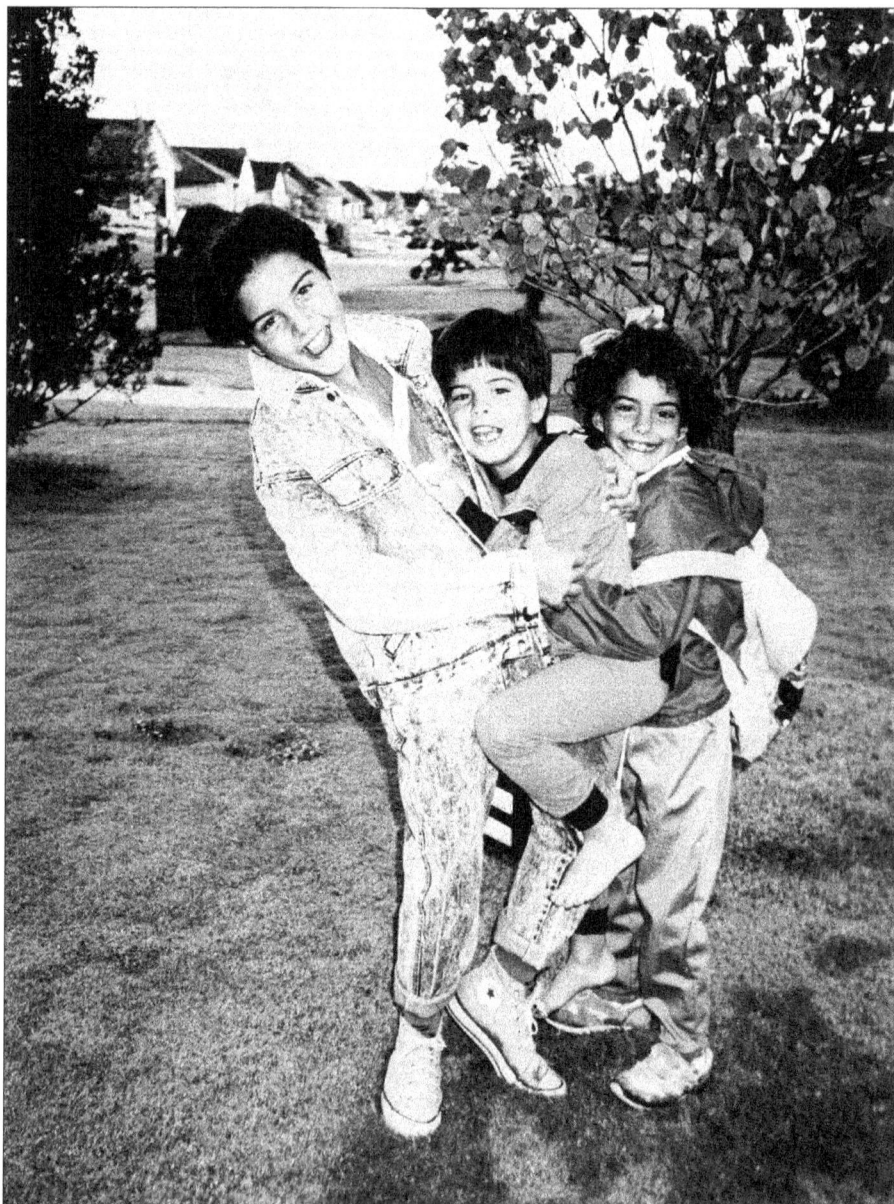

Lisa, Michael, and Tracy Truels

HAPPY DAYS

I wish my kids would not grow up
I like them just the way they are
One believes in Santa Claus
The other says she needs a car!

I like to watch them as they play
They yell and scream and sometimes fight
They remind me of another day
When I was small and all seemed right.

My little girl makes pretty sounds
Her music fills the house
Our little Beagle – she's a hound –
Wrestles with a plastic mouse.

My little boy plays with his swords
And builds a little toy for fun –
He captures all the evil hoards
And shoots them with his laser gun!

My teen-age girl has other thoughts
Of clothes and style and handsome men
Her jeans must all be acid-washed
Our little pup is her best friend!

My wife is busy in the galley
Baking Christmas pie
Oh, how nice it is to see
That twinkle in her eye!

I like things just the way they are
I'm really quite content
I'd like to put time in a jar
So happy days would never end!

CHANGING FACES

"Those aren't love handles," I said. "My belt's just a little tight!"

I was sitting quietly in the doctor's lounge one Friday afternoon, eating a left-over bagel from the morning food tray, when Herb Silverstein, the plastic surgeon, walked in.

"Why the gloom, Dr. Truewater?" Herb asked. "It's Friday afternoon – the week-end is almost here. Cheer up!"

"I'm not really somber, Herb," I replied. "I'm more puzzled than anything."

"Dr. Truewater, are you puzzled?" Herb said. "I'm surprised. Tell me more."

"I was thinking about yesterday's malpractice reform rally at the state Capitol," I told Herb.

"Quite a turnout," Herb said. "Over a thousand doctors turned out to protest the tripling of malpractice insurance in just three years."

"The rally was a success," I answered. "Hopefully, the legislators got the message, or there won't be enough doctors around for the trial lawyers to sue!"

"No, what bothers me," I continued, "is that I ran across Dr. Culbert Trudeau, the general surgeon, who I hadn't seen in five years, and said hello."

"Good for you," Herb quipped. "What's the problem?"

"Well, when I said hello, he didn't answer me," I continued. "He just walked on."

"That sounds like Dr. Trudeau," Herb retorted.

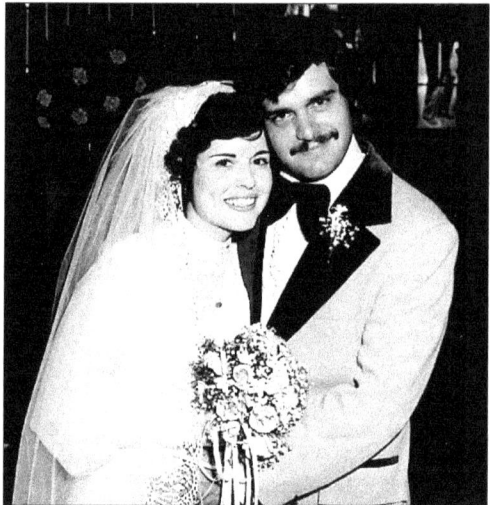

"No, no," I replied. "I mean, we used to scrub together at the Heart Palace up north. "After I caught up with him, he said he didn't recognize me with my sunglasses on."

"I mean, have I changed that much in five years?" I asked Herb.

Herb looked at me without saying a word.

"Herb, answer me," I replied angrily.

"Do you want an honest answer?" Herb asked.

"Of course," I said. "I can handle the truth."

"Well, the truth is, you look different than you did five years ago," Herb replied.

"How's that?" I asked.

"Well, let's face it, Dr. Truewater," Herb answered. "You've gained a little weight, and you're five years older."

"And?" I asked.

"And you've got jowls, Dr. Truewater," Herb explained.

"Jowls?" I said. "I've got jowls?"

"And love handles," Herb added, as he looked down at my waist.

"Those aren't love handles," I said. "My belt's just a little tight."

"Your hair's turning gray, and you've got saddlebags," Herb added, as he looked under my eyes.

"Well, I was taking out a ruptured appendix late last night," I added. "My eyes always swell up a bit if I haven't had a full night's sleep."

"And a double chin," Herb added.

"Alright, alright, I've had enough of the truth," I said.

"Besides, you're speaking like a true plastic surgeon – always looking for more work."

"Here, let me show you my wedding picture," I said, as I pulled out an old, worn-out picture from my wallet."

"See, I haven't changed that much," I said confidently.

Herb perused the faded portrait of me and Margaret taken 30 years ago on our wedding day, as we stood before the matrimonial altar.

"Your wife Margaret looks good," Herb began.

"And?" I asked.

"And who's that hippie next to her with the long hair?" Herb chided. "Is that her first marriage?"

"That's me!" I replied angrily.

"Oh, yeah," I recognize the nose," Herb joked.

"I guess I do look different," I added, as I looked more carefully at my old wedding picture. In those days, my inseam matched my waist – size 28 – and I weighed 40 pounds less.

"It's kind of funny," I said in a more philosophical tone. "Here we are – doctors who are supposed to have the answers – and we still don't understand the aging process."

"The textbooks tell us that aging involves a decreased ability of the body to repair itself. As humans, we are constantly repairing our DNA and re-configuring ourselves. As we grow older, enzymes involved in the transcription of proteins make more mistakes, which results in an accumulation of altered proteins and a subsequent loss of proper function. In short, we fall into a state of disrepair," Herb explained.

"Well, I'm not falling into disrepair and I'm not suffering a complete loss of function!" I answered.

"I'm a little older, and a little wiser, that's all!"

"I think as doctors, we are more work-oriented and goal-oriented," Herb continued. "We figure, as long as we're still doing the work, that everything's the same – and that time sort of stands still."

"Sometimes, we're so busy with our careers and saving lives, that we don't realize that our kids are growing up and getting ready to leave the house. And the last one we ever think will get sick is the doctor himself!"

"You're right again, Herb," I said, as I finished my bagel and stood to leave. "It's important to spend quality time with our family, and to take stock of our own life situation. Time marches on, and it's important to face up to the transient nature of our existence."

"By the way," I added. "Do you do facelifts?"

TIME TRAVEL

I wish I could
Jump back in time
And say hello
To friends of mine!

I'd like to travel
To a day
When I was young
And liked to play!

I'd say hello
To Mom and Dad
And thank them for
The time we had.

I'd say hello
To brother Jim
And tell him how
I think of him!

I'd see that girl
Who smiled so sweet
And tell her now
I think she's neat!

I'd do these things –
Don't ask me how
If I knew then
What I know now!

I LOVE YOU WITH ALL MY COLON

As a general surgeon, I am sometimes frustrated that other, more glamorous areas of surgery get more attention. The field of general surgery is a busy, bustling specialty, generating more revenue for the hospital than many other specialties.

Contrary to popular opinion, general surgeons spend just as many years in training as most surgical specialists. Yet the general surgery wards are often the last ones to be renovated.

Last year, the gynecology ward and the cardiology and cardiac surgery wards at Holy Christian Sinai Hospital both received new carpets, new color television sets, and new furniture.

What did they do for general surgery? We got two new fluorescent light fixtures in the hallway to replace the 20-year-old incandescent fixtures, mostly because patients complained of getting lost in the dark.

I came up with an idea to remedy the situation, and approached Rodney Rooter, the head of Holy Christian Sinai Hospital Marketing.

"I've decided that the field of general surgery needs a facelift, Rodney," I began.

"How so, Dr Truewater?" Rodney asked.

"We need a marketing pitch," I told him. "You know, something to increase our visibility in the community."

"I think general surgeons are quite visible in the community," Rodney replied. "And we much appreciate the revenue they bring to the hospital."

"Of course," I answered. "It's just that we rarely get mentioned on the TV or radio. For example, the cardiac surgeons have a red badge shaped like a heart that says, 'I LOVE YOU WITH ALL MY HEART.' Now that's something people can identify with," I said.

"And the kidney transplant team has a kidney-shaped badge that says, 'I LOVE YOU WITH ALL MY KIDNEY,'" I said.

"Well-spoken, Dr. Truewater," Rodney Rooter replied. "Holy

Christian Sinai Hospital spends hundreds of thousands of dollars a year to increase name recognition with the public. We want people to think of Holy Christian Sinai Hospital every time they see a kidney or heart."

"I'd like to see that same name recognition on behalf of general surgery," I began, with a glow in my eyes that often accompanies my greatest inspirations.

"Just what are you getting at, Dr. Truewater?" Rodney retorted, looking at me suspiciously.

"I've got an idea for a marketing strategy that'll blow your hat in the creek," I began proudly.

"Let's hear it, Dr. Truewater," Rodney answered. "I'm all ears!"

"From a physiologic standpoint," I began, "the kidney or even the heart can't hold a candle to the colon. Why, the colon absorbs hundreds of gallons of water and nutrients a day. If you were to smooth out the absorptive surface of the colon on a flat surface, it would occupy the size of a tennis court," I beamed.

"Why would you want to flatten out the colon over a tennis court?" Rodney asked, somewhat confused.

"Colon cancer kills over a million Americans per year," I continued, ignoring Rodney's question. "We've got to increase the visibility of the colon among the population at large."

"We do?" Rodney asked.

"As a general surgeon, I'm proud to work with the colon," I continued. "Why, the colon even affects how you feel."

"The colon affects your disposition?" Rodney asked.

"Of course," I answered. "If the colon malfunctions, you can get constipation or diarrhea and …"

"Say no more, Dr. Truewater," Albert interrupted. "I'll grant you that the colon is an underrated organ, but what does this have to do with marketing?

"I was ready to move in for the kill. The grand moment had finally arrived. It was time to present my plan to increase the visibility of general surgery at Holy Christian Sinai Hospital.

"What I am proposing, Mr. Rooter," I began, "is to market a brown, cylindrical badge with the words, 'I LOVE YOU WITH ALL MY COLON.' At the bottom of the badge would be the words, 'Holy Christian Sinai Hospital.'"

I proudly showed Mr. Rooter a somewhat quickly sketched prototype for my cylindrically-shaped badge. His mouth hung open in disbelief.

For several moments, Mr. Rooter said nothing, his eyes wide open with what I perceived to be appreciation for my brainstorm. I even fancied Mr. Rooter wondering how a physician, with little marketing experience, could come up with such a firecracker scheme to market Holy Christian Sinai Hospital.

"Dr. Truewater," Rodney slowly began after further reflection. "Let me begin by saying that I have the highest regard for your abilities as a general surgeon. In fact, I think you're one of the finest physicians on the Holy Christian Sinai Staff."

"Furthermore, I want to say that the colon, which you work with on a daily basis, is an extremely important part of the human body."

"However," Rodney continued, "and I hope you don't take this too personally, Dr. Truewater, but you simply can't market a part of the body where the sun don't shine. It's not the kind of image that this hospital is trying to promote."

"How about something with the liver or gallbladder, Dr. Truewater?" Rodney asked in his most sympathetic tone.

"You see, Dr. Truewater," Rodney continued, "in marketing we target programs that connote wholesomeness and purity, in keeping with the hospital's image. The kidney cleanses the blood and removes the impurities. The heart is muscular and strong, pumping thousands of gallons a day. The colon—well, the colon just doesn't lend itself to the image of wholesomeness and purity that we're trying to promote."

"But the colon is involved with waste disposal," I added. "It's ecologically correct."

I must admit I was somewhat deflated by Mr. Rooter's initially cool response to my marketing proposal. On the way back to my office, I thought about the often-unheralded general surgeon. Like the defensive line players in football, someone's got to do the dirty work, even if the colon doesn't grab the spotlight.

When I returned to the office, my patient, Mrs. Ivy was waiting for her post-operative evaluation. She had ruptured her colon two weeks earlier, and almost died from peritonitis. I examined her, found her recovering nicely from her surgery, and gave her a return appointment for two weeks.

"Before I leave, Dr. Truewater," Mrs. Ivy replied, "there's just one thing I'd like to say."

"What's that, Mrs. Ivy?" I asked.

"Thanks for saving my life, Dr. Truewater," she replied. "I mean that from the bottom of my heart."

"Thank you, Mrs. Ivy," I replied, "for letting me be your physician."

As Mrs. Ivy left the office, I realized she had taught me a valuable lesson. The greatest gratification in medicine comes not from medical school, or the marketing department, or even one's perceived self-image, but rather from a doctor's own patients.

Appreciative patients are worth their weight in gold. Maybe being a general surgeon isn't so bad after all!

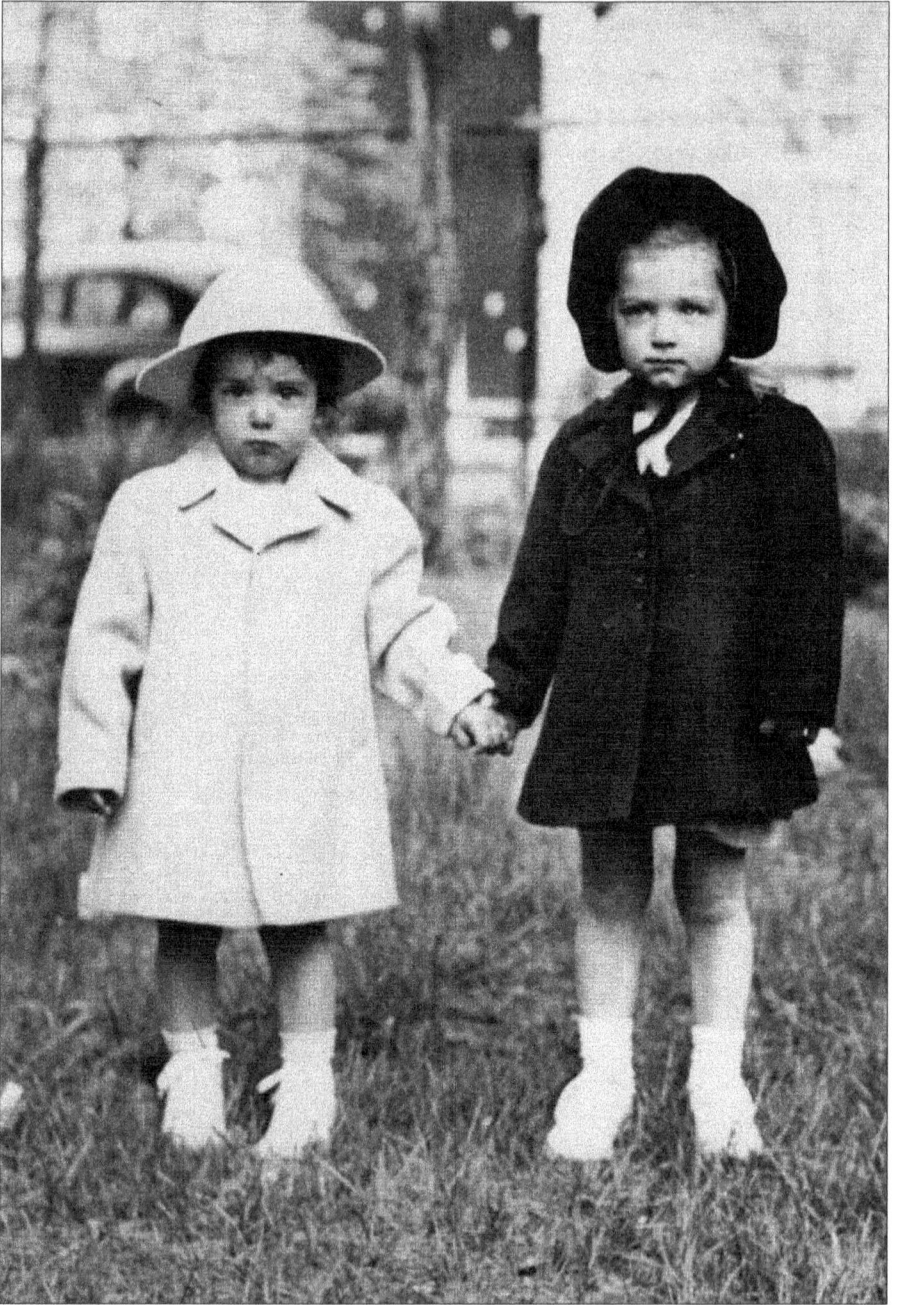

Bill and Karen Truels, 1948, in Chicago

THE ORPHANS

I walked upon a London street
'Twas cold and dark and wet
I saw two orphans sitting there
Up against a step.

The older boy had loaned his coat
For his little sister's ware
The raindrops fell upon his head
But he didn't seem to care.

His rain-proof hat was on her head
He loaned her that as well
But if the raindrops bothered him
His face would never tell.

The two of them sat fast asleep
I thought that I would cry
They seemed to have an inner peace
That money couldn't buy.

I've often thought about that pair
As through the world I've been
True love means giving all you have
And finding peace within!

THE PICK-UP TRUCK

I promised to buy my daughter a car on her sixteenth birthday, if she did well on her report card. In one semester, she went from a "C" student to an "A" student, and on her sixteenth birthday she reminded me of my promise.

"Happy Birthday, Lisa!" I greeted her at the breakfast table. "Your Mother and I bought you a nice chocolate cake with sixteen candles for your birthday party."

"Forget the cake, Dad," Lisa replied. "I'm waiting for that car you promised me on my birthday!"

"Oh, that!" I replied, hoping she might have forgotten my overly generous offer, made in a moment of weakness.

"I'll even make it simple for you, Dad," Lisa replied. "I'll tell you what kind of vehicle I want."

"Let me guess," my wife responded. "Our little darling wants a yellow Chevrolet Camaro with a convertible top!" Margaret exclaimed.

"Not a chance!" I quickly interjected. "My spoiled daughter wants a red Corvette with a removable T-top!"

"You're both wrong!" Lisa responded. "Remember, we've got to save money for college. Nope. What I want is an old Ford pick-up truck with five on the floor, a nice stereo, an oversize gas tank, and air conditioning."

Margaret and I were stunned, and could think of nothing to say.

"What would a girl want with an old Ford pick-up?" I asked incredulously.

"You looking for some action on the street?" Margaret added.

"Maybe," Lisa responded coolly. "But there's nothing that beats an old pick-up for convenience and durability. Why, anytime I need to move, I just throw everything in the pick-up and take off!"

"Are you planning to move?" I asked. "Is there something you're not telling us?"

"Well, no," Lisa responded. "It's just that I'll be starting college in a couple of years and most college kids move an average of once a year. A pick-up would come in mighty handy."

"Your Father and I could rent a trailer and help you move when the time comes," my wife responded. "You don't need a pick-up."

"There's more to it than that, Mother!" Lisa exclaimed. "Why, every time me and the gals want to go somewhere, we'd just pile in the back of the pick-up and head on out!"

"Isn't that illegal?" Margaret asked. "I mean, to drive with a bunch of kids in the back of a pick-up, that sounds awfully unsafe. After all, someone could fall out the back of the truck!"

"It may be unsafe," I replied, "but the state of Oklahoma only requires the two people in the cab to wear seat belts. I guess they figure that if you're stupid enough to ride in the back of a pick-up, you deserve to die!"

"You people don't have any sense of fun!" Lisa pouted. "Living in Carter, Oklahoma, isn't exactly the greatest experience in the world!" she complained.

"What's wrong with driving to Sayre on the week-ends?" Margaret asked. "That's what your Father and I did!"

"And with the rodeo in Elk City this September, you and your girlfriends could drive the pick-up and watch the barrel racers," I added.

"Then, you'll get me a pick-up?" Lisa pleaded.

"Sure," I said. "It certainly would be less expensive than a sports car."

"I would like just a few more options on it, though," Lisa added. "For example, I've always wanted a gun rack."

"A gun rack?" Margaret exclaimed. "I suppose next you'll want a shotgun, so's you can round up the boys!"

"Hardly, Mother," Lisa replied. "No, I'd just like some place to hang my dressage whip."

"Why not just throw it in the cab with you when finish riding for the day?" Margaret asked.

"Besides," I commented, "I'm not sure that's the kind of image you want. What would the boys think of a girl that drives a pick-up truck with a whip on the gun rack?"

"I've already talked about it with Ralph," Lisa responded. "Ralph says he likes girls that drive pick-up trucks – they're more aggressive and fun to be with."

"I always thought that men, with their testosterone, were supposed to be the aggressive ones," I replied.

"You'll find that estrogen has a little kick to it as well," Lisa responded.

"I guess times haven't really changed that much," I commented. "Margaret, do you remember that old 1947 Ford pick-up truck we used to go courting in?"

"I sure do!" Margaret replied. "Complete with an overhead hat rack, a brass spittoon, and a set of bull horns on the hood!"

"The only thing different," Margaret added dryly, "is that nowadays the girls do all the calling!"

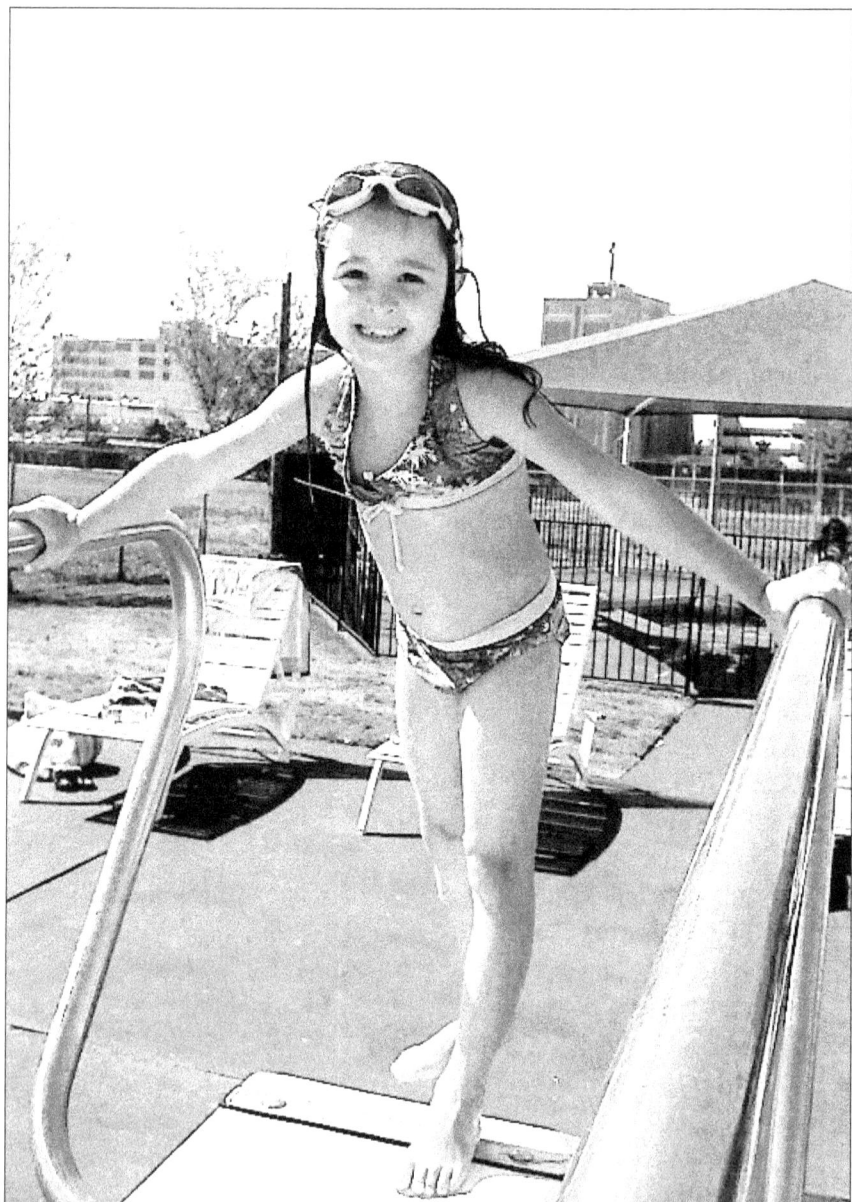

Jaedn

TIME PASSAGES

I regret the passage
Of each and every day
My children growing up
And moving far away!

I wish I had a camera
I'd freeze each day in time
We never would grow old and gray
We'd never say goodbye.

But life is always changing –
Will nothing every last?
The flowers of each newborn spring
Are but echoes of the past!

So treasure every moment
Heed the children's pleas
Take time each and every day
To count your memories!

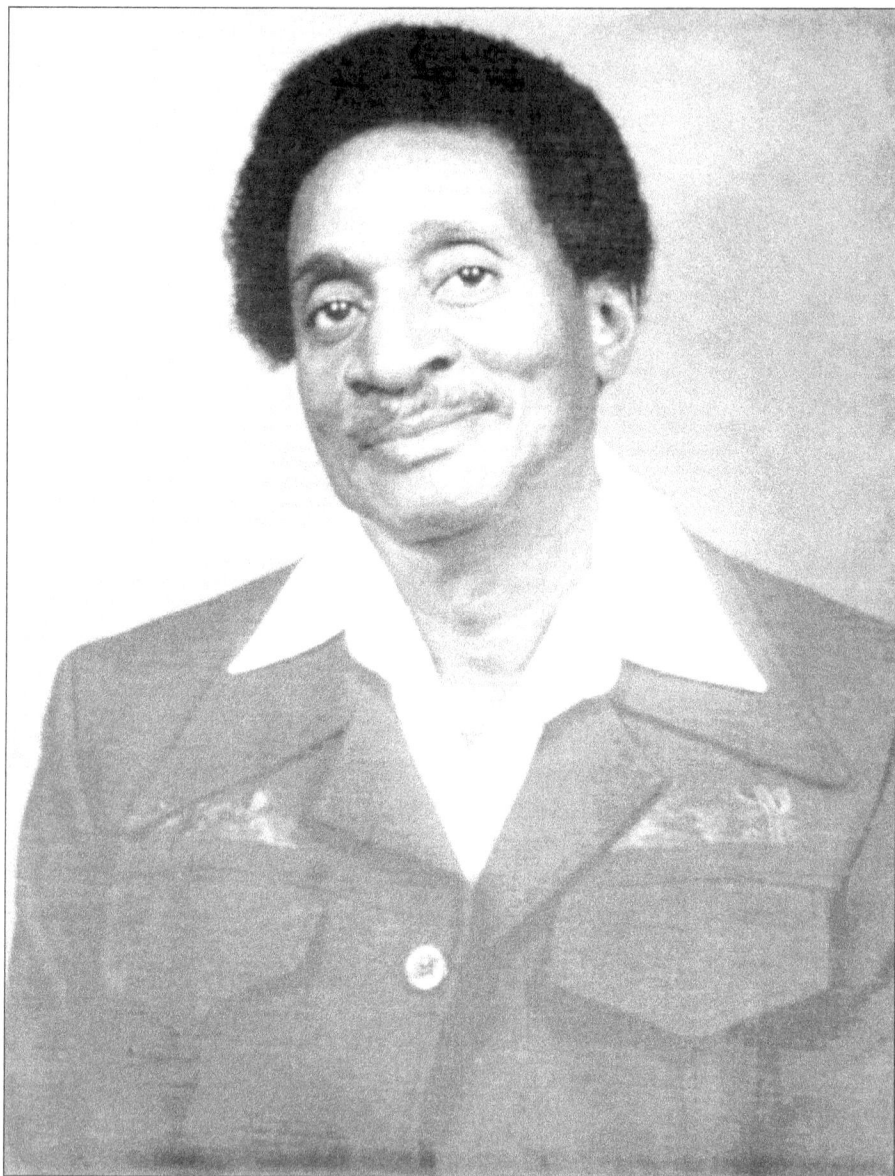

Cecil Eaves, age 57, underwent cardiac transplantation on October 8, 1989, at the Oklahoma Transplantation Institute, Baptist Medical Center, in Oklahoma City.

THE HEART DOCTOR

He who would replace a heart
To give someone a brand-new start
Toils long into the night
To spare someone from death's cold bite.

That same heart which beats so strong
Once did sing a different song.
Full of strength and vitality
It pulsed with hope and destiny.

What a tragic twist of fate
That one man's death is another's break!
Are we ruled by powers on high
That never tell the reason why?

Years ago, from ages past,
The sacrificial heart was cast
To please the fickle gods of earth
The heart did symbolize rebirth.

The nimble fingers quickly sew
To bind with string the heart and soul
Who would ever think that they
Could be joined in such a way?

And when this man, part old, part new
Leaves the operating crew,
He'll journey out upon his own
And wonder what these gods have sewn!

How can a man whose time was done
Receive a heart that is so young?
This is the miracle of rebirth
That God has placed upon the earth!

For if a man can give his all
To spare another from his fall,
Perhaps mankind could learn to share
And rid the earth of its despair!

THE GOOD OLD DAYS

I was sitting in the doctor's lounge last week with Rocky McSquealy, the prominent general and vascular surgeon, reminiscing about the good old days, while we waited for our gallbladder case to start.

"Residents don't have it like we used to, Dr. Truewater," Rocky began.

"How do you mean?" I asked.

"Well, in my hey-day, we worked from sun-up to sunset, took call every other night, and worked over a hundred hours a week," Rocky continued.

"That's true," I replied. "I understand the federal government has mandated an eighty-hour work week for residents, and that even counts being on call at night."

"I think the worst rotation I had was in 1974 during my rotating internship – I rotated on pediatrics 24 on, then 24 off – except that when you were off call, you still put in a 12-hour day! It added up to 120 hours a week. I resolved never to become a pediatrician and never to start another scalp vein!"

"Rotating internships don't exist anymore, either," Rocky replied. "They're considered a waste of time. Now you have a computerized match system – kind of like letting a video game determine your career choice and location. I know one resident who ended up in Alaska – he must have pissed off somebody!"

"Well, my residency was kind of rocky," I replied. "I suppose a prominent surgeon like you must have had it made."

"Hardly, Dr. Truewater," Dr. McSquealy replied. "I mean, as a third-year medical student, you stand with your mouth agape, looking at all the horror going on around you – people getting shot, dying and all that."

"Then, as a fourth-year student, you think you're hot stuff because all the other medical students presume you've got it together – king of the hill, you know."

"I agree, Rocky," I interjected.

"As a fourth-year student, I had a little moxie. I had sutured a few wounds, even delivered a few babies. And I knew that in a few months I'd get my degree and get past all those monthly exams. I figured I was in the driver's seat."

"That feeling didn't last long, Dr. Truewater," Rocky interrupted. "The next year, as a surgical intern, all the junior residents and attending physicians were complementing me about how smart I was, and what a good surgeon I would make. So I signed up."

"Sounds to me like you made the right choice," I replied. "I mean, look at you now – a busy general surgeon with lots of referrals."

"I thought it was a good choice, too," Rocky continued.

"As a first-year resident, I was getting to fix inguinal hernias and even got to take out a few gallbladders. And if there was a problem, my second-year resident was there to back me up. Things seemed pretty rosy."

"So, what happened, Rocky?" I asked.

"I became a second-year resident," Rocky McSquealy smiled glumly.

"I was now in charge of writing orders and managing patients. It seemed like I couldn't do anything right. During Grand Rounds in the lecture hall, my attending physician cross-examined me in front of all the other residents and medical students – even my chief resident was critical, and said I just couldn't do anything right – he called me the worst blankety-blank surgeon he'd ever seen! And my chief resident insisted on doing all the cases while I was delegated to first assist!"

"So, what happened?" I asked, as I noted Rocky's voice quivered a bit when he relived the good old days.

"Well," Rocky mused, "I went to the Surgery Department chairman and turned in my resignation – took off my badge and put it on his desk – just like the movie *"Top Gun"*. I told him I didn't have what it takes to be a surgeon. I think I had actually convinced myself that these naysayers were right."

"So you resigned?" I asked in disbelief.

"Not exactly," Rocky answered. "You remember Dr. Shrilling."

"I sure do," I replied. "Chief Shrilling was feared by all the medical students for his verbal grilling of any medical student who hadn't memorized Schwarz's textbook of surgery before starting his rotation. When I was a resident, he kept calling me Nate – which I thought was good, because if I ever did anything wrong, I figured it would go on Nate's record! We lived in fear of that man."

"Well, it turns out Dr. Shrilling had another side to his personality," Dr. McSqualy continued.

"He looked me square in the eyes and said, 'You don't get it, do you, McSqualy?'"

"Get what?" I asked Dr. Shrilling.

"You're going through a hazing, just like some pissant college fraternity, Dr. McSqualy. You've got to understand that surgery isn't some cozy nine to five job – it's a 24 hour a day job. You're dealing with sick patients, some of whom will die from their injuries or disease."

"You're getting up in the middle of the night to see a patient with a gunshot or appendicitis or bowel obstruction or gangrene. And every time you have a complication, you've got unhappy patients, angry family members and malpractice lawyers circling overhead like a bunch of hungry vultures, ready to charge you with incompetence or neglect, threatening you with bankruptcy under the pretext of improving the quality of care, while they fly away in their private jets. It's a cold, cruel world out there, doctor, and surgeons have got to be tough enough to handle it."

"Temperament is also important – the ability to keep your cool while everybody else is losing theirs – we look for that."

"Truth be told, McSqualy," Dr. Shriller added, "You're doing an excellent job. You're a fine surgeon, you've got great judgment, and you get along well with your patients. That's a combination that's hard to beat!"

"Then, why all the flack?" I asked Dr. Shrilling.

"Let's just say it's like being in a crucible – a trial by fire. It toughens you to adversity and prepares you for the road ahead, where you, as a surgeon, are making life and death decisions."

"Besides, McSqualy," Dr. Shriller added, "It's tradition. It's all about tradition. It all goes back to those early surgical gurus who set the table for everybody else. Now get out there and get back to work before I get accused of playing favorites!"

"And that was the end of the discussion," Dr. McSqualy added. "I finished my surgical residency in due course and here I am today."

"So, what do you think of the good old days?" I asked Rocky.

Rocky thought for a moment, as he twirled the cup of coffee in his hand.

"I've got mixed emotions, Dr. Truewater. "I mean, for all the apparent shortcomings of the new system, with residents working fewer hours under less punitive conditions, I'd have to say that the new surgeons coming out – both male and female – are pretty darn good."

"Maybe the new generation isn't so bad after all," I added. "And with more emphasis on the importance of the family, maybe there won't be so many divorces!"

"Well spoken, Dr. Truewater," Rocky answered, as we put on our caps and headed back to surgery.

Maybe the good old days weren't so great after all!

THE SURGEON'S TOUCH

I heard Tom Watson, one of the top golfers in the world, during a TV interview today in preparation for the PGA golf tournament.

"How hard is it to play out there today, Tom?" the TV announcer asked candidly.

"Extremely difficult!" Tom replied. "The greens are smooth as glass! You need the deft hands and light touch of a surgeon to play out there today!" Tom added.

Now, I respect Tom Watson and his opinions. I've got every one of his golf tips on video tape, and review them once a month. But, try as I may, I find absolutely no correlation between expertise on the golf course and technical expertise in the operating room. Let me give you an example.

Dudley Balbano is probably the best general surgeon in town. He's so good that one day he was first assisting a cardiovascular surgeon on a coronary bypass, when the cardiovascular surgeon felt weak and had to drop out – it was only his fifth heart that day. All of the other cardiovascular surgeons were either operating or on angioplasty standby and couldn't come. So, you know what happens? Dudley finishes the operation himself! He's that good!

Well, Dudley has been taking golf lessons for five years now at Partridge Creek Golf Club. According to Tom Watson, Dudley's deft surgical hands and light touch should make him a great golfer, right?

Well, Dudley has the bad habit of never hitting the golf ball more than six inches off the ground. When he tries to correct for it, he smashes his club into the ground three inches behind the ball, inflicting pain and suffering on his deft hands. One day, Dudley had to cancel three surgery cases because his wrists were injured from golfing the day before!

But that's not all. Dudley's "surgeon's touch" ought to make him an excellent putter, right? Wrong again. When Dudley putts, he either leaves the ball six feet short or six feet past the hole, no matter how long the putt.

"I'm absolutely terrified of three-foot putts," Dudley confided to me one day. "Everybody expects you to make them. It's a lot of pressure."

I thought to myself. Here's a surgeon who cross-clamps the aorta without trepidation on a patient with a ruptured aneurysm in hemorrhagic shock, and he's afraid of a three-foot putt!

On the other hand, take the case of Brad Thornberry. Brad is probably the best golfer among the general surgeons. He has the lightest touch around the greens. He hits the longest drives. Even Tom Watson would be impressed to see Brad play, with his deft hands and surgeon's touch.

Being such a good golfer, you would think that Brad would be one of the best surgeons, too. Right? Wrong again. The first time I scrubbed with Brad, he opened up the skin, soft tissue, muscle, and peritoneum, all with one stroke of the knife.

"Oops!" Brad said. "She's a little skinnier than I thought!"

As far as deft hands are concerned, Brad is the only surgeon I know who can tie air knots and make them work.

"It looks like I can see spaces between those knots," I told Brad one day on a ventral hernia repair.

"Those are just as good as square knots!" Brad replied. "I've never had a recurrence yet!"

"They just don't look as pretty," I replied.

"Pretty is as pretty does," Brad answered.

Needless to say, the general public also holds the notion that a surgeon's deft hands provide an advantage in golf, especially in putting. One Sunday afternoon, I was playing in a putting contest during our annual Holy Christian Sinai Church fund raiser.

As luck would have it, Chuck Pepper and I made the semi-finals that year. Chuck is an excellent plumber, and did all the plumbing for the church expansion two years ago. The final putt was a thirty-footer, downhill, with about a four-foot right-to-left break – the hardest kind for a right-handed golfer. If ever you needed the right touch, this was the time.

"Let's see that surgeon's touch!" my friends yelled sarcastically.

I went first. My putt looked perfect. It started out right of the hole, then gradually broke into the hole, just lipping out at the last minute.

Chuck putted next. His putt had the perfect speed and direction, dropping into the center of the cup for a victory. I reached out my hand to congratulate him. You'd think the man would be ecstatic.

Instead, he politely shook my hand and angrily left. As he walked off, I heard him mutter to his wife, "I knew I could have been a surgeon!

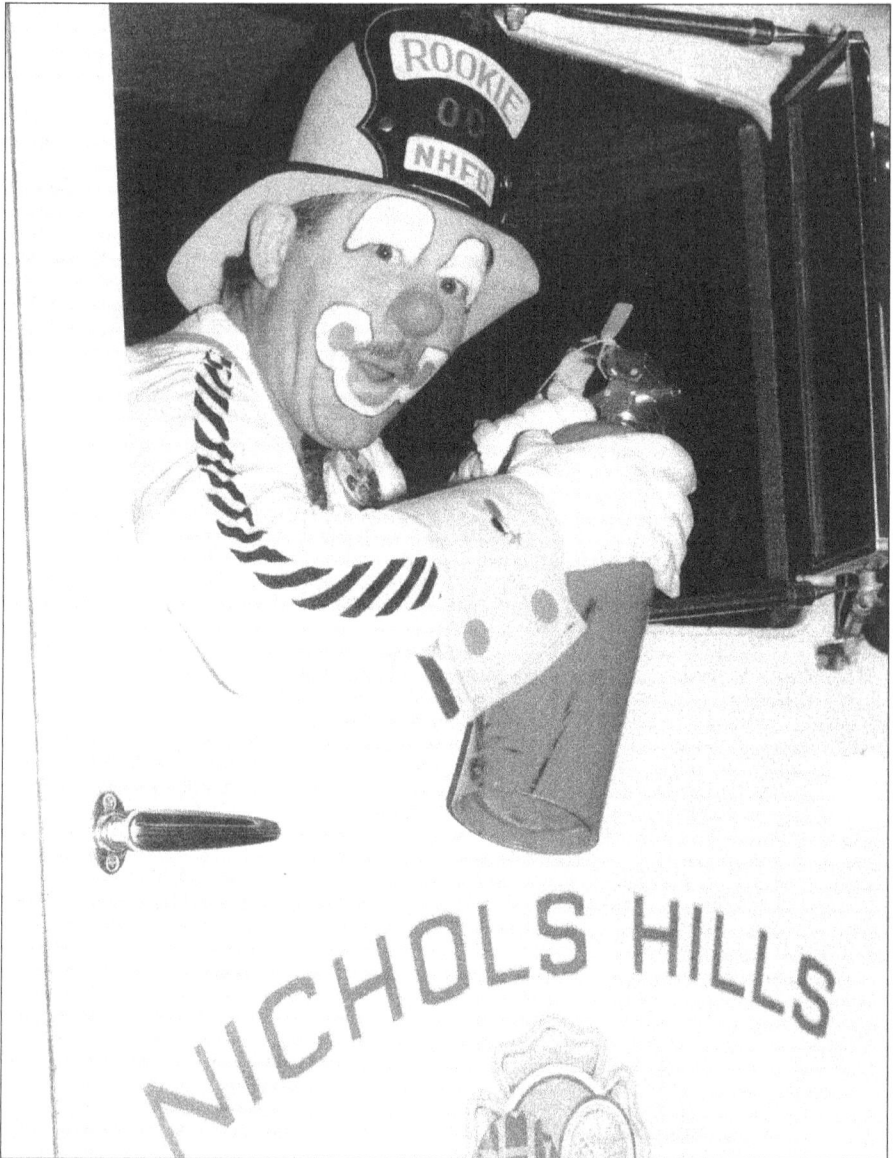

Mike Billingsley, RN, is a firefighter for the Nichols Hills Fire Department. His clown name is "Ricky the Clown". Mike also works at the Baptist Burn Center teaching preventive burn education.

THE CLOWN

Today I felt the pain again
Like when you lose a long-time friend
Reality will come around
And once again I'll play the clown.

I've played before the kings and queens
And filled their minds with happy dreams
I've played before the orphan child
And seen his face light up with smiles.

I can imitate most anyone
Even though it's just for fun
I can play a boy or grandpa too
Or a sailor on the ocean blue.

People wish they could be me –
Gay and fun and so carefree!
It must be nice to be a clown –
Then you never have to frown!

But in order for a laugh to feel
You must know what it does conceal
For Nature's ways are much too sly –
You cannot laugh if you cannot cry!

I think of all those days of yore
The times we ran along the shore
I think of how life used to be
And still how much you mean to me!

And so I feel the pain anew
Each time my thoughts turn back to you
I'd like to live my life again
And do the things we did back then!

Thus I while my time away
Dreaming of another day
Until reality comes back around
And once again I play the clown!

THE EMPATHY BELLY

I happened to walk past the pre-natal education class last week, and caught my first glimpse of the "empathy belly." Ruth Job, the neonatal instructor at Holy Christian Sinai Hospital and a long-time friend, waved hello.

"Would you like to try one of these on, Dr. Truewater?" Ruth asked. "It might improve your understanding of female patients," she added.

The "empathy belly" looked like some sort of primitive art object. The idea was conceived by a woman in California. It consisted of a lead shield, weighing about 35 pounds. On the front of the shield were two large breasts, which sat above a swollen, "pregnant" abdomen.

"Like some sort of medieval costume," I replied.

"The 'empathy' belly is designed to make men feel the suffering we women go through when we're pregnant," Ruth replied. "I'm taking some over to Will Rogers High School tomorrow."

"Why would take these to a high school?" I asked. "All you'd do is get a bunch of laughs and snickers from the students."

"Once one of those young bucks straps on an empathy belly for a couple of hours, he'll think twice about getting some young girl pregnant," Ruth answered.

"Sounds like a good idea," I replied. "It'll make men feel the responsibility and physical stress women endure while pregnant. Mind if I try one on?" I asked.

"Be my guest," Ruth replied.

I slipped off my suit coat and strapped on the empathy belly. The additional weight was more than I expected.

"This thing makes my back hurt," I said.

"Get used to it," Ruth replied. "Now, whatever happens, wear this for four or five hours, and you'll learn to understand pregnant women a whole lot more than any medical textbook could explain."

As I headed to the parking lot, I realized that I had forgotten my suit coat at the prenatal class, but decided to pick it up in the morning. I thought what a clever idea this empathy belly was, and wondered why I hadn't thought of it first. As I drove home, I tried to think up some other idea that might at first seem trivial, but might actually have serious educational value.

Unfortunately, I was so wrapped up in my thoughts that I wasn't paying any attention to the speed limit. I was ten miles over the limit and, sure enough, a friendly policeman stopped me.

"Let's see your driver's license, buddy," the policeman began.

I reached for my wallet, but suddenly remembered it was in my suit coat back at the hospital. As I fumbled around, the policeman noticed my empathy belly. His mouth hung open in disbelief.

"Now I've seen it all," he replied.

"It's O.K., officer," I began. "You see, I'm a doctor and...."

"I don't care who you are," the officer snapped. "If you can't find your driver's license, you're coming with me to the station."

As I rode with the officer in the police car, I must confess I was beginning to panic. What if they put me in jail overnight? Would the other prisoners think funny thoughts about me? Would I survive the night? I could just see the headlines the next day in the Daily Oklahoman: "Famous Doctor Arrested for Impersonating a Woman." My practice would be ruined! And what would my wife think?

When I got to the station, I was allowed to make one phone call. I called my wife, Margaret, and told her to come down right away to the police station and get me out of jail.

Now, you'll have to understand that the first thing my wife does when I come home each night is to jump up and greet me with a hug and a kiss. I admit it's a little old-fashioned, but we're the sentimental type.

When Margaret arrived at the jail, she greeted me with her usual hug and kiss. With my hands cuffed behind my back, I was unable to stop her. I will never forget the look of shock on her face as she bounced off my swollen abdomen and landed on the floor.

"Bill Truewater!" she exclaimed. I know I'm in trouble whenever Margaret uses my full name. I braced for the worst.

"Bill Truewater," she continued angrily, as she struggled to her feet. "They say it's possible to be married to someone, and still never really know them. I've put up with a lot of your eccentricities, but this takes the cake! Of all the years we've been married, I never once suspected that..."

"I can explain everything," I interrupted. "This is called an 'empathy belly', and it's used in prenatal classes to teach men what it's like to be pregnant. Ruth Job, the prenatal instructor convinced me to try it for a few hours. That's the honest truth, so help me God!" I cried pitifully.

Fortunately for me, Margaret, and even the police officers believed my story, and I was a free man once again. The next morning, I happily returned the 'empathy belly' to Ruth and picked up my suit coat and wallet.

"How'd it go last night, Dr. Truewater?" Ruth asked.

"Rougher than expected," I replied. "If the world had to rely on men becoming pregnant, there'd be a lot fewer babies. That 'empathy belly' really helped me understand what women endure when they're pregnant."

"Great!" Ruth replied.

"And it did something more," I added.

"What's that?" Ruth asked.

"I've resolved to never become pregnant!"

MY LAST WISH

There's just one thing I ask of thee –
Come, my son, and hear my plea.
I'm healthy now, my mind is strong
But I may leave before too long.

Don't get me wrong – I hope to see
The day your girl is big like me.
I've lived a life that's full of pride –
Remember when we camped outside?

We did the things that families do
Back when your Mom was with us too!
I've no regrets, my life's been good
I've lived the life I hoped I would.

But when my time for dying comes
There's just one thing I ask of thee –
After all is said and done
Let me go with dignity!

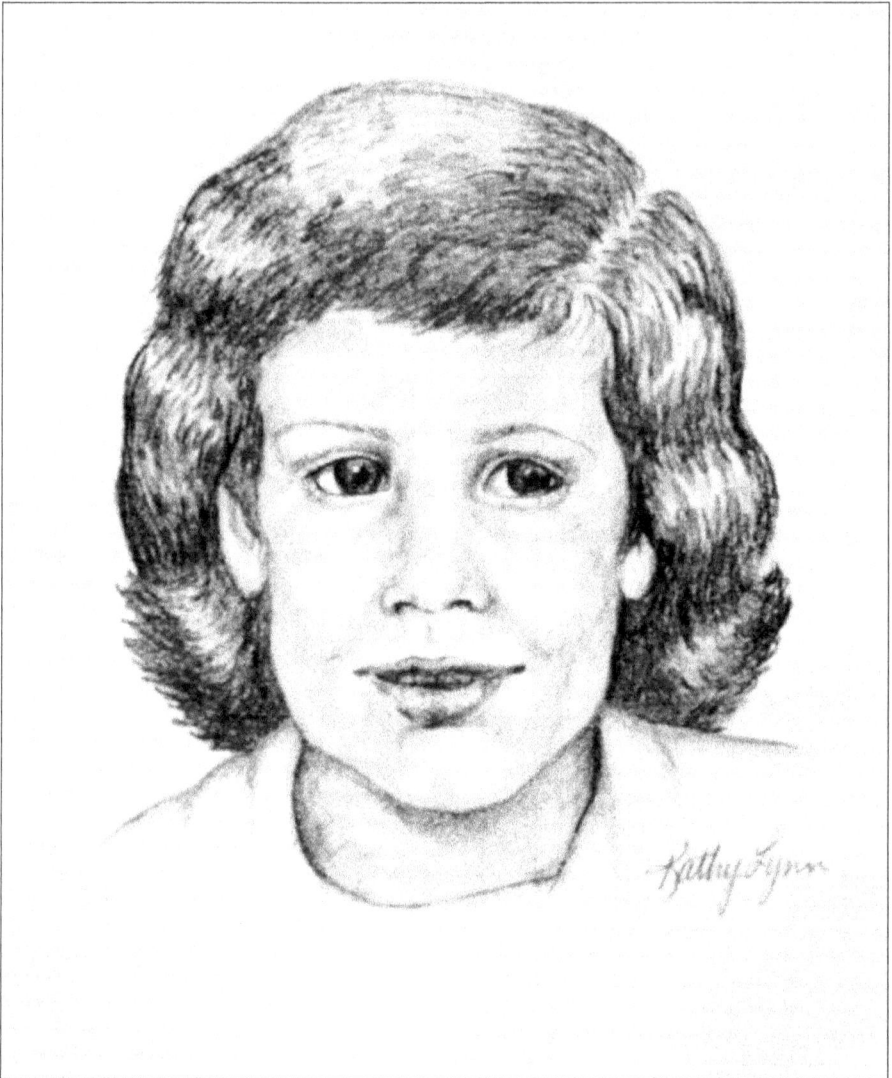

Jori Sine, daughter of Joe and Mary Sine, died of a malignant brain tumor when she was five years old. Jori's speech was slurred during the final stages of her illness, but the courage of this brave little girl was an inspiration to all.

JORI

I know you're sad
But please don't cry
And wipe that tear
Back from your eye!

I'm only five
I know that's true
But I've a word
To share with you

My eyes are big
My hair is brown
And I'm the cutest
Girl in town!

I'd love to talk
So clear and true
But the words
Will not come through.

I've grown old
Before my time
But I can still
Make letters rhyme.

Some will grow
So big and strong
Others fade
Before too long.

And who's to say
I ask of you
Because my days
Are numbered few

That I can't give
A gift that shines
And sees you through
The troubled times.

My gift is love
A gift so plain
A gift so pure
Like fields of grain.

A gift that smiles
And has no price
A gift that warms
The coldest ice.

Recall the love
I gave to you
Don't give up
When you are blue!

God gives us all
A place and time
To show our gifts
To all mankind.

Share that love
To all who come –
Let them know
All men are one.

I know you're sad
But please don't cry –
And wipe that tear
Back from your eye!

GREMLINS

"You seem a little down today, Dr. Truewater," Jess Barker, the urologist, said to me as I sipped coffee in the doctor's lounge.

"One of my patient's died, Jess," I replied. "I had just finished removing a colon cancer. I was closing the incision, when suddenly he developed a ventricular fibrillation."

"That's pretty unlucky," Jess replied.

"We went through the full cardiac resuscitation, but couldn't revive him. I felt pretty bad about it."

"Sounds like a good case of Murphy's Law in action," Jess responded. "If something can go wrong, it will."

"Chuck Yeager, the test pilot, talks about it in his book," Jess continued. "He calls them 'Gremlins' – little glitches that happen that are totally unexpected, totally unpredictable, and can sabotage your entire operation."

"Were there any other risk factors besides cancer?" Jess asked.

"My patient was about fifty pounds overweight and a chain smoker," I replied.

"I tell you, Truewater, we do it to ourselves. We cause a lot of our own misery, our own health problems," Jess said. "If our society could practice a little more preventive medicine, we'd all be a lot healthier for a lot less money."

"What does Woody Allen say?" Jess continued. "Sudden death – it's nature's way of telling us to slow down!"

"Granted, my patient was overweight and a chain smoker," I said. "But he still didn't deserve to die."

"Of course not. None of us deserves to die, Truewater," Jess answered. "But it happens anyway."

"And don't blame yourself, Truewater. Those 'Gremlins' can strike at any time. Some things are just beyond our control, not only as physicians, but as human beings."

"By the way, Dr. Truewater, how old was your patient?"

"Not very old," I replied. "He was only forty-seven."

"Isn't that about your age, Dr. Truewater? Jess asked innocently.

"Me? I asked. "Why, I'm forty-seven, too."

I paused to reflect for a moment.

"I guess that's what bothers me," I confessed.

"When I started in practice, I was younger than most of my patients. I'd look at their charts to check how much older they were. Lately, I've noticed that my age is catching up to my patients!"

"Watch out for those gremlins, Truewater," Jess joked.

"But I've got a confession to make as well," Jess added. "When I started in practice, it seemed like my prostate patients were all old. Lately, they seem to be getting younger."

"As a matter of fact, Truewater," Jess confided, "I've noticed a few prostate symptoms myself. Now, that's a little unsettling."

"Furthermore," Jess continued, "you've just had a patient die that was the same age you were. That makes you sit up and take notice."

"Of course, I've had patients die who were my age or younger," I replied. "But when you first start out in practice, you feel like you're invincible, like it can't happen to you."

"It reminds me of those rookie fighter pilots in those World War II. movies," I continued. "They always thought it was the other guy who got shot down – not them."

"It happens to all physicians, eventually," Jess continued. "You take care of patients for years. Each year, a certain fraction of them die. That's to be expected. Their congestive heart failure or their cancer, or whatever, overtakes their body's ability to combat the problem, and they die. That's what they teach you in medical school."

"Then one day it finally hits you," Jess continued. "You have a patient die, and for some reason, it's not like all the others."

"Whether it's someone you know, or someone who's your age, it suddenly hits you. You're faced with your own mortality, and it's kind of scary."

"You ain't seen nothing yet, Truewater," Jess said. "Wait until you have your first heart attack followed by your first coronary bypass – talk about facing your own mortality."

"I'm not planning to have a heart attack, Jess," I continued. "I don't smoke and I'm not overweight."

"Don't forget Murphy's law, Truewater," Jess rebutted.

Just then, the infectious specialist, Dr. Alice McWilliams, spoke up.

"I've been listening with some interest to your conversation, gentlemen," Alice began. "I have a different perspective. You see, instead of being younger, I'm older than most of my patients. And instead of worrying how much longer I have to live, I take Helen Keller's approach – I thank the Lord for each and every day I'm alive."

"That's not a bad philosophy," I replied. "Instead of looking at the glass as half empty, you look at it half full."

"That way," Alice continued, "each new day becomes a gift from God. Of course, death is a tragedy – there's no getting around that. As physicians, we deal with death or the possibility of death on a daily basis."

"But I also look on life as a blessing. I don't feel like I'm owed or deserve so many years on this planet. I just take them as they come and make the most of it."

As I left to start my next case, I felt reassured by Alice's advice. Sometimes you can learn more about medicine – as well as life – talking in the doctor's lounge than you do in medical school!

REMEMBER ME

Remember me
When all the days and months have turned to years
And all the busy dramas of your life
Have tempered all the heartache and the strife.

Remember how we used to run and play
"Time was on our side!" we used to say
The sky was always clear and fresh and blue
And every day we whispered, "I love you!"

Remember me, when all your life is done
And all the battles fought that should be won
Remember when we frolicked in the blue
For that is how I'll always think of you!

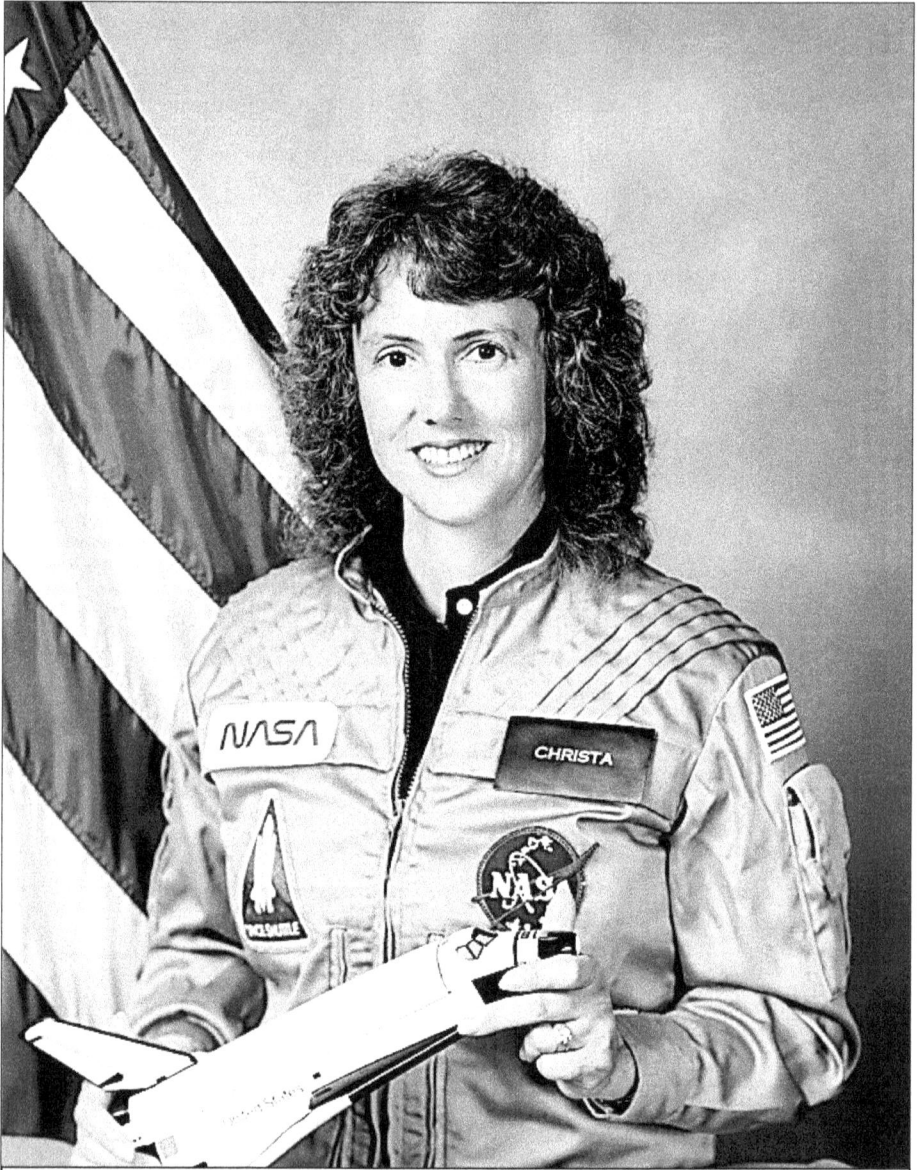

Christa McAuliffe, a school teacher-astronaut from Concord, New Hampshire, died in the space shuttle Challenger tragedy on January 28, 1986. It is reported that the astronaut, sitting next to her, Greg Jarvis, from Hermosa Beach, California, told Christa, "Take my hand, we're going down."

A TRIBUTE TO CHRISTA

It's been a real struggle
Just to get this far
I'll be the first school teacher
To reach upon a star!

I wish to thank my friends
For all that they have done
I hope this trip to outer space
Will be the greatest fun!

I know there is a danger
It's foolish to deny
But I'd also be a fool
To live and never try!

I think about my future
To view the world from space
A world without boundaries,
Color, creed, or race!

Imagine all the lessons
I could teach my class
Mountains, storms, and oceans
That dreams could not surpass!

I'll be their best example
Of what they ought to be
Reach out for that rainbow
And it will set you free!

One thing that I leave with you
Hold your head up high
Better to have lived and failed
Than never to have tried!

It's been a real struggle
Just to get this far
I'll be the first school teacher
To reach upon a star!

TO CHRISTA

Take my hand
We're going down
Our ship of life
Has run aground.

All our hopes
And all our schemes
Are but the stuff
Of what we dream.

We'll make our peace
With hands that bind
Our luck, our fate
Has not been kind.

We'll never part
I promise you
And when I go
I'll think of you.

So take my hand
And don't be sad
Let's thank the Lord
For what we had!

LIVING ARTIFACTS

I was sitting in the surgery lounge, munching on a cookie, waiting for my anesthesiologist to finish an earlier case, when Herb Silverstein walked into the lounge.

"Welcome, Herb!" I said. "I thought you were retired. What's happening?"

"I'm retired, Dr. Truewater," Herb began, "But I like to come back and visit every so often. I kind of miss the old stomping grounds."

"It doesn't seem that long ago that you were doing those plastic reconstructions for spina bifida patients," I said.

"That was ten years ago," Herb answered. "I've been fully retired five years now."

"By the way," Herb added. "What happened to the donuts they used to have in the surgery lounge. I see you're just munching on cookies these days."

"Conflict of interest," I answered.

"Conflict of interest?" Herb asked. "What do you mean?"

"Well, the Eli Lilly rep used to bring donuts on Monday morning until the federal government declared that this was a conflict of interest," I said.

"The government was afraid that, if we ate a 15-cent donut for breakfast from Eli Lilly, then we would be biased toward using Eli Lilly products. So now we eat cookies that the hospital brings from the cafeteria."

"That's so silly," Herb answered. "After all those contributions the Congressmen receive from 'disinterested parties', you'd think they'd let us have a 15-cent donut without arousing claims of favoritism."

"It's a brave new world," Herb added.

"I still remember the time you got mad about your surgery instruments," I began.

"That was at the old Presbyterian Hospital on 12th Street," Herb interrupted. "I tended to be a grouch in those days, and I complained to Nurse Martin for the umpteenth time about my surgical instruments."

"I made the mistake of telling her that these surgical instruments were worthless."

"Nurse Martin replied, 'Alrighty then', picked up the whole box of instruments, walked over to the window, opened the window, and calmly threw the instruments out the second-floor window onto the Burford Hollies that adorned the front of the old Presbyterian hospital!"

"I think you started the feminist revolution all by yourself that day, Herb," I quipped.

"Yep, those were the good old days," Herb laughed.

Herb looked around the newly expanded doctor's lounge and, wishing to change the subject, he said, "I remember when this lounge was half this size. I guess they had to make room for all these new computers."

"Yes, they've done a nice job of renovating the old surgery lounge," I said. "With these new computers, we can dictate and sign our medical records while we're waiting for the next case to start."

"Progress," Herb replied cynically. "I remember when this hospital had a home for unwed mothers at the south end of the campus. Then they ran an adoption agency for the newborn babies. That was true compassion."

"Herb, you're going back fifty years," I replied. "Why, you probably knew the founding fathers of Holy Christian Hospital."

"As a matter of fact, I knew Dr. Spencer and Sister Coletta – nice, compassionate people," Herb answered. "But they were much older than me."

"That makes you sort of a living artifact, Herb" I quipped.

"A living artifact? Hmm. That reminds me of another Oklahoma story," Herb laughed. "You probably don't remember Jim Thorpe."

"Jim Thorpe? Of course I know about Jim Thorpe," I answered. "We studied him in Oklahoma history – Oklahoma's greatest athlete, an Olympic champion – he also competed in football, baseball, basketball, lacrosse and even ballroom dancing, and is heralded by the Sac and Fox Indians."

"But have you heard about the controversy?" Herb asked.

"What controversy?" I asked.

"Well, Jacobus Franciscus 'Jim' Thorpe is buried in Jim Thorpe, Pennsylvania. It seems that Jim grew up in the Sac and Fox nation in

Oklahoma, and Jack Thorpe, his son, would like to bring his body back to Oklahoma, to be buried next to his family."

"But can they do that?" I asked.

"It seems that the Indians are declaring Jim Thorpe's remains to be an artifact, and wish them to be removed to the reservation in Oklahoma, under the Native American Graves Protection and Repatriation Act," Herb stated.

"You know, when Jim Thorpe was alive, he was dishonored for taking money as an amateur athlete in minor league baseball. He won the Olympic decathlon and pentathlon in 1912 in Sweden and was awarded two gold medals by Czar Nicholas II. and King Gustav V. of Sweden. He wasn't allowed to recover those gold medals until 2022!"

"Today, we name our Rehab facility after Jim Thorpe!"

"Well, how long do you have to be dead to be declared an artifact?" I asked.

"Jim Thorpe died in 1953 – that would be 70 years," Herb answered. "But it doesn't have to be that long – after all, you just declared me to be a living artifact!"

"I was joking," I quipped.

"But think about the poor people in Jim Thorpe, Pennsylvania," I added. "They would have to rename the town."

"Let me think," Herb replied. "I guess they could rename it Joe Paterno, Pennsylvania. Have you seen Joe, lately? He's another living artifact – they call him 'Joe Pa' – one of the greatest living football coaches. I wouldn't be surprised if he helped forge the Liberty Bell!"

"That would be a great honor for Joe, to have a town renamed after him," I replied, "except his reputation went south instead of north!"

"Well, I've got to go start my case," I concluded. "It was nice of you to drop by, Herb – you're always welcome here, you know. It's like having a history lesson."

"I appreciate that, Dr. Truewater," Herb answered – "Even if I am a living artifact!"

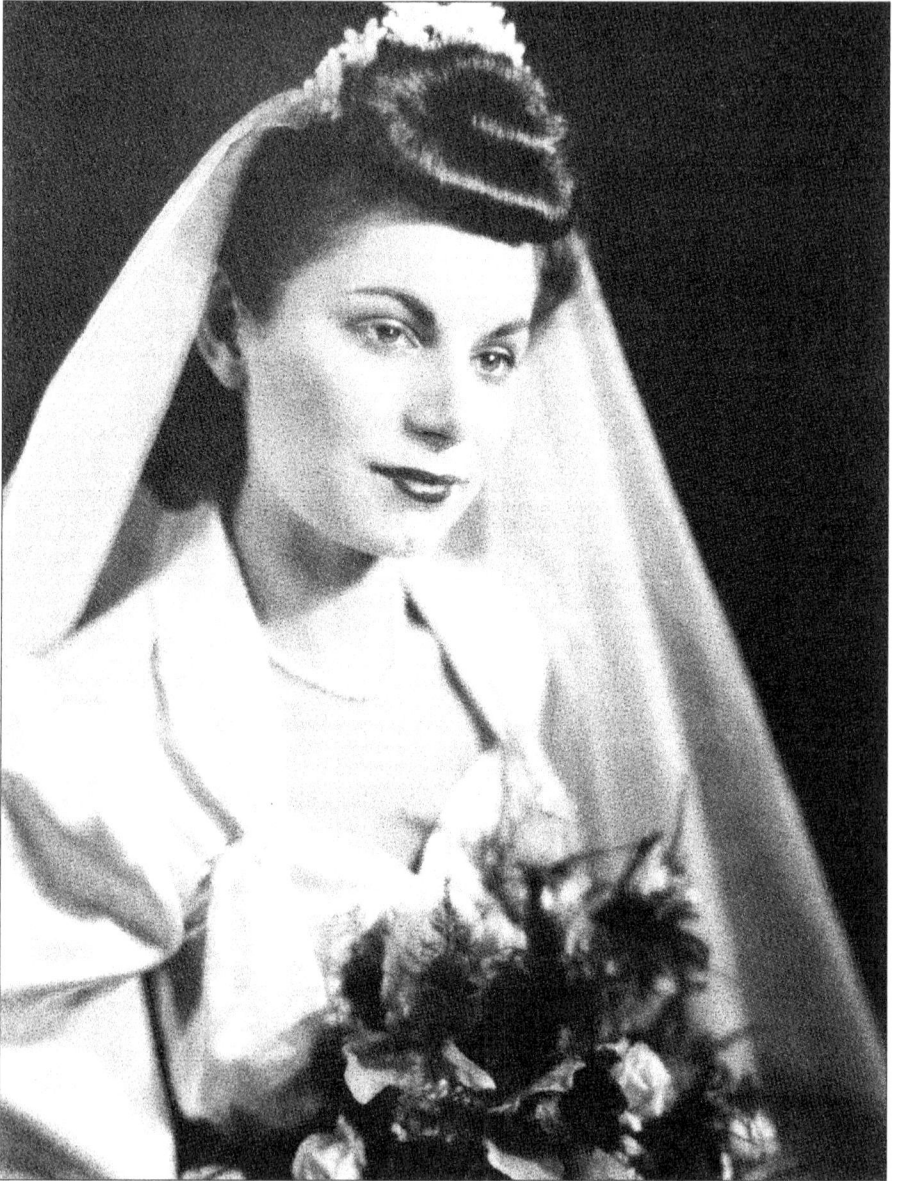

Georgia Kokonas Truels

TO MOM

I miss you, Mom
I knew I would
I'd bring you back
If I but could.

I think of days
When I would play
And you would call
Me from the fray!

"It's time to eat!"
You'd yell to us
"So come inside
And quit the fuss!"

We'd sit around
The glowing fire
And you'd remove
Our wet attire!

We had the time
To run and play
Tomorrow seemed
A long, long way!

But now the days
Go by so fast –
My thoughts of you
Are in the past.

And when I look
At your old chair
Sometimes I think
I see you there!

It seems a shame
That I can't play
And hear your voice
Above the fray!

I wish that we
Would never cry
I wish that we
Would never die!

The last days when
You felt the pain
I wish that I
Could live again.

I'd talk about
A love so true
I'd take the pain
Away from you!

But through it all
Our love will shine
And carry us
Through tougher times.

I know not where
We come or go
We play the game
And never know.

I miss you Mom
I knew I would
I'd bring you back
If I but could!

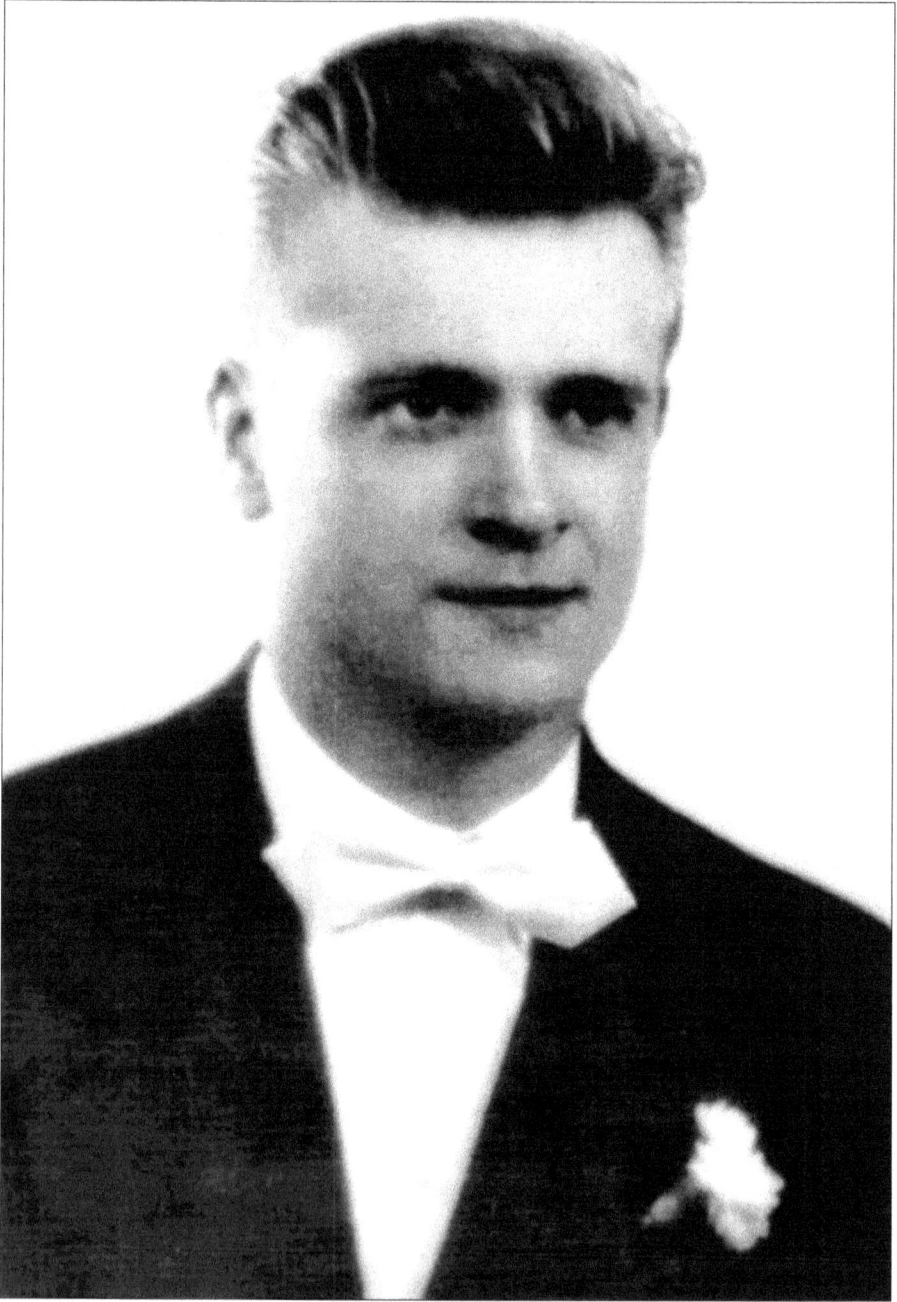

Ed Truels

TO DAD

Remember when we went out fishin'
At the break of dawn?
We'd sit in that old wooden boat
And fish all morning long!

We'd talk about the things
A Father tells his son
We'd relive all those football games
We really should have won!

We'd talk about my friends at school
And problems of the day
Somehow you knew just what to do
And just the thing to say!

I still can see those stripers
Jumping at our bait –
With plastic worms and minnows
We never had to wait!

Perhaps the greatest things in life
Are never really known
Until we view them from the past
When we are all alone!

Today, I brought my son with me
He likes to fish her too
You know I really miss you, Dad
I'll always think of you!

A NEAR-DEATH EXPERIENCE

We were all shocked to hear that Jack Arnold, the prominent, if not obstreperous, cardiologist, had a cardiac arrest. Jack was rushed to the emergency room and revived, to most everybody's relief. Being a close friend of Jack's, I was anxious to visit him in the hospital.

"Hello, Jack," I greeted him, as I entered the hospital room with a bouquet of flowers.

"Save those for the funeral, Dr. Truewater," Jack quipped. "I'm allergic to flowers."

"Sorry about that," I replied.

"You're forgiven, Truewater," Jack answered smiling. "Actually, I'm glad you came to visit me. I just feel darn lucky to be alive."

"Sounds like you had a close call, Jack. Tell me what happened."

"It's the strangest thing, Truewater," Jack began. "One of my elderly cardiac patients, Marge Abercrombie, was going through a list of 27 medications from three different HMO doctors, when I suddenly felt sick."

"Happens to me all the time," I said. "That's why I take frequent breaks between patients."

"No, this was different," Jack responded. "I began feeling nauseated and dizzy. Then I broke out in a sweat. The next thing I knew, I hit the floor. I remember my patient asking if it was her fault."

"They rushed me from my office to the Holy Christian Sinai Hospital Emergency Room. Dr. Morgagni actually said that I looked dead when I came through the door."

"I've heard Dr. Morgagni say that about other doctors, Jack," I interjected. "He said that to me one time when I was up all night operating on a trauma patient. It's just a figure of speech he uses."

"This was no figure of speech, Truewater," Jack replied. "For several minutes, I didn't have a recordable pulse or blood pressure."

"That's kind of scary," I replied. "Sickness is something that's only supposed to happen to patients, not doctors. It's sometimes hard to think of ourselves as patients."

"I wasn't doing too much thinking at the time, Truewater," Jack answered. "I was having my own near-death experience."

I had read a number of books about near-death experiences, and I was curious to know if Jack had seen any visions or long-deceased relatives during his sojourn into the unknown – something that might give me a clue into the nature of the universe, or which religion I should choose.

"Just out of curiosity, Jack," I began, "Do you remember anything about your near-death experience?"

"As a matter of fact, I do," Jack answered with a smile on his face. He closed his eyes as he tried to remember the vision.

"I saw a long, dark tunnel with a light at the end."

"That's the Nothingness, the Void," I said excitedly. "Just like the novel, Moby Dick, by Herman Melville."

"Then I remember a giant woman coming slowly towards me wearing soft, white clothing," Jack continued.

"My God," I replied excitedly. "Sounds like the Virgin Mary or maybe your Guardian Angel. This could be really big."

"Then I saw a man with a clipboard standing next to her, wearing a long, white gown and calling my name, Jack Arnold, over and over again."

"That must be St. Peter, checking the roll call," I interjected. "My God, Jack, you made it to the Pearly Gates of St. Peter! Is that when they called you back?"

"Not quite," Jack answered. "The woman with the white gown had two bright, shiny discs, one in each hand, and slowly began moving towards me."

"The Scales of Justice," I replied excitedly. "They really do exist. Did she weigh your good qualities on one side against your bad qualities on the other?"

"Not hardly, Dr. Truewater," Jack replied. "My bad qualities might break the scale, if you know what I mean."

"Besides, after that second shot of epinephrine, I began waking up. I realized I was in the Holy Christian Sinai Hospital Emergency Department, and that the man with the clipboard and the white robe was my HMO gatekeeper, Dr. Morgagni."

"My God, I hope you paid your premiums," I quipped.

"But, what about that long, dark tunnel you saw, you know, the Void?" I asked.

"Turned out to be that long hallway to the waiting room," Jack answered. "They need to spruce it up with a few fluorescent lights."

"And what about your Guardian Angel, the giant woman with the white clothing, and the metal disc in each hand?" I blurted out.

"More like an Avenging Angel," Jack replied cynically. "It was Nurse Patterson coming at me with the defibrillator paddles. I can still remember her saying, 'Get ready for the shock of your life, Dr. Arnold!'"

"That's when she hit me with 300 joules – twice. I might add. "Talk about coming back to reality – I must have jumped three feet off the table. I still don't think she likes me."

"That electroshock probably saved your life, Jack," I reminded him.

"In a way, Nurse Patterson was your Guardian Angel – she converted your heart rhythm from a ventricular fibrillation to a sinus rhythm."

"Don't get me wrong, Dr. Truewater," Jack answered. "I'm extremely grateful for the excellent care that was rendered by Holy Christian Sinai – it literally saved my life!"

"It's just that these near-death experiences are a little too close for comfort – I could have died, you know."

"In a way, Dr. Truewater, I guess it puts everything into perspective. Maybe it's Nature's way of preparing us for the future."

"You're right, Jack," I answered. "Every once in a while, we are confronted with the vastness of the universe, and our own relative insignificance."

"It teaches us humility," Jack replied. "But it does something else."

"What's that?" I asked.

"It makes us appreciate our friends even more," Jack added, with a tear in his eye. "Because we know we're not alone. Thanks for stopping by, Bill."

"My pleasure, Jack," I answered. "That's what friends are for!"

HAPPY FATHER'S DAY!

I almost made it. I bent over the bed to kiss my wife goodbye before heading off to the golf course.

"Happy Father's Day," my wife whispered as I started to leave, putter in hand.

"That's right," I replied. "I almost forgot. This is Father's Day. How nice of you to remember. I'll be back around noon."

"Where are you going?" Margaret asked, now beginning to wake up.

"I've got a little golf contest with some of the guys," I answered.

"What about the Bridge Walk?" Margaret asked.

"What Bridge Walk?" I asked.

"You know," Margaret replied. "The Oklahoma City Chamber of Commerce Charity Bridge Walk. They're reopening the Canadian River Bridge and donating the proceeds to the future Holy Christian Sinai Hospital Chest Pain Center."

"What Chest Pain Center?" I asked.

"You could take Michael," Margaret added. "All you do is walk one mile across the bridge, and the sponsors donate ten dollars for the Chest Pain Center."

"Why don't I write a check for ten dollars to the Chest Pain Center?"

"It's a fitness thing," Margaret replied. "Besides, it's good publicity for the hospital, and it's a good chance to be with your son – you know, male bonding."

"For the moment, I'd rather get my male bonding on the golf course," I replied. "Besides, if I can't play golf once a week, I might get chest pain myself. You know, I'm under a lot of stress at work, being a surgeon and all."

"I understand," Margaret sympathized. "As a surgeon you're constantly under pressure, making life and death decisions on a daily basis. It's a terrible burden, and creates a lot of stress."

"Exactly," I replied. "I'm glad you understand," I added, as I picked up my putter and headed for the garage.

"But, what about Father's Day?" Margaret added testily.

"My idea of Father's Day," I answered, "is to go out and play a relaxing round of golf. After all, I'm the father and today's my day."

"Exactly," Margaret replied. "And leave me to take care of the kids."

"Look," I said, "precisely what is my role as Father? I'm the provider – I put the meat on the table, so to speak. And I do spend time with the kids."

"It's just that I've got a one-dollar Nassau bet going on the front and back today," I continued. "And Jim says he'll spot me a stroke on each side, with fifty cents for each greenie, and a dollar for each skin."

"Sounds more like Indian casino gambling than golf," Margaret replied sarcastically.

"Besides," she added, "your role as modern father encompasses more than just putting meat on the table. You're also a family man, to say nothing of certain chores that need to be done around the house."

"You don't want your kids to grow up and say they never saw their father because he was too busy being a doctor or playing golf," Margaret chided.

The shame approach worked. I put my putter back in the corner of the bedroom, and prepared to attend the Charity Bridge Walk.

Needless to say, Michael tired out about half way across the bridge, and I ended up carrying him on my shoulders the rest of the way. When we got home, I was completely exhausted.

"How was the bridge walk?" Margaret asked innocently.

"Let me put it this way," I replied. "For a while, I was worried I'd become the first patient in the Holy Christian Sinai Chest Pain Clinic. I ended up carrying Michel the last half mile, and it must have been 90 degrees in that hot Oklahoma sun."

"This Fatherhood thing is beginning to wear thin," I joked.

"It's a lot better than being single," Margaret added. "In fact, that's what marriage is all about – sharing the responsibility."

"You're right," I replied. "After all, what did I have when I was single – just two things, really."

"And what were those?" Margaret asked.

"Time and money," I quipped. "That's all I had – time and money."

"Very funny," Margaret retorted.

"Don't get me wrong," I added. "You're absolutely right about sharing the responsibility. Becoming a father adds yet another role to my life."

"I can remember when my father took me fishing one Sunday morning at Lake Thunderbird instead of playing golf – that was the first fish I ever caught, and one my best childhood memories."

"As a physician, I sometimes get so caught up in my career that I neglect my role as father and husband."

"That's easy to do," Margaret replied.

Just then, my son Michael came running up to me with the newspaper.

"Dad!" Michael said excitedly. "*The Revenge of the Teen-Age Mutant Ninja Turtles* is playing at the show tonight. Can we go?"

I thought about my upcoming day – repairing an inguinal hernia, taking out a gallbladder, and seeing about ten patients in the office. And I thought about Michael's upcoming day – spending seven hours at school, studying geography, English, and mathematics, preparing for his own career. Maybe a little relaxation was in order for both of us!

"I'd love to see *The Revenge of the Teen-age Ninja Turtles*," I said, as I winked to Margaret.

"After all, that's what being a father is all about!"

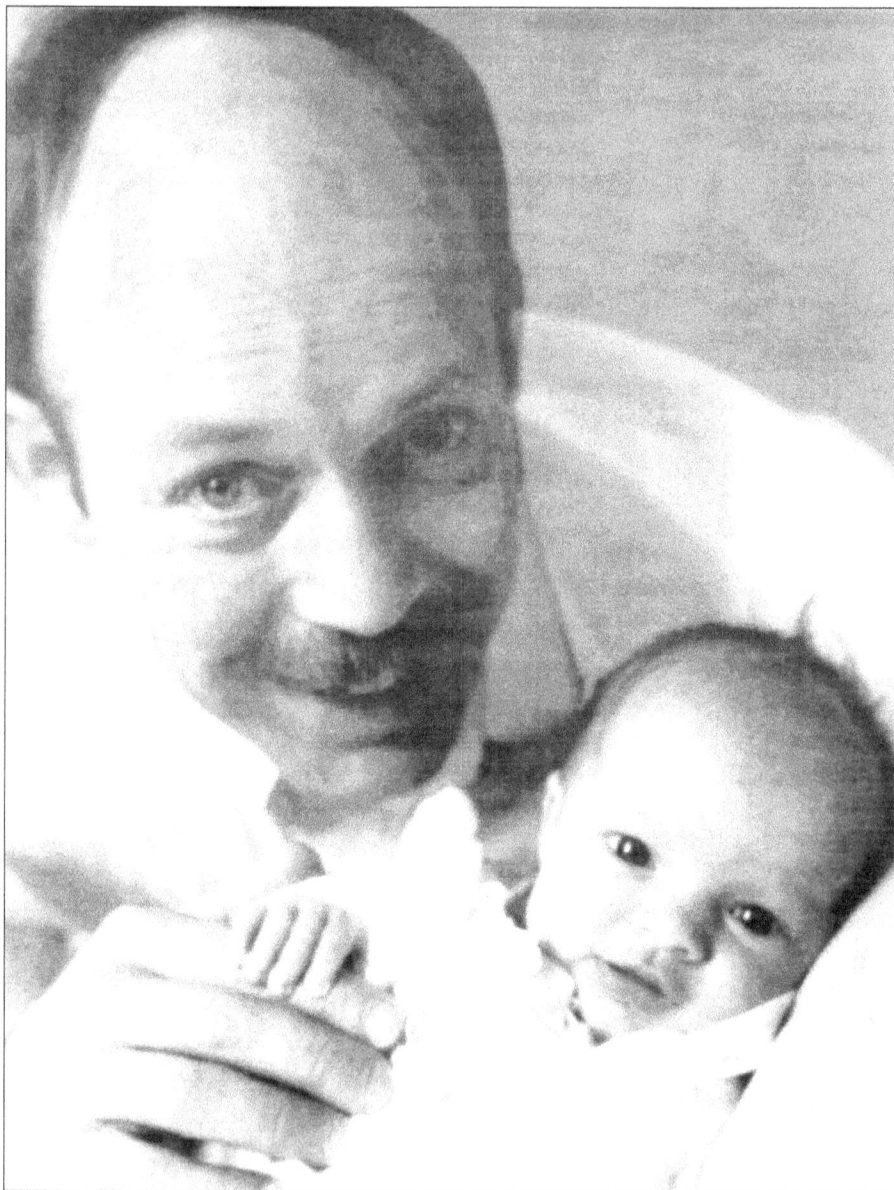

Dr. Johnnie Jones died in 1987 of a brain tumor at the age of 38. He is survived by his infant daughter, Julienne, and his wife, Cami, who is an R.N.

A FATHER'S WISH

I tuck you in your bed tonight
My little girl with eyes so bright.
I only wish that we could go
Together in life's picture show.

The backward flips, the forward rolls,
The roller skates, the swimming holes –
The first day that you go to school
And learn about that golden rule.

I'd like to see you climb that bus
And watch the kindergartners fuss!
I'd like to be there as you grow
And greet you with a father's glow!

I'd like to see you on your date
With eyes so big they captivate!
The pretty dress of blue and red
The velvet bow upon your head.

But fate has cast a different lot
For we shall be together not.
The life force which in you does play
Decreases in me every day.

O how I wish that I could be
More than just a memory!
I know not where we come or why,
I only think and then I cry.

We never know how long we'll stay
So make the most of every day.
Never look back with remorse
Nature always takes its course.

Live each day as if your last –
Never dwell upon the past
For when your days on earth are through
I'll be waiting there for you!

ARE YOU A LOOKER?

*"The Greek philosophers divided the world into
earth, air, fire and water.
I divide the world into lookers and flushers."*

I was sitting in the Doctor's Lounge on Monday morning, sipping a cappuccino in order to wake up, and munching on a strawberry tart from the pharmaceutical rep.

"That's a nice bronze tan you've got there, Dr. Truewater," Herb said. "You must have been out cutting the grass this weekend."

"No, I'm allergic to cutting grass, Herb. Makes me sneeze all the time. But I did play some golf."

I gazed at Herb's fair-complected skin, as he put on his blue surgery cap, with the bottom edge folded up an inch to keep from looking like Cro-Magnon man, with the big forehead.

"Actually, you look a little pale yourself, Herb," I replied. "Maybe you need to get out of the operating room and get a little more sun."

"I did get some sun," Herb answered. "I just don't turn dark like some people I know."

"You know, it wouldn't be a bad idea," I replied, "to check your stools."

"Why would I want to do that?" Herb laughed.

"You are a looker, aren't you?"

"I beg your pardon," Herb replied in disbelief.

"What's a looker?"

"Well, the way I see it, there are basically two groups of people in this world – the lookers and the flushers."

"I still don't get it," Herb replied.

"The lookers are basically scientifically oriented," I continued. "They check their stools before they flush. If the stools are dark, they may be losing blood and be anemic, causing them to look pale. That's why you should always check your stools."

"And the other group?" Herb asked.

"The flushers are people who are prim and proper and sort of deny their humanity. They want everything to be clean and neat."

"They don't look before they flush."

"Well, that's sort of a simplified view of the world, Dr. Truewater," Herb replied.

"You think all the world is divided into flushers and lookers--you must have skipped Philosophy 101 and the thoughts of the great Greek philosophers," Herb added.

"It's one way of looking at the world," I replied.

"The Greek philosophers divided the world into earth, air, fire and water. I divide the world into lookers and flushers."

"For example, in my area of wound care, where I debride wounds on a daily basis, I've got a realistic view of the world, without all the frills and deception. I'm a looker."

"And how would you classify me?" Herb queried.

"Well, you're a plastic surgeon, Herb. That makes you a romantic – you want everything to be pretty and nice, clean and proper. You avoid the unseemly aspects of human existence. You view the world through rose-colored glasses. That makes you a flusher."

"In fact, a recent article has come out that divides people into 'ploppers' and 'swooshers.'"

"People with firm, round stools have been shown to be healthy, happier people than those with more loose, liquid stools."

"I didn't know you could define happiness by the caliber of one's stools," Herb replied dryly.

"But I've got another explanation for your behavior, Dr. Truewater."

"What's that?" I asked.

"Most doctors are achievement and goal oriented. Ever since they were toddlers, their parents praised them for their accomplishments. That's how they were raised, and that's why they became doctors."

"What's that got to do with being a looker or a flusher?" I asked.

"Well, according to Sigmund Freud, when you were a toddler, and first learned to use the toilet, your parents praised you for your accomplishments."

"And?" I asked.

"And you became a looker," Herb replied.

"Ever since then, Dr. Truewater, people have been clapping at your achievements."

"Are you suggesting that my desire to achieve, in fact my entire professional career, dates back to my toilet training?"

"Exactly, Dr. Truewater," Herb answered.

"I never did understand psychology," I answered.

"Anyway," I continued, "what's important is that you check your stools. If they're dark, you may be losing blood and have a colon cancer or stomach ulcer, which can cause anemia and make you look pale."

"I appreciate your concern, Dr. Truewater," Herb replied.

"In fact, our chief of surgery died not very long ago of colon cancer. Since the age of 50, I've gone to the gastroenterologist every two years for a colonoscopy."

"By the way, Dr. Truewater, how would you classify a gastroenterologist?"

"I guess someone who does colonoscopies would be a looker *and* a flusher," I replied.

"Ah, the best of both worlds," Herb quipped, as he put on his mask and headed back to surgery.

WHERE'S GRANNIE?

Whenever you're in a hospital, never let anything bad happen on Sunday afternoon. Now, I have nothing against Sunday afternoon. That's the day most people are out enjoying themselves. It's the Lord's Day of rest. People are taking time off work to relax, and contemplating the deeper questions of our existence.

Which is why you should never get sick on a Sunday afternoon. You see, the regular doctors, nurses, and technicians are out relaxing and enjoying the beauties of Nature.

In fact, the most embarrassing thing that ever happened to me as a physician occurred on a Sunday afternoon. I lost my first patient – my first dead patient, that is – on a Sunday afternoon. Allow me to explain.

Presley Watkins' elderly grandmother died suddenly from a heart attack after being hospitalized for abdominal pain. Her real name was Lottie Smith but Presley always referred to her as "Grannie".

"Dr. Truewater," Presley began, "I'd like you to get an autopsy on Grannie, so that medical science can learn more about heart disease."

"I think that's a good idea, Mr. Watkins," I responded. "I'll have Nurse Riley call the pathologist."

"Now, you'll have to understand this was a Sunday afternoon. Nurse Riley was a "float" nurse, which meant that she did not normally work on that floor.

"Nurse Riley," I said, "let's call the pathologist, Tommy Agee, and get an autopsy on Mrs. Smith."

"No problem, Dr. Truewater," Nurse Riley replied.

The following day, I finished rounds early, and decided to drop by the pathology department to check on Mrs. Smith's autopsy.

"Hello, Tommy," I began. "I'm curious to find out what you found on Mrs. Smith's autopsy yesterday."

"Hello, Dr. Truewater," Tommy replied. "Who's Mrs. Smith? What autopsy?"

"You know," I answered testily – "Didn't Nurse Riley call you yesterday about performing an autopsy on an elderly lady who died of a heart attack yesterday – Lottie Smith?"

"I didn't do any autopsy yesterday, Dr. Truewater," Tommy replied. "And I didn't receive any phone calls from a Nurse Riley. In fact, there are no bodies in the morgue."

"She must have gone to the funeral home," I answered.

"My next step was to check medical records for Mrs. Smith's chart. After searching for about 15 minutes, the medical records clerk, Alice, came to me with a perplexed look on her face.

"Dr. Truewater," Alice began. "I can't seem to locate the chart on Mrs. Smith. Our computer says she died yesterday, and all input was terminated."

"Don't worry, Alice," I responded. "Let's be patient. I'm sure the chart will show up."

When I got to the office, I called the Rosethorn Funeral Home, but Mrs. Smith was not there, either. In fact, no one seemed to know exactly where Mrs. Smith had gone!

Just then, Presley Watkins, Mrs. Smith's grandson called the office.

"Dr. Truewater," Presley began, "did they find out what Grannie died from yet?"

"Not yet," I answered. "We're having a small problem, Presley," I continued.

"What's that?" Presley asked. "Perhaps I can help."

"Let me be honest about this, Presley," I stammered. "We can't seem to find Grannie. I guess you could say we've temporarily misplaced her. I'm sure it's only a temporary thing."

"Can't find Grannie?" Presley asked in disbelief. "You mean, like rolling back the stone in the Bible?"

"No, no, nothing quite that dramatic, Presley, I'm afraid," I said sympathetically. "I'm sure this is just a temporary thing. The hospital's a big place with lots of nooks and crannies. Sometimes things get lost," I explained.

"Things get lost?" Presley asked in disbelief. "Dr. Truewater, we're talking about real people here. Don't they have a computer to keep track of things like this?"

"Yes, there is a computer to keep track of the patients," I answered, "But once they die, the computer terminates all input – sort of a safety factor built into the software, ever since they discovered that some dead patients had been accidently charged for services not rendered."

"You don't think they could have accidentally sent Grannie home?" Presley asked.

"No, no," I replied. "The volunteers would have noticed something wrong when they took Grannie to her car. I'm sure this is just a temporary glitch. Let me get back to you in a few hours, Mr. Watkins," I concluded.

About thirty minutes later, the phone rang. Tommy Agee, the pathologist, was all excited because he had tracked down Grannie.

"We found Grannie!" Tommy said excitedly. "She's at the University."

"Good," I replied. "I understand Grannie had always wanted to go to the University."

"The University is running a research project on coronary artery disease," Tommy continued. "But before that, Grannie had to comply with Oklahoma State Law and go to the Medical Examiner's morgue downtown, since she died less than 24 hours after admission."

"When the Medical Examiner released her, she had to go to the Rosethorn Funeral Home to receive a special latex injection. From there, she went to the University for the special cardiac autopsy."

"Sounds like Grannie had a busy night," I exclaimed in disbelief.

"What happened to the medical record?" I asked.

"Everything was documented correctly in the chart," Tommy continued. "But, you see, it was Sunday afternoon. I went for a walk along Lake Hefner, and checked out to Dr. Kiston for a few hours."

"The 'float' nurse was new at her position," Tommy continued. "Ever since nursing school, she had been taught to always send the chart with the patient. When Grannie died, the 'float' did everything correctly, except for inadvertently sending the chart with Grannie on the gurney. Without the medical record, we couldn't find out just where Grannie went."

"Just as I suspected, Tommy," I said.

"What's that, Dr. Truewater?"

"If you ever get sick in a hospital," I replied, "don't do it on a Sunday afternoon!"

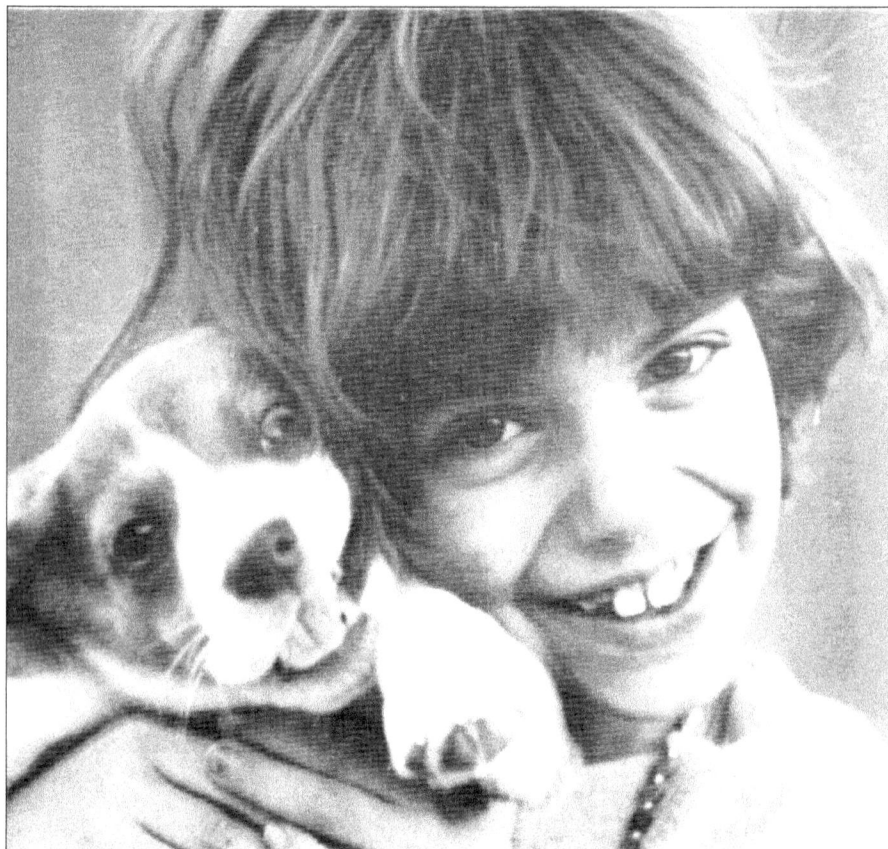

Tracy Truels with furry friend.

THE RACER

The little girl smiled with delight
As she watched the puppies jump and fight
"Pick the one you like the best-
Before the others take the rest!

"Skip that one," the old man said,
"The others all are better fed."
Then with a limp he tried to race
And fell down flat upon his face!

"I want that one" the girl then cried,
"He may not live," the man replied.
"I'd like to try to help him out –
That's what life is all about!"

"I'll call him 'Racer' – that's what I'll do –
He'll be the fastest of the crew!
I'll feed him good and make him tall –
I'll show him love is meant for all!"

But as she slowly walked away
With Racer on that happy day,
The old man wished them both good cheer
And then his eyes welled up with tears.

For as the girl with Racer played
He saw her slowly limp away
Never would she run or race--
Never would she take first place.

He wondered how it came to be
That life was never trouble free –
Some people seem to get the breaks –
Others only get the aches!

Then he smiled and saw the key –
"That girl will my teacher be!
For even though she was so small,
She taught me love was meant for all!"

THE CANDY MACHINE

There's a certain candy machine on the first floor of the Doctor's Office Building that is absolutely driving me crazy. It's not that I mind paying fifty cents for a candy bar – actually, the price is quite reasonable. It's just that I'm a creature of conscience, and I don't want to saddle myself with any more guilt than befalls a man of my stature. Let me explain.

As a physician, I am looked upon as a role model for my patients. Thus, I am expected to follow my own advice. When I tell my patients to stay away from saturated fats and simple sugars, I'm sure they expect me to follow the same recommendations.

One of my patients, Hamp Adkins, came to me last week for some simple dietary advice.

"Tell me, Dr. Truewater," Hamp began, "How can I lose weight and keep it from coming back? I don't want any of those fancy fad diets. I just want a simple, wholesome diet that I can follow every day."

"No problem," I told Hamp. "Stay away from simple sugars like candy and cake. Eat plenty of bran, stay active, and avoid saturated fats to help protect your coronary arteries."

"That almost sounds too simple," Hamp replied.

"It is simple," I answered. "It's just that we Americans are always trying to complicate our lives with food we don't really need."

Hamp thanked me for the advice and left the office, content that he had found the formula for a happy, healthy diet.

Now, I don't pretend to be perfect. Most of the time, I'm able to follow my own advice and live by the same guidelines that I set for my patients. Every once in a while, though, temptation sets in, and I find myself yielding to my darker instincts.

Such an occasion occurred last Saturday morning. I had finished doing some dictation at the office, and was preparing to leave the building. The lobby was devoid of patients, and as I walked past the candy machine, a particular candy bar happened to catch my eye.

"Just one time isn't going to matter," I told myself. "Lighten up. Enjoy life a little. In one hundred years, who's going to know the difference?"

Without fully realizing what I was doing, I yanked two quarters out of my pocket and thrust them in the machine. My mouth was already salivating as I punched the "D5" selection and watched the giant corkscrew advance my candy bar towards the hopper.

I quickly checked the lobby for any witnesses to my dastardly deed, then pushed my hand into the hopper, my heart now pounding in my chest. Ecstasy was only a bite away.

But alas! Something went wrong. My candy bar had hung up on the corkscrew. There it was, dangling precipitously in front of my eyes, as if taunting me for so easily yielding to my baser instincts.

"Very well, then," I thought to myself. "Perhaps there is a God in heaven after all, and this is His way of telling me never to eat candy bars. Yes, that was it – sort of like divine intervention."

I thanked my lucky stars for sparing me from the evils of the flesh and sheepishly walked out the door.

As I headed to the parking lot, I thought about how I would tell my friends about the last time in my life I ever tried to purchase a candy bar and how God intervened. I would tell them how I fought temptation. But would they really care?

Then, I had second thoughts. I thought about the fifty cents that I was losing – that wasn't right for the machine to keep the money. One small tap on the glass and that candy bar would fall into the hopper. Not that I would eat it for myself – of course not. I would give it to my kids – that would be better than letting the machine keep it.

As I walked back to the candy machine, I thought how important it was for mankind never to become a slave to his mechanical devices. I tapped the glass gently, but the candy bar would not fall.

"This is silly," I thought to myself. "All I have to do is leave a note on the glass. I could say something like, 'Dr. Truewater lost fifty cents in this machine.'"

But this wouldn't work either. My patients would have written proof that their doctor didn't follow his own advice and avoid sugar. Besides, what kind of doctor would complain about losing fifty cents in a candy machine? They would think my practice was on the rocks.

This was now becoming a matter of principle, of mind over matter. I kicked the machine gently and watched the candy bar start swinging. I was getting desperate. Five kicks later and I almost had it. By now, I had broken a sweat as I alternated my kicks with taps on the glass, watching the candy bar slowly move forward. The prize was almost mine – after all, I had paid for it.

"Doctor Truewater, excuse me, is that you, Dr. Truewater?" the man asked as he gently tapped my shoulder.

As I slowly turned to answer the voice, my worst nightmare came true. It was Hamp Adkins, the very patient who I had counseled against eating sugar! And here I was, pounding on the candy machine – caught in the very act, as it were, of sugar lechery.

"I'm glad I caught you, Dr. Truewater," Hamp began.

"I can explain everything," I replied defensively, trying to think up some excuse.

"I just stopped by to pay my bill," Hamp continued, as he handed me a check. "Thought I'd save myself the postage."

"Well, thank you, Hamp," I replied, hoping that he wouldn't comment on my antics with the candy machine.

"That crazy candy machine did the same thing to me last week," Hamp confessed. "After I left your office, I decided that one more candy bar wasn't going to kill me. After all, in a hundred years, who's going to know the difference?"

Hamp kicked the machine twice in just the right place, and dislodged the stubborn candy bar, then handed it to me.

"Thanks, Hamp," I replied.

As I walked back to my car, I realized that patients sometimes understand a whole lot more than doctors give them credit!

LIFE'S BATTLE

Somehow it seems a little strange
That in my body's cells
A tumor grows inside of me
And in my body dwells.

You know that it's a real shame
The two of them should fight
Someday I hope they'll get along
And make my future bright!

As for me, I'll never give up hope –
You're a fool if you do –
There's so much life I've yet to live
Before my days are through!

From the old man in his rocker
To the newborn baby's cry
All of life is just the same –
We battle 'til we die!

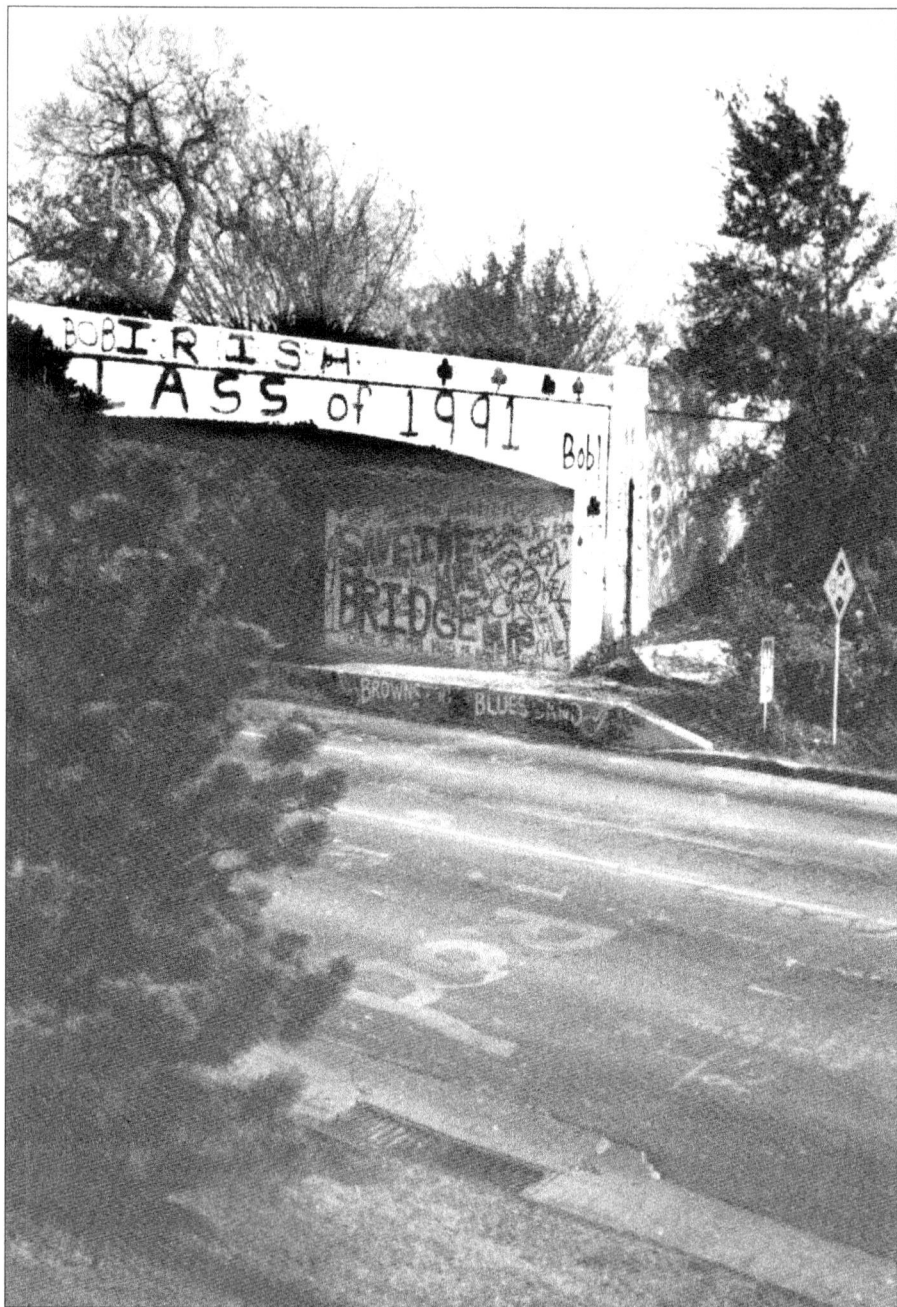

Graffiti Bridge on Western Avenue in Oklahoma City.

GRAFFITI BRIDGE

There's a place called Graffiti Bridge
Up upon the Western Ridge
In a sleepy part of town
That's the scourge for miles around.

Imagine driving past a bridge
With nasty words scrawled over it!
"Lisa loves Mike" and "OSU's the best!"
The ugliest landmark in the West!

Years ago when life was simple
The railroad bridge was an example
Of life the way it ought to be –
Clean and smooth and wrinkle-free!

But then the students spoiled our park
By coming here to share their art
Spray-painted words in green and blue
Tell us of a different view.

Some say the bridge allows expression –
Provides an outlet for aggression
It gives a place to congregate
For those who like to stay out late.

I'd like to see the bridge remain
As a symbol of our pain
The world's not perfect, as you know
People come and people go.

One day those kids may go to war
Then they'll really learn the score!
Some may give their lives that we
May live in a democracy.

Then they'll look back on those days
Of football games and panty raids
When the worst thing that you ever did
Was desecrate Graffiti Bridge!

THE WHITE COAT CEREMONY

"Dr. Truewater, I just have one question," Herb began, as I sat in the doctor's lounge, waiting for my case to start.

"No, problem, Herb," I replied. "Is this a philosophical issue or scientific?"

"A little of both," Herb replied, as he stared at my white lab coat with 'Dr. Truewater, General Surgeon' stenciled on the chest pocket.

"It has to do more with appearance than anything," Herb continued, as he stared at the prescription pads, scissors, cell phone, stethoscope and other paraphernalia I had stuffed in my pockets."

"Something wrong with my appearance, Herb?" I asked defensively, as I stared at his non-descript gray scrubs, with the words "Plastic Surgeon" stenciled on the pocket lapel.

"Let me be blunt about this, Dr. Truewater," Herb responded.

"Why the white lab coat?"

I stammered for a minute, unsure just how to respond.

"Let me guess," Herb continued, before I had a chance to reply.

"You just got back from the rat lab, where you're working on a cure for cancer, and now you're getting ready to make rounds on your patients in the hospital, and save more lives in surgery."

"Well, not exactly," I answered. "You don't have to be doing research in a rat lab to wear a white lab coat."

"I guess the best way to describe things would be to say that it's clinical."

"Clinical?" Herb asked.

"Yes, clinical," I answered.

"When you're working with patients who are ill, they want to know that somebody with a scientific bent is trying to solve their health problems."

"Well, if I was a rat in a lab," Herb replied, "I would expect to see the lab technician, who was doing research on my body for the good of mankind, to be wearing a white coat."

"But why wear the lab coat in the hospital, Dr. Truewater?" Herb grinned.

"It's professional," I answered.

"Professional?" Herb asked.

"Yes, professional," I continued. "You see, if you're sick and in the hospital, you want somebody who looks like a doctor to be taking care of you. You don't want some businessman, who looks like he just walked in off the street, to be in charge of your life."

"In fact, there's even a White Coat Ceremony at the University of Oklahoma, where incoming freshman medical students get frocked with a white coat by the Dean of Students as their introduction to medicine."

"I get it," Herb replied sarcastically. "First you get frocked. Then you meet your attending and get de-frocked in front of your fellow students, when you're asked on rounds to recite Halsted's six principles of wound closure."

"It's just a tradition, Herb--sort of a welcoming ceremony."

Besides," I added quickly. "The white coat provides protection."

"Protection?" Herb asked. "Protection from what?"

"Bodily fluids," I replied, as I looked at a small drop of blood on the hem of my coat from a recent dressing change.

"You never know when someone's going to vomit or bleed or whatever. We're in a hospital, you know."

"You sound like Dr. Strangelove," Herb replied. "Wasn't he the one who talked about preserving precious bodily fluids?"

"Could be," I replied. "But, you know, you don't look so great yourself in those dingy gray scrubs, Herb."

"My white lab coat is so old that it's turned yellow," Herb grinned.

"By the way," I added, as I looked at the day's surgery schedule. "Why are you wearing scrubs?"

"That's simple, Dr. Truewater," Herb replied.

"Scrubs are necessary in surgery. They're a necessary part of a surgeon's attire," Herb added, as he munched on a doughnut from the pharmaceutical rep.

"But you're not on the surgery schedule today, Herb," I said.

"True enough," Herb replied defensively, choking briefly on his doughnut.

"But I put these on in the morning so I don't have to wear street clothes. It's just more convenient to wear scrubs – even when I don't have surgery that day."

"Besides," Herb added, as he sipped on his cappuccino, it looks more professional."

"Professional?" I asked.

"People expect surgeons to wear scrubs. It's important to look like a surgeon, you know," Herb replied. "There's less explaining to do."

"I remember as a senior in college at Northwestern when one of the Nerds who went to medical school came back to visit us wearing scrubs," I added. "I think he was trying to impress his former colleagues—kind of like that Western song, '*How do you like me now?*'"

"After all, clothes make the man," Herb added.

"I rest my case," I said, as I hung up my white coat in the doctor's lounge, and headed back to surgery.

As I walked back to the operating room, I realized that it's not enough to pass four years of medical school, followed by four years of residency, with oral and written exams. You've also got to look like a doctor!

But even more important than looking like a doctor is acting like a doctor – showing compassion for your patients and concern for their recovery. One of the most successful doctors I ever met worked in a small town, and wore blue jeans and tennis shoes – he looked like he was about to go fishing! But his patients loved him because they knew he cared about each patient personally.

THE GOOD OLD DAYS

Do you remember
When life was simple
Coke was a dime
And gum was a nickel.

Old time cars
Were once brand new
With rear jump seats
And whitewalls too!

Saddle shoes
And bobby socks
Rock and roll
And record hops.

The Fourth of July
Was a day to play
With baseball games
That went all day.

For twenty-five cents
You could buy hot dogs
Or ride the subway
All day long.

The dollar
Was the standard then
People never heard
Of yens.

The dollar is now old –
No longer backed by gold!
Now we print more every day
To keep the national debt at bay!

We never spent
More than we earned
A balanced budget
Was our concern!

Now the government
Spends so much
That our grandchildren
Will feel their touch!

We had our problems
That was true –
But way back then
We could solve them too!

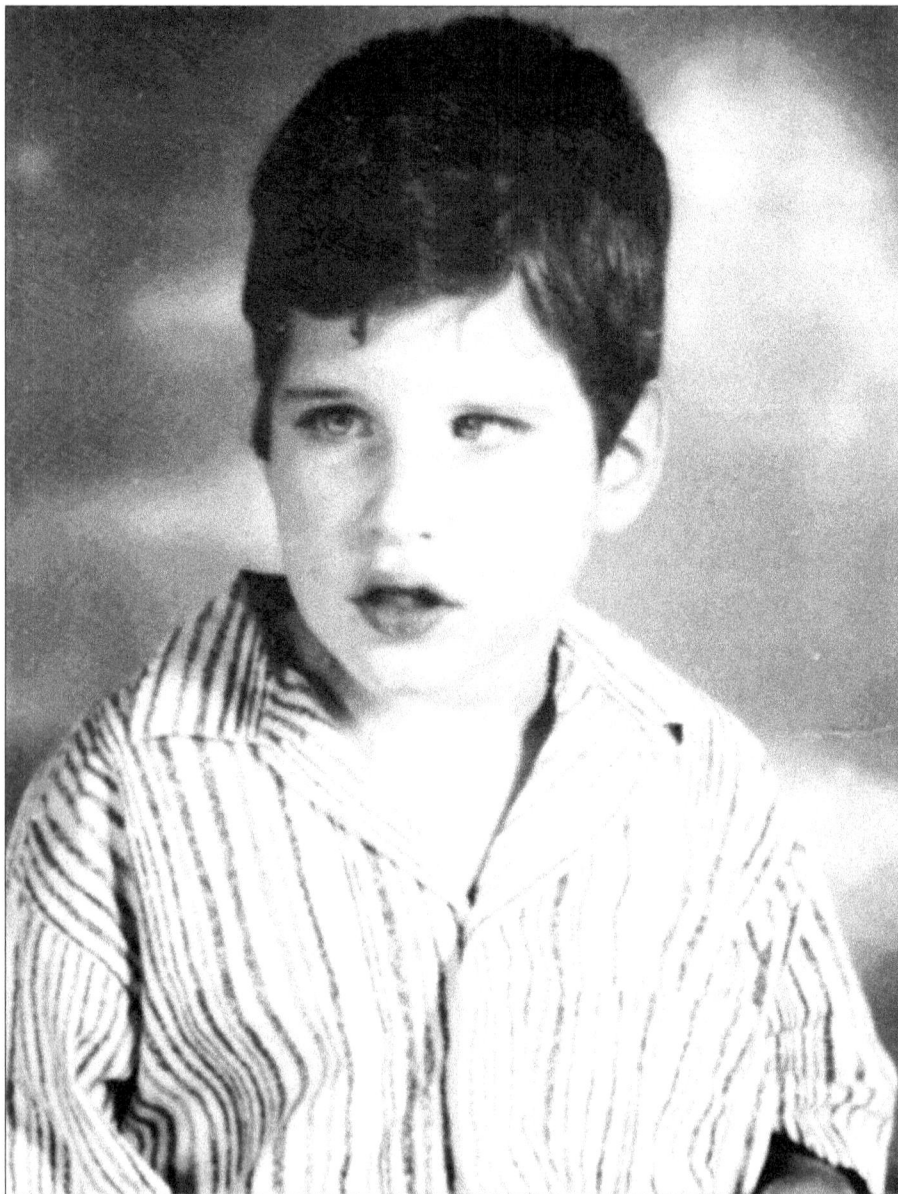

Isaiah Daniel Spencer, age 9, suffers from cerebral palsy.
Danny is cared for by his mother, Paula Spencer.

MY SPECIAL CHILD

Do you like my little boy?
He's cute enough for me.
I know he's not the perfect thing
That others want to be.

His eyes, you see, are turning in –
He may not ever walk
His brain can't keep the signals straight
He may not even talk.

He'll never be a doctor
Or a lawyer or a king
He'll never rule the world
Or fight for anything.

No, he's just my precious boy
He loves me every day
And each night when the sun goes down
We fold our hands and pray!

The gift of life is very dear –
A treasure from above
Thank you for my special child –
God shower him with love!

TORNADO ALLEY

Oklahoma weather is notoriously unpredictable and sometimes downright violent. Cold fronts from the North, dry mountain air from the West, and warm, moist air from the Gulf of Mexico all meet over Oklahoma, creating some of the most unpredictable and hazardous weather the world has ever known. Thus, it comes as no surprise that Oklahoma has produced some of the best meteorologists in the world.

In fact, the weathermen in Oklahoma are so highly trained that even though I'm a doctor, I can't for the life of me figure out what they're saying. For example, it's not unusual to be quietly listening to my favorite Chicago baseball team, minding my own business, when my radio starts beeping, and the program is interrupted by Jerry France, the world-renowned meteorologist, who views himself as the self-appointed Protector of the Realm.

My favorite baseball player, Andre Dawson, is just getting ready to hit a game-winning home run and Jerry France comes blaring over the radio with a weather alert.

"Sorry to interrupt your programming," Jerry begins humbly, "but we've just received a weather advisory from the National Severe Storm Center in Norman, Oklahoma."

For the first couple of years I lived in Oklahoma, I would always run and get out the state map from the glove compartment of my car, place it on the kitchen table, and meticulously try to identify the proposed path of destruction.

By the time I finally finished the above maneuver, however, the baseball game would be over, and Jerry France would be back on the radio with a new set of coordinates. When I found out that most Oklahomans have never seen a tornado, I decided to lighten up. Eventually I found myself ignoring the weather reports and periodically looking out the window to determine my survival status.

That was before the tornado struck. One night in May, 1986, I was invited to a roast duck dinner in Edmond, Oklahoma, along with several other guests, who included Sister Carmen at Holy Christian

Sinai Hospital. As sister Carmen recited the dinner prayer, and before Jerry France even had time to get on the radio and give his first set of coordinates, we all heard a clap of thunder followed by a loud roar. Within a minute, the walls of the house literally began to shake and my ears began to pop from the sudden drop in air pressure caused by the oncoming tornado.

We all ran into the closet and feared for our lives as the house next door was literally blown away. The roaring sound of the tornado was deafening, and even the concrete floor began to vibrate beneath our feet. I found myself wishing I had told my wife that morning how much I loved her. I thought of things I wished I had done, but never found the time. Fortunately, the tornado spared our house, and we all declared that it was an Act of God that none us us were killed.

The tornado affected all of us differently. I now viewed weatherman Jerry France as the Protector of the Realm, like many other Oklahomans who have experienced firsthand the destructive forces of Nature. When I saw Sister Carmen several weeks later, we greeted each other and relived our close encounter with the Almighty.

"You may not know this, Dr. Truewater," she began, "but God was talking to us that night."

"I couldn't hear Him above the roar of that tornado!" I replied jokingly. "Besides," I added, "Our Lord sure has a funny way of communicating – a thunderstorm would have been more than sufficient to get my attention!"

"That's not what I mean," Sister Carmen replied. "That tornado was God telling me to quit putting off for tomorrow what I ought to do today. All my life, I've been wanting to help elderly people by developing an extended care facility. The Lord was telling me that it was time to get the rest of my life underway. I'm temporarily leaving Holy Christian Sinai Hospital in order to devote my entire schedule toward the creation of such a facility."

I must admit that my interpretation of the tornado was far less profound. Maybe I was overlooking something. Perhaps I was not tuned in to the deeper vibrations of our universe. I viewed the tornado as a chance experience – a simple case of being in the wrong place at the wrong time. While the destructive forces are real, I did not imbue them with any sense of intelligence or purpose.

And what kind of God would maneuver a destructive tornado to destroy seventeen houses and cause millions of dollars in property damage, just so Sister Carmen would get the hint to build an old folks home? Why couldn't He just whisper it to her in some quiet moment of prayer?

But the tornado did teach me one thing – an acute awareness of my own human condition – frail, without sufficient time, and too often without sufficient purpose. Perhaps we would all do well to take timeout and listen to our inner voice. Seize the moment! Obey that impulse! Don't let the triviality of our daily life consume our deeper aspirations, for who knows when the next tornado will strike!

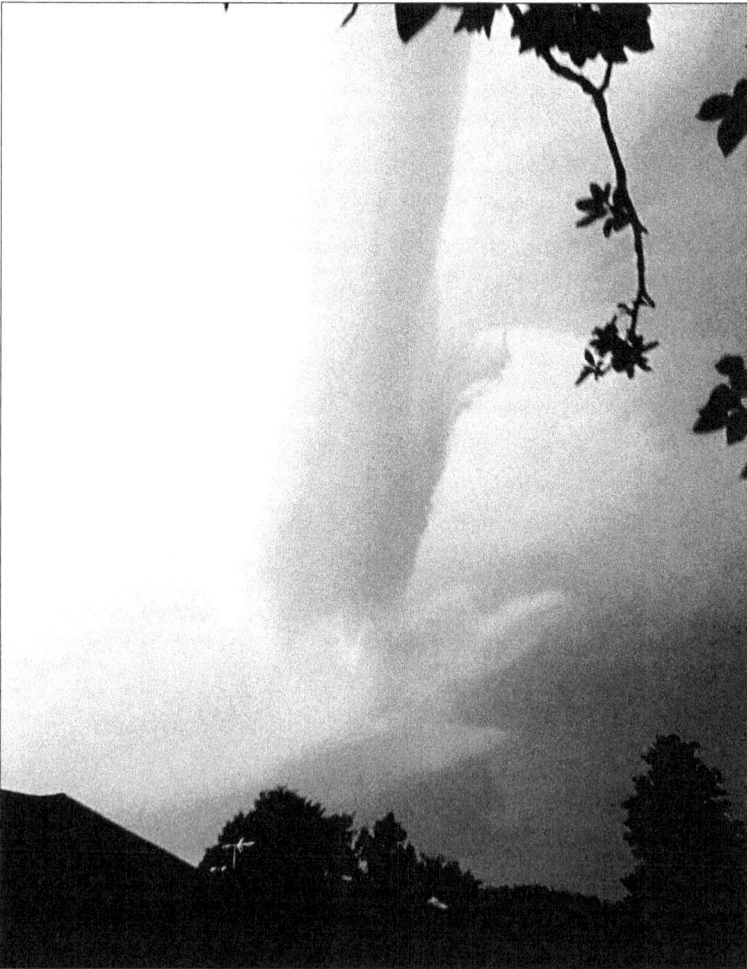

Taken from my front porch, May 29, 2012

WILL I SEE YOU AGAIN?

After you're gone
Will I see you again?
Will we dwell in a place
Where life never ends?

Will we go to a land
With streets lined with gold
Where we never grow hungry
And we never grow old?

Will your soul and my soul
Come together as one?
Will we join hands again –
Will we play in the sun?

Will we go to a world
Where peace rules the state--
Where there's no room for war
And no room for hate?

As I think of our love –
How great it has been –
If I were with you
I'd be happy again!

THE HOLY CHRISTIAN SINAI GOLF CLASSIC

I just finished playing in the sixth annual Holy Christian Sinai Golf Classic, which the doctors play every year to help raise money for charity. Deke Brumbaugh won this year. Deke Brumbaugh wins every year.

Deke is a psychiatrist at Holy Christian Sinai. He teaches the virtues of "positive thinking" and "positive mental attitude" to his patients. "You're a winner if you think you're a winner!" Deke loves to tell his patients.

Each year, Deke brings in three outside "guests" to play in the Golf Classic.

"They're boys from my Sunday School class, who don't get to play much golf," Deke says, whenever someone asks him who's going to be on his team this year.

Now these "boys" as Deke calls them average about 6'2" in height, weigh about 160 pounds, and have 28" waists. In the golfing jargon, they're known as "flatbellies".

"But Deke," someone usually objects, "Those boys from your Sunday School class were hitting the ball 300 yards! Are you sure their handicaps are 20?"

"They're real gorillas," Deke explains, "but they lack finesse around the greens. You should see them try to chip and putt!"

"We were playing in the group behind you, Deke," I added. "I saw one of those 'gorillas' sink a 30-foot putt and another one chip in the hole from off the green!"

"That's the fun of playing in a tournament!" Deke exclaims. "You never know when someone's gonna' get lucky! That's what positive thinking is all about!"

Last November, the Golf Classic Planning Committee met to plan this year's tournament. Inevitably, the subject of Deke Brumbaugh's Sunday School team came up.

"It's not fair to the other players," Chris Tomason complains. Each year, Deke brings in three unknowns from his Sunday School and wins the Golf Classic!"

"That's not all," Mary Carter adds. "Deke doesn't go to Sunday School. In fact, he doesn't even go to church! Deke's brother teaches golf at the University. Those 'Sunday School Boys' are members of the second-string golf team!"

Now, Bill Hadley is the pragmatist in the group. He loves playing the devil's advocate and he is obviously not a golfer.

"There's another side to this story," Bill begins. Dr. Bill Hadley is an oncologist who heads the weekly Tumor Board and he's always trying to get the radiation therapists, surgeons, and oncologists to get along with each other. Bill loves to tell the other side to a story. No matter what opinion you express, Bill Hadley will always defend the other side.

"Each year Deke Brumbaugh pays $200 in entry fees," Bill explains. "That money all goes to charity. And that's $200 more to feed the poor than if Deke didn't play. Besides, does it really matter who wins? It's the fun of going out there and playing golf, eating hot dogs, sipping an occasional beer, and raising money for charity. That's what the Golf Classic's all about!"

"Well, I care who wins!" Ray Sturgis, the neurosurgeon interjects. "I pay my $50 each year, I'm one of the best golfers out there, and I'm tired of coming in second place to a bunch of flatbellies who aren't even affiliated with Holy Christian Hospital. I say we can the suckers!"

"I say we let it ride," Bill Hadley responds, before anyone else can second the motion. "Besides, Deke Brumbaugh contributes to the Holy Christian Sinai Research Foundation every year, and I'd hate to risk losing his support!"

Before concluding their session, however, the Committee came up with a unique solution. Instead of making trophies for first and second place, all the trophies read, "Winner, Holy Christian Sinai Golf Classic".

That way, everybody came out a winner – Ray Sturgis' team finally won, we raised more money than ever for the Holy Christian Sinai Charity, and Deke Brumbaugh's positive thinkers never knew the difference!

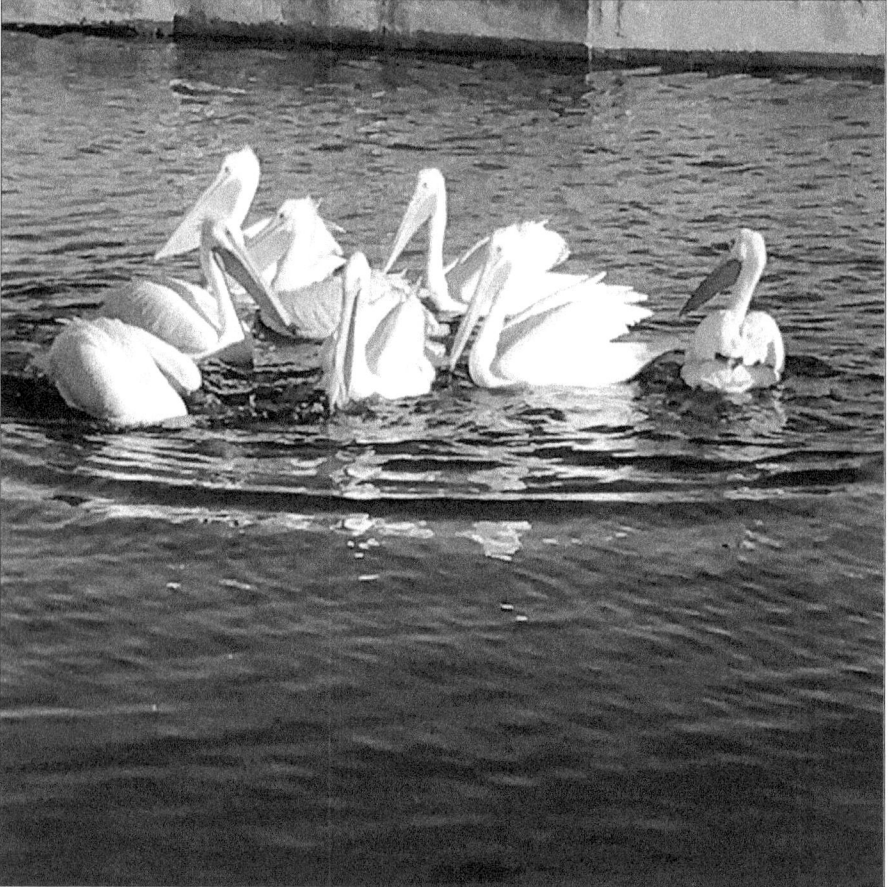

Pelicans visit Lake Hefner in OKC.

TO LAUREN

You didn't have
To take your life
We could have talked
And made it right.

I know that school
Was very hard
But you were always
Such a star.

You often were
So very serious
Some even said
You were mysterious.

A little joy
A little smile
Might have made
Life more worthwhile.

I think you fell
In love too hard
When you broke up
Your life seemed marred.

No single boy
Is worth that much
You still had
You father's touch.

I will miss you
Like a Dad
I'll always think
Of what I had.

If you can hear me
Where you are
You will always
Be my star.

NO PAIN, NO GAIN

I walked into the surgery lounge looking for a quick cup of coffee when I saw Herb sitting in the lounge chair with his leg propped up. He had a cast that extended from his foot to his thigh.

"What happened, Herb?" I asked.

"I was on the roof hanging Christmas lights when I slipped off the ladder and broke my leg," Herb replied.

"Now, what's a 60-year-old plastic surgeon doing on the roof of his house?" I asked. "You're supposed to hire a handyman to do that kind of thing. And don't tell me you can't afford it."

"I'm a fixer-upper, Dr. Truewater. And I'm kind of handy around the house."

"I can see that," I answered, as I stared at Herb's total leg cast.

"Does it hurt?" I asked, as I tapped on the cast with my knuckles.

"Ouch! Don't touch that cast, Truewater!" Herb snarled.

"Of course it hurts. Pain is nature's way of telling us that something's wrong."

"I suppose so," I replied. "I know that in physiology class we were taught about Pacinian corpuscles and "A", "B", and "C" pain fibers that lead to the thalamus and then to the other pain centers in the brain. The pain stimulus is nature's way of telling us to withdraw or pull away from, say, a hot object to avoid being burned."

"Exactly," Herb replied.

"Pain is nature's way of protecting the organism from harm," Herb added, as he sipped on his cappuccino coffee. "It's just that simple. Pain serves a useful purpose."

"But is it really that simple?" I asked.

"How do you mean, Dr. Truewater?" Herb replied.

"Well, my personal trainer tells me, 'No pain, no gain' – like, in order to really advance, you must endure pain. He talks like pain is a good thing."

"I would get a new trainer, Dr. Truewater," Herb quipped. "I can't believe you're paying him to hurt you."

"And the philosopher Frederick Nietzsche argued that which doesn't kill you makes you stronger," I added.

"I would get a new philosopher," Herb replied. "Besides,

Nietzsche had a nervous breakdown, which didn't make him any stronger."

"I guess what I'm driving at, Herb, is that as physicians, we deal with patients who are in pain. I mean, why do we suffer? Why did it hurt, for example, when I tapped your cast?"

"You touch my cast again, and I'll kick you with my good leg!" Herb threatened.

"Besides, who are we to question Mother Nature or God, for that matter?" Herb added. "I mean, look at Job in the Bible. Job suffered, to be sure, but in the end God made it right."

"God made it right?" I asked. "I mean, the poor man suffered from painful boils, lost his family and friends, and suffered in isolation."

"True enough, Herb replied. "But maybe God intends for us to suffer, Dr. Truewater, say for punishment or for some greater good that we don't yet comprehend, but that God comprehends. I believe that all things work for the Greater Good."

"You make it sound like we're on some medieval earthly plane, enduring pain and suffering and hardship as we climb upward, in order to arrive at some more perfect place, like Shangri-La or heaven, where there is no pain and suffering," I replied.

"Well, certainly as physicians our goal on earth is to relieve other people's diseases and pain, in order to arrive at a better world for all," Herb added.

"And I think it's important to keep a positive attitude about pain. I mean, look at me. I'm in pain as we speak from this broken leg. I could whine and moan, but I'm not going to do that. The way I look at it, I'm paying the price for doing something stupid, like falling off the roof. There's a lesson to be learned here, and I choose to be upbeat about it."

"Hand me my pain pills, will you, Dr. Truewater? I left them on the counter by the coffee pot."

"Of course, Herb," I replied, as I passed off his narcotic pain pills.

"In fact, look at these pills," Herb replied. "They're derived from the poppy Papaver Somniferum. God gave us narcotics to deal with our pain, you see? God isn't just going to let us suffer without relief."

"I suppose not," I replied. "But what about cancer patients who are in pain? You're not going to tell me they did something wrong, and now they're paying the price?"

"Of course not, Dr. Truewater. I believe cancer to be a malfunction of our controller genes, for whatever reason, be it a virus or a failure of our immune system to eradicate random mutations. As the cancer grows, it causes chronic pain."

"Similarly, as we get older, our ability to repair ourselves declines. Our joints and bones become brittle, and we must deal with chronic pain."

"But why does this happen?" I asked. "Why do we experience pain for no apparent reason?"

"I mean, is the pain-pleasure response that our bodies generate simply a matter of chemical mediators in the brain, or is it part of a larger pattern of our universe, where everything is a balance of opposites, like the Chinese yin-yang or the physicist's matter and anti-matter?"

"Your questions are getting to be a pain, Dr. Truewater," Herb replied, as he rested his hand on his total leg cast.

"Let me just say that, while there is a God, there is also a certain randomness in the universe, and a certain set of physical laws, which our material bodies must obey."

"When I fell off the roof, that was a chance occurrence. Gravity took over, and I hit the ground at 18 feet per second and felt pain. On the other hand, when I kissed my wife, I felt pleasure."

"As such, we must learn to accept this dualism – namely that without pain, there can be no pleasure."

"I suppose so," I replied. "But I'd rather just take the pleasure and forget the pain."

"Bishop Berkely claimed that our view of the world was a function of our perception. And particle physics teaches us that the influence of the observer can affect the outcome. I believe that by maintaining a positive attitude, our very perception of pain, and for that matter our very perception of the world will improve."

"Cancer specialists tell us that people with a positive outlook can live longer," I added.

"But what about death, Herb? What will your attitude be then?"

"I will be smiling," Herb replied, as he looked down at his total leg cast – "Just as I smile today, despite the pain."

THE EAGLE PILOT

The Eagle pilot showed his jet
To all the people gathered 'round
"This plane can carry seven tons
And travel twice the speed of sound!"

Then he saw a little boy
Sitting in a wheelchair
His little eyes were opened wide
As he dreamed of flying in the air.

The pilot stepped down from his plane
And came up to the boy
He shook his little palsied hand
And made him jump with joy.

"Here's an Eagle Air Force Patch
That's worn by all the crew
It's something you can show your friends –
This one is just for you!"

"I don't know how to thank you!"
The little boy then cried,
He kissed the Air Force pilot
As tears flowed from his eyes!

"I dreamed that I could fly through space
And sail in the blue
Now every time I wear this patch
I'll fly this plane with you!"

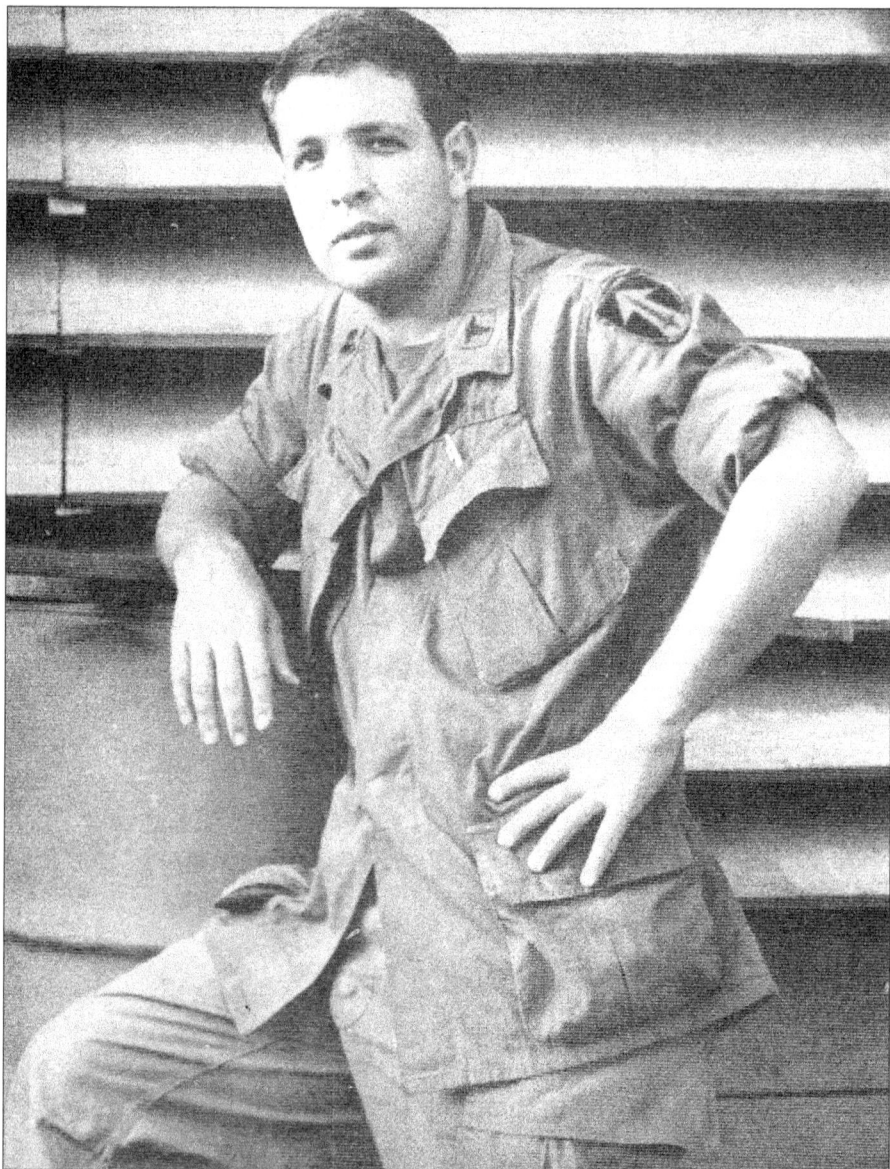

Captain Norman Paul Singer, M.D., son of Joseph and Ann Singer from Oklahoma City, graduated from the University of Oklahoma Medical School in 1967. He was killed in Xaun Loc, Viet Nam on May 18, 1969 at the age of 29. Dr. Singer was also an artist, and designed and constructed "The Old Rugged Cross" for the Sisters of St. Anthony. A tribute to Dr. Singer may be seen at the Cowboy Hall of Fame.

SAYING GOODBYE

Why must people say goodbye
Instead of just hello?
Wouldn't this be a nicer place
If no one had to go?

Why do people die?
It doesn't seem quite fair
Why do we grow old and gray
And vanish in the air?

The Lord must have his reasons
For this changing of the guard
Evil ones are laid to rest
But good folks still die hard!

I'm sure this is a better world
With new replacing old
But if we never said goodbye
It might not be so cold!

CHANGING THE WORLD

Our medical school was going to change the world. With the Viet Nam War raging, and the country divided, we were going to cast off the bonds of the establishment, and create a new world of peace, prosperity, and brotherhood.

To prove our sincerity, our first official action was to refuse the complementary black bag that was customarily provided free by one of the drug companies. Our second official act was to refuse the complementary stethoscope provided by another drug company as yet another expression of our independence from the military-industrial complex. Instead, we each went out and spent about $125 to purchase our own black bags and stethoscopes.

Next, we set out to change the medical school curriculum. The first two years of medical school training typically involved little patient contact. This seemed ludicrous to us, since we were in training to be physicians. Besides, after sixteen years of textbooks, things were getting a little boring.

I remember our class president, Paul Woodward, pleading for more patient contact.

"Things have got to change," Paul told the administration. "Medical students today are insisting on patient contact--it's the most important part about being a physician--we've got to stay in touch with the people!"

Paul would make rounds with the third and fourth year medical students at six o'clock in the morning before classes started for the first year medical students.

"It's absolutely amazing how much you can learn by making rounds in the morning!" Paul told us. "Why, I actually saw a patient today with a butterfly rash on her face--the malar rash of lupus. You see something like that once and you never forget it!"

Accordingly, several of us in the dorm would wake up at five in the morning in order to accompany the juniors and seniors on rounds. That evening, we would swap stories with our fellow classmates.

"I saw five cases of pneumonia, two patients with the nephrotic syndrome, and one patient with herpes," I announced proudly at the dinner table that night. "It sort of puts everything you read in the textbooks in perspective," I added. "That's nothing," Mary Strothers added. "I saw a baby with meningitis which developed from an untreated otitis media."

Mary was from the gifted and talented section of our class and was planning to be a pediatrician. She had already made a name for herself at the University of Missouri at St. Louis, where she helped determine the amino acid sequence for growth hormone.

"There's nothing like a little clinical perspective to crystallize what you read in the textbooks," Paul Woodward, our class president added. "If only I could get that through the heads of our medical faculty!"

Last month, I attended the twenty-year reunion for our medical school class. I was curious to see what my colleagues had been doing. I noticed Mary Strothers standing by the hors d'oeuvres.

"Hello, Mary!" I exclaimed. "It's me, Bill Truewater. How are things going?"

"Well, it's good to see you, Bill!" Mary replied. "Things are going quite well! I'm involved in Dr. Watson's DNA sequencing program at Harvard. In twenty years, we hope to have the entire DNA sequence for the entire human genome!"

"That's fascinating!" I replied. "I was reading just the other day where colon, breast, and lung cancer were all tied in to the P51 chromosome site. But tell me," I asked, "I thought you were going to be a pediatrician. What happened?"

"Well, things change, Bill," Mary replied. "After two years as a pediatrician, I got tired of all the clinical contact. I missed my research."

Just then Paul Woodward walked by.

"Hello, Bill!" Paul began. "How's life treating you?" "Fine," I answered. "What're you doing these days?" "I'm a radiologist in a small hospital near Carbondale. I love it!"

"Do you remember when we used to get up early as freshman in order to make clinical rounds?" I asked. "Remember how we said all that patient contact reinforced our textbook knowledge?"

"I sure do," Paul replied. "But when I got into my junior and senior years, working 14 to 18 hours a day, and not sleeping every third night, I sort of burned out on patient contact. Like I say, I'm a radiologist, and I love it."

But the crowning blow was Atley Reeson. Atley led the campaign in 1969 against accepting the black bags and stethoscopes from the drug companies.

"Atley Reeson!" I exclaimed. "What're you doing these days? You look as fit as a fiddle!"

"Good to see you, Bill," Atlee replied. "I've been doing a lot of traveling these days. I'm the designated medical spokesman for a new anti-viral agent called Virokil. It gives me a chance to see the world plus it pays well."

"But what about changing the world, and doing away with the military-industrial complex?" I asked. "Remember when we weren't going to accept any gifts from the pharmaceutical companies?"

"Well, that was probably a little immature on our part," Atlee responded philosophically. "After all, the pharmaceutical companies weren't to blame for the Viet Nam War. Besides, times change. We're no longer at war and it's time to forgive and forget."

"Ironically," Atlee added, "this new antibiotic may do more good for the third world than any revolution."

When I returned to work the next day, an office full of patients was waiting, as well as my first year medical student preceptor, Jerry McDowell.

"Nice to meet, you, Dr. Truewater," Jerry began. "These sessions are the only clinical contact I have all week."

"That's good," I replied. "But I'd hate to see you burn out. When you're a medical student, the hardest thing to do is to study. And when you're a busy physician, the hardest thing to do is maintain patient contact!"

After my student left, I thought back to my first year in medical school twenty-five years ago. "Medical students are still anxious to make patient contact their first year," I thought to myself. "The more things change, the more they stay the same!"

IF I KNEW THEN

If I knew then what I know now
I'd do some things I didn't know how –
I'd speak the words I was afraid to say
Not save them for another day.

I'd be happier then, and thank my friends
For supporting me right 'til the end.
I'd smile more often, don't you see
Things aren't as bad as they appear to be!

I wouldn't be nearly so shy
I wouldn't be afraid to cry!
I know I'd have more confidence-
My car would have much fewer dents.

I'd be an expert, don't you see
At the age of twenty-three –
But learning from hard blows we face
Is how we learn to run the race.

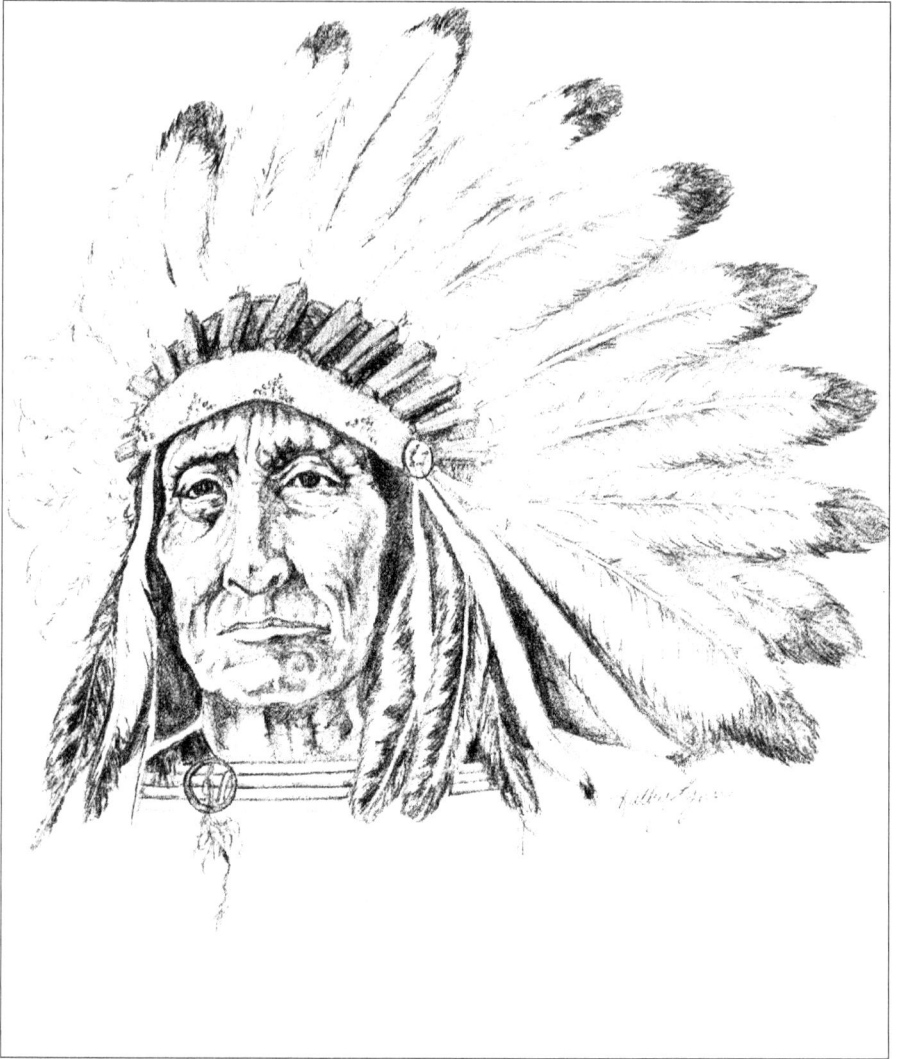

THE NATIVE AMERICAN

"My people once owned all this land,"
The American Indian proudly said,
"We cultivated all this soil
Along the river bed."

"The corn grew nearly six feet tall
We had more than we could eat
The deer ran wild in the woods
We never lacked for meat."

"The river then was full of fish
They frolicked in the stream
As kids we fished here every day
Our life seemed like a dream."

"Now the fish have all but died
Pollution fills the air
I still come out here every day
But no one seems to care."

"I sit along these river banks
These cars look kind of queer
I dream about the days gone by –
Of corn and fish and deer!"

DEATH BY MEDICARE

I have been hounded and harassed by Medicare, but last month was the final straw. Against my will, Medicare stopped my medical reimbursements in a most unusual fashion. They pronounced me dead. At first, I thought this was some sort of intentional attack, but subsequent events have led me to believe that basic incompetence was at the heart of the problem.

It all started when my claim for financial reimbursement, after treating an elderly man following a car accident, was denied. Usually, Medicare follows some complicated formula for reimbursement, which always turns out to be the same – take half my bill and label it the "allowable charge." Then, lop off another 20% and tell the patient that my charges are in excess of the "community standard", which was calculated twenty years ago and never revised.

This time, however, the reimbursement was zero. I decided to handle the matter personally and called my Medicare representative, Hiram Holler.

"Mr. Holler," I began, "my name is Dr. Bill Truewater." I explained the situation, including the zero reimbursement, and, after a few minutes on terminal hold, Mr. Holler returned with my file.

"Dr. Truewater," Mr. Holler began. "I have very bad news."

"How's that?" I replied.

"Well, our records show that you died two months ago," Mr. Holler replied sympathetically. "All Medicare reimbursements will be made to your estate."

"I admit that I haven't been feeling well lately," I answered, "but I had no idea it was that serious. Just out of curiosity, what was the cause of my death?"

"Even if I had that information, Dr. Truewater," Hiram responded angrily, "I'm not at liberty to reveal it – that's confidential patient information."

"But I'm the patient," I responded. And I'm not dead! Can't you tell I'm still alive? I'm officially requesting an appeal!"

"I've never had this happen before," Mr. Holler continued. "In the past, our computer has declared patients dead before their time, but this is the first time it's happened to a doctor."

"Surely Medicare has a protocol for reversal of their decision," I continued, periodically pinching myself to verify my existence.

"Have no fear, Dr. Truewater," Mr. Holler responded. "We'll send a committee out this week."

"A committee?" I asked.

"Yes," Mr. Holler continued. "We have a Verification Committee consisting of five standing members that conduct interviews with the supposed dead person. If the Committee determines by at least a majority vote that the person is, in fact, alive, then a Petition for Reinstatement of Benefits is filed on behalf of the formerly deceased."

"That sounds good to me," I responded. "I always do well with interviews. In fact, it was a strong Medical School Admission Interview that got me into this mess. And when I took my oral exam for my surgery boards, I once again rose to the occasion."

"Oh, it won't be anything that difficult, Dr. Truewater," Hiram Holler assured me.

"Will there be a physician on this Verification Committee to check my blood pressure or other vital signs to determine viability?" I asked, as I cradled the phone on my shoulder to check my own pulse.

By now I was convinced that the cause of my death would be a heart attack sustained while talking to an insurance company on the telephone.

"No, nothing like that, Dr. Truewater," Hiram assured me. "No, the most difficult thing you'll be asked to prove is that you're Dr. Truewater, and not some imposter trying to collect benefits."

"How do I prove I'm Dr. Truewater?" I asked.

"Just be yourself," Hiram replied. "We'll need letters of recommendation from responsible politicians in your community."

"There are no responsible politicians in my community," I answered.

"But I've got five friends who'll verify that Dr. Truewater is alive and well, and living in Oklahoma City. And I've got a birth certificate with my foot print from Edgewater Hospital in Chicago," I added.

"Good," Mr. Holler replied. "You'll also need a current Visa or Mastercard as a further help for the Verification Committee."

"What for?" I asked.

"Well, there's a $500 fee for performing the life resurrection process."

By now, I was getting frustrated. Why should I have to prove I'm alive to an organization that for years has belittled my claims and represented my charges as "above reasonable and customary standards for the community", yet refused to send me a copy of "reasonable and customary charges" based on current physician fees?

"I've got an idea, Mr. Holler," I began.

"Go ahead, Dr. Truewater," Hiram answered.

"What would happen if I didn't appeal my death decision?" I asked.

"Why, that's absurd, Dr. Truewater!" Hiram indignantly replied.

"Does that mean I wouldn't have to sign that Medicare form at the beginning of each year, stating that I am guilty of a felony and could go to jail if I mis-code my claim forms?" I asked.

"Why, yes, I suppose so," Hiram answered.

"And, if I remain deceased, does that mean I wouldn't have to provide my patients with a list of other physicians who would perform the same surgery?" I asked.

"Why, yes, I suppose so, Dr. Truewater," Hiram replied again. "Dr. Truewater, I'll personally see to it that this matter gets straightened out within the next six months," Hiram continued.

"That won't be necessary, Hiram," I replied. "I'm not going to appeal the decision. I'd rather die a quick Medicare death than watch my Medicare reimbursement drop 10% a year for the next ten years because the government can't balance the budget!"

As I hung up the phone, I had one final thought. Since Medicare had declared me legally dead, could I file for my own death benefits?

Author's note: This actually happened to one of my patients. A Medicare committee, consisting of five members, actually visited her house, and conducted an interview to confirm that she had not died!

MY FIRST NEEDLESTICK

About two months ago, I stuck myself with a needle in surgery – nothing major, mind you, but a surgeon worries nowadays when something like that happens. Then one week later, I developed a fever, lost about five pounds, and even noticed a lump in my neck. The conclusion to me was inescapable – I had AIDS!

Now you must realize that I'm the kind of person that sometimes worries too much about my health. As a medical student, it seemed like every time I read about a new illness, I would develop all the symptoms. As a student, I had diagnosed myself, at one time or another, as having scarlet fever, lupus erythematosus, mononucleosis, tuberculosis, and even leukemia – all of which proved unfounded.

But nevertheless, I was convinced I had AIDS. Not that I hadn't taken all the proper precautions. I was wearing my safety goggles with the special side shields to prevent an errant drop of blood from sneaking past my peripheral vision. I was even wearing two sets of gloves, though I'm not at all convinced of the virtues of such a practice.

But perhaps I hadn't taken enough precautions, I thought to myself. I ran into Ted Danstrom, the plastic surgeon, in the doctor's parking lot, and rather casually approached the subject.

"Tell me, Ted," I asked, "what precautions do you as a plastic surgeon take to prevent AIDS?"

"Abstinence!" Ted responded with tongue-in-cheek.

"No, I don't mean that," I replied. But before I could elaborate on my question, I saw Dr. Hadley Upper, the infectious disease specialist, parking his car.

As I walked toward Hadley's car, I kept wondering how I could ask him discreetly about the fever, weight loss, and the small lump in my neck.

"Hello, Hadley!" I exclaimed.

"Hello, Dr. Truewater!" Hadley responded.

I decided to get right to the point. "Hadley," I began, "what are the first signs of AIDS?"

"Simple," Hadley replied. "Fever, weight loss, and sometimes a small lump in the neck. As a surgeon, it's important for you to recognize the symptoms. We're seeing more and more AIDS patients these days, you know, Dr. Truewater."

Hadley's answer was hardly reassuring, but I needed to get more information. "What precautions can I take as a surgeon, then, Hadley?" I asked.

"Well, good eye protection is important," Hadley replied. "I'm not so sure about double gloving, though. They've found that one third of the gloves used outside surgery can't even hold water, let alone protect against a virus. The same thing goes for condoms."

By now, I figured I was a goner. I would never live to see my kids grow up and take drugs. I could just see the headlines two years from now – "DR. TRUEWATER, FIRST OKLAHOMA SURGEON TO DIE FROM AIDS DUE TO A NEEDLESTICK!"

I finally broke down and confided my story to Hadley Upper about the needlestick in surgery two months before.

"At least, if I did get AIDS, it would be an on-the-job injury," I moaned.

"Not necessarily," Hadley replied brusquely. "Did you document your episode of the needlestick in the chart after it happened?"

"Well, no, not at the time," I responded. "In fact, I really didn't think it was that important when it happened," I answered defensively.

"And then, of course, there would always be the usual questions about your private life," Hadley continued.

"Questions about my private life?" I queried. "What about my private life? Did I do something wrong? I'm on my second divorce – I mean, my second family," I explained. "Is that a problem?"

"No, no," Hadley reassured me. "Just the usual questions about your sexual preferences and drug history."

"Well, I'm a straight arrow in that regard," I replied.

Needless to say, Hadley had done little to allay my anxieties about contracting AIDS from a needlestick. Although I realized that the odds were extremely small, I was still reluctant to share the problem with my wife. When I returned home that evening she had only one question.

"Tell me, Bill," she began, after the kids left the kitchen, "Why did you use a condom last night? You know I had a tubal ligation two years ago."

"You can't always be sure about tubal ligations," I replied calmly. "Sometimes the tubes can grow back together. It's always better to be safe than sorry."

"But why two condoms?" she asked.

"Some of the condoms have been found to have holes," I explained.

Fortunately, my story has a happy ending. My AIDS titer was negative, as was the Mono spot test. But the cat scratch titer was positive. I had totally forgotten that I had been scratched by my neighbor's cat several weeks earlier! I had all the symptoms and signs of cat scratch fever! After about a month, the lump in my neck went away, and my activity level returned to normal.

The only regret I have is that we still haven't found a cure for AIDS. The anxiety which I endured was only a small microcosm of the ominous fate awaiting thousands of men, women, and children each year until a cure is found!

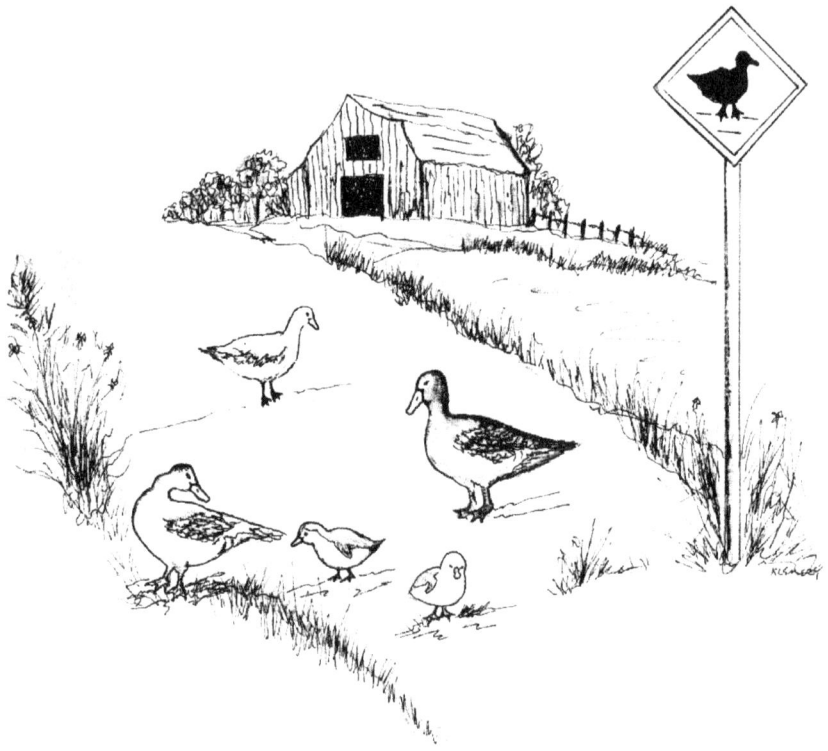

STOP FOR THE DUCKS

I'm speeding down the lake road
Rushing to my job
The little ducks cross single file
Everyone must stop!

They're never in a hurry
They never like to rush
Why must all these busy cars
Stop for crossing ducks?

But as I sit and watch them walk
I think about my life
Why must everything we do
Be filled with war and strife?

Why can't I hold my head up high
And walk with measured pace?
There's no need to run around
And dash from place to place!

And as I leave, my mind's at peace –
I've forgotten all the fuss
For all I really had to do
Was stop and watch the ducks!

REVEREND NORMAN NEAVES

"More than anything else, bar none, I want Kipp to feel that I love her as deeply and purely as I was capable of doing and that truly I felt blessed to be her husband."

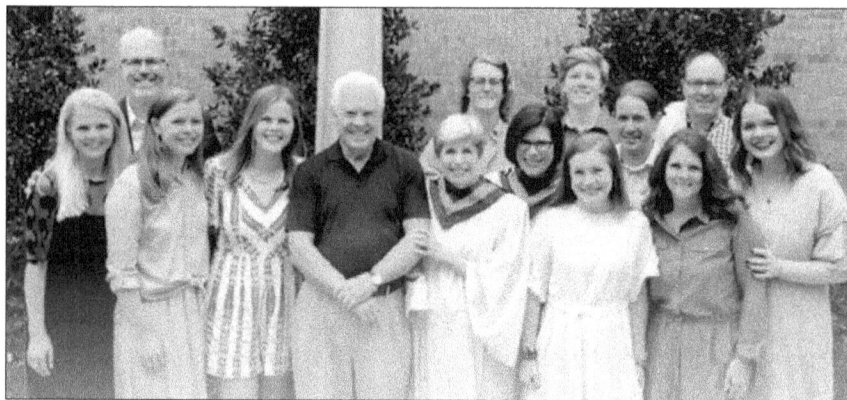

What childhood events shaped you?

I had two brothers and a mom who grew up on an Oklahoma farm and a father who was a traveling salesman. We lived on a modest income in a one-bedroom home – the bedroom is where my grandmother slept.

We learned basic and strongly individualistic principles from our mother and started throwing papers in the third grade at 2:30 every morning and again every afternoon after school. We played very competitive Little League baseball and later high school football and track, and was on a track team that broke a nineteen-year-old state record in the 880 relay that still holds today. We were a very hardworking and patriotic family who stood together through thick and thin.

I attended Oklahoma City University, Duke University and Drew University. I have a bachelor's degree in history and philosophy, a master's degree in systemic theology, a doctoral degree in organizational behavior and applied strategic concepts, and another honorary doctorate in divinity.

Why do bad things happen to good people?

There are many classical and creative answers to that question, far more than I can do justice to in this short interview. I would not presume to have a definitive answer as that would presume upon the mind of God which no human can appreciably define, but I would suggest that perhaps its meaning is wrapped up in the idea that finally the whole point of our existence has not to do with our comfort so much as with the development of our character, not with what happens to us so much as with how we handle what happens to us and how we develop as a human being through our encounters with all of life's experiences.

Good things happen to bad people and bad things happen to good people, both good and bad things happen to all people, and it seems to me what finally matters is what we do with what happens to us and who we become in and through them.

Is the universe friendly?

That's not something any of us can answer definitively, is it? To do so would presume we sat on a loft out beyond space and time and could make such judgments from our lofty perch. We're all but mere human beings and none of us can be definitive about such things. But what we can do is "faith" it. And what does that mean? It means on the basis of how we size up things and how we receive what billions have come to regard as revelation in an invaluable writing such as the Holy Bible, we can get a hint and even more that there is someone behind the great scheme of things and that this being who is God himself is an utterly gracious and good being and that he created everything (even all that is beyond our supposed sophisticated scientific presumptions, way beyond those!)…and that finally what he had made is indeed a good and wonderful and beautiful and blessed realm that we can trust completely and that indeed is "friendly."

What advice do you have for someone with a spouse with a chronic illness?

The answer to that doesn't lie in cookie cutter piece of wisdom, as if one could go along mouthing words of theological or philosophical import. I mean, all you'd have to do would be to refine and memorize your little words of advice or supposed wisdom and then go around delivering it to those in such need. But that would miss everything, wouldn't it? I mean, here's a person who is struggling and anxious and afraid and all we must give to them at that time is quasi-philosophical neatly packaged words of wisdom. It misses, doesn't it, it really misses big time.

What the person might need most of all is someone who will come alongside them simply as a friend, someone who is more into listening and empathizing than someone who needs to start talking and explaining and fixing things. A warm and heartfelt hug can communicate so much more than a philosophical dictum, eyes that are soft and sincere and maybe even tearful, a person who allows himself or herself to be in the same boat as the person hurting and struggling. There's so much reassurance there, so much that is communicated out of the heart and soul rather than out of the head and mind, and I've learned over the years that that is what counts most of all. Now, please, I don't mean to say that words of faith aren't relevant at all. Not at all. But sometimes we mistake that that is what really gets through to someone suffering as you suggest rather than those words that can come across as empty and beside the point.

How would you like to be remembered?

That's a simple one for me, Bill. I'm not into legacies all that much, it's not what my life is all about. But there is one simple set of deep feelings inside of me that are almost too deep for me adequately to express, but I'll share it like this. More than anything else, bar none, I want Kipp to feel that I love her as deeply and purely as I was capable of doing and that truly I felt blessed to be her husband. And then right after that, the same thing for my three kids, too – I hope they'll know that despite my imperfections and shortcomings, the one thing that means more to me than anything else is that they also know that my feelings of love for them, each one, go down inside of me, deeper than anything else along with my feelings for their mother. Those four people are the core and crux of my life. But right behind them are their spouses and our six grandchildren and three dogs that we have had in life, Boomer and Mac and Little Buddy. It's amazing to me that dogs can get so deeply inside of us like they do, but those three have.

Finally, I just hope that others will know that I gave everything I had to the creation of the Church of the Servant, that I gave it my very best, and that even though I'm human and certainly didn't do everything perfectly and things I wish I could do over, I will always count it my greatest blessing along with my family that I got to be a helper alongside the Lord in bringing into being a place where people are loved and enjoyed and celebrated and where the Good Lord himself is honored and deeply loved.

THE ANESTHETIST

It's not an easy job
Giving anesthesia
So that the surgeon can do her work
And the patient feels no pain.

The anesthetist must have the physical skill
To establish the correct airway
That provides the precious oxygen
We all need to survive.
She must provide the wind to ventilate the patient's lungs,
And supply the correct medicine at the correct dosage
To prevent hypotension and hypoxia.

The surgeon is the captain of the ship
But the anesthetist is the navigator
Whose job it is to make sure the ship returns to shore
For each and every patient.

To comfort and assure the patient
Who is worried and apprehensive and even scared
That he won't wake up –
A fear of death that we all have
Which is magnified before each surgery.

At times, the anesthetist must even re-assure the nervous surgeon
That her patient is doing well
And that she may safely proceed with the surgery.
The anesthetist, working quietly and diligently,
And at times unnoticed,
Is literally the wind beneath the surgeon's wings.

*Dedicated to LaDora Castoe, nurse anesthetist, who worked 30 years, and
Dr. Frances Oakes, anesthesiologist, who worked 40 years at Deaconess Hospital,
providing anesthesia of the highest quality to over 100,000 patients.*

NEVER SAY NEVER

"Are you ready for those 'never' events, Dr Truewater?" Herb asked, as we sat in the doctor's lounge waiting for our laparoscopic gall bladder case to start.

"What's a 'never' event, Herb?" I asked.

"Something that's never supposed to happen," Herb replied.

"Well, that could cover a lot of things, Herb," I answered. "You know, like people are never supposed to shoot each other, or commit adultery – things like that."

"Those aren't on the approved list," Herb said.

"What list?" I asked.

"The National Quality Forum has identified 28 medical occurrences as 'never events' – things that should never happen in a hospital," Herb explained.

"What kind of events are 'never events', Herb?" I asked.

"Well, for example, according to the National Quality Forum, patients should never be allowed to attempt suicide in a hospital."

"Of course not," I replied. "That would be inappropriate. Better to do that at home."

"But, according to the National Quality Forum," Herb added, "If a patient attempts suicide in a hospital resulting in serious disability or death, then the hospital is legally and financially responsible."

"That sounds bizarre," I answered.

"It gets worse, Dr. Truewater," Herb added. "Medicare and the private insurance carriers are imposing the doctrine of 'strict liability' on the hospitals."

"Strict liability?" I asked.

"It means that no matter what you do to protect someone from an injury, you're responsible for the consequences. Strict liability is usually reserved for dangerous activities, like skydiving or raising alligators. Now, the legislators and lawyers are applying it to hospitals."

"They're classifying going to a hospital as a dangerous activity?" I asked.

"You could put it like that," Herb replied.

"For example, if a patient gets a pressure ulcer when he's in the hospital, that's classified as a 'never event' – something that should never happen."

"But that's crazy," I answered. "We all know that in certain situations, such as a trauma patient with an unstable neck injury, you can't rotate the patient, and pressure ulcers can occur despite using an air bed. And certain patients, like morbidly obese diabetic patients who refuse to turn, or patients with terminal illnesses who are wasting away – you'd have to suspend them on wires to prevent a pressure sore!"

"It gets even better," Herb added. "There is a growing list of 'never events' that are being considered."

"For example, some lawyers have proposed that a patient should never fall in a hospital. If an elderly patient, who's unsteady on his feet, doesn't use his walker on the way to the bathroom and falls down, why, they're proposing that the hospital's responsible. Medicare won't pay the bill to fix his broken hip. And the family can sue the hospital for negligence!"

"In other words," I said, "you can fall down at home, and Medicare will pay for it, but if you fall down in the hospital, why, that's a 'never event' and Medicare won't reimburse the hospital!"

"Exactly!" Herb replied. "Following the Deficit Reduction Act of 2005, a quality adjustment in the DRG reimbursement payment for certain hospital-acquired conditions has been mandated. And the National Quality Forum has identified 28 events as 'never events' that should never happen."

"For example," Herb continued, "a chest infection following coronary bypass grafting occurs about once every hundred times. That's being proposed as a 'never' event. Others on the prospective list include infection from vascular catheters, deep vein thrombosis and pulmonary embolus – the experts have determined that those events should 'never' happen in the hospital!"

"I think I'm getting it now, Herb," I replied. "One way to save money is for the insurance carriers to hold the hospitals to a standard of perfection, and then simply refuse to pay for any complications!"

"But if big-ticket items are being targeted," I continued, "Such as ventilator-associated pneumonias or hospital acquired staphylococcal septicemias, won't that drive the hospitals out of business?"

"Dr. Truewater, you simply don't understand that these government bureaucrats are basically good-hearted people with the best of intentions," Herb replied slyly.

"The whole idea of refusing to pay for certain complications is to improve the quality of care which, in the long run, will decrease the cost. The government figures that if they don't pay for certain complications, they'll be less likely to happen. By holding hospitals to a higher standard, the complication rate will fall, and hospital costs will decrease."

"And by classifying certain occurrences as 'never events'," I quipped, "such complications might decrease and eventually disappear altogether!"

"Everybody wins, Dr. Truewater, including the lawyers, who helped draft the legislation, because patients will be allowed to sue the hospital for a 'never' event!"

"But, wait," I added. "I've got a better idea."

"Let's expand the list, Herb!" I exclaimed.

"Expand the list, Dr Truewater?" Herb asked. "Why, it's already too long!"

"No, I mean, think about it, Herb. Our government has determined, after years of research and statistical analysis, that it has the power to declare that certain medical events, such as pulmonary emboli or catheter infections, or even falling down should never occur inside a hospital."

"That's correct," Herb replied.

"Well, if that's the case, then why not declare that people should never die inside a hospital – or outside a hospital for that matter?"

"Furthermore, if the government has the power to say that certain events should never happen, why can't the doctors give the government a list of 'never' events that should never happen?"

"Imagine the possibilities, Herb," I continued. I was on a roll.

"Let's hold the government responsible for death, suffering, poverty, wars, and famine, and declare such calamities 'never events' that must never be allowed to occur – either inside or outside a hospital! And, if the government failed to prevent these 'never events' from occurring, citizens would simply refuse to pay their taxes until the government straightened up its' act! Why, wars would end, people would prosper, no one would die, and eternal happiness would be found on earth!"

"Dr. Truewater," Herb quipped, "I think you've just entered Never-Never Land! You should know that you can't use logic against the federal government. Now, let's go and take out that gall bladder before the government decides that cholecystectomies are a 'never event'!"

WAKE UP WITH A SMILE

Isn't it great
To wake up in the morning!
To smell the fresh air
And see the birds soaring!

The dew on the ground
The sun in the sky
The wind through the trees
The bird's lullaby!

Each day that we live
Marks the time of our birth –
The day that our God
Created the earth!

For on that Great Day
When our planet was born
God smiled on it all
And created the morn!

And like our Creator
Through all of life's trials
Isn't it great
To wake up with a smile!

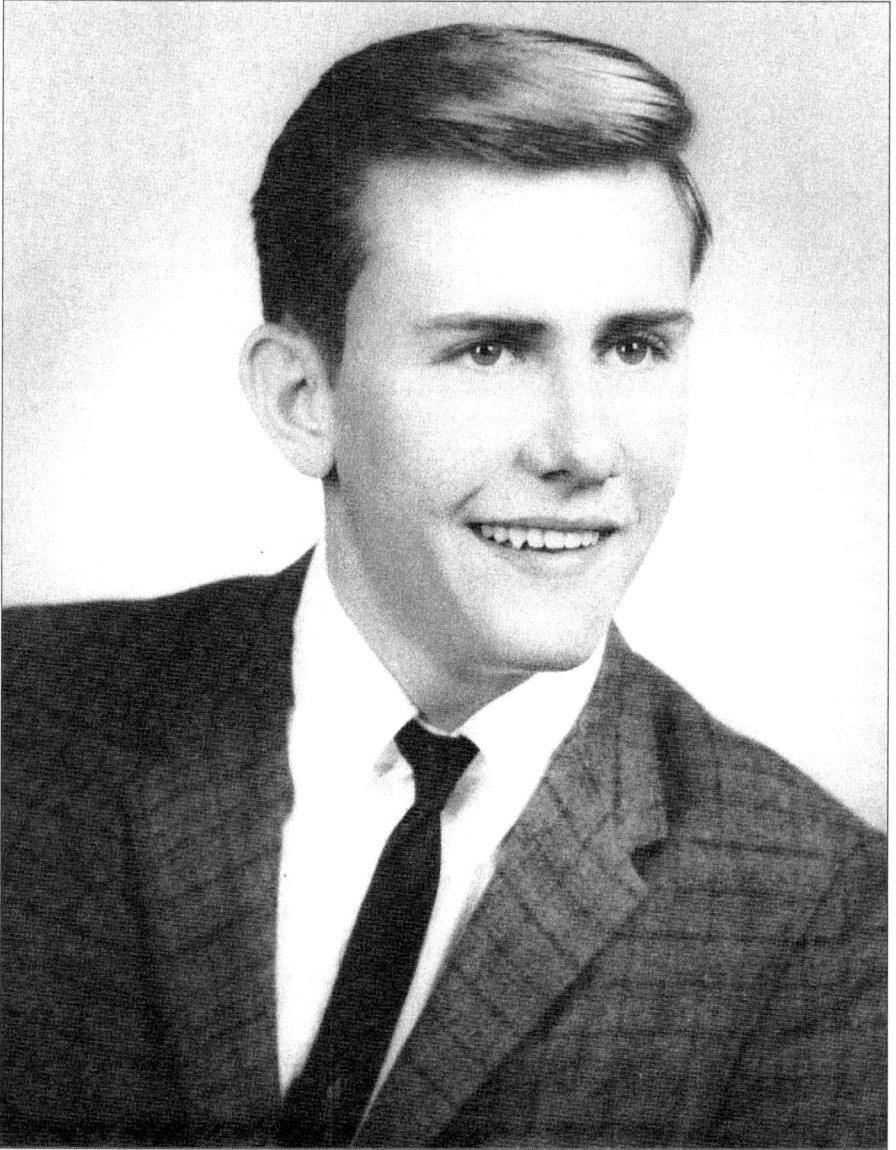

Jimmy (James) William Bettis, son of Margaret and Willis Bettis of Tulsa, Oklahoma, was killed in action on March 12, 1968, in Viet Nam. Jimmy was twenty years old. He is survived by two sisters, Jo Ann Montgomery and Margaret Bettis Truels, and one brother, Ronnie Bettis.

THE WALL

I take a trip to Washington
And there I see The Wall –
A tribute to our fighting men
Who fought and gave their all.

I see the list of warriors
Written there in stone
Men who fought their country's wars
All through the land are known.

God gives every one of us
Before we're even born
A name that we will call ourselves
In honor or in scorn.

Throughout our lives the job at hand
Though difficult to do
Is live each day the best we can
And to our name be true.

I see the people view the wall
And find the name they know
The soldiers died to keep us free
They loved their country so!

I've seen walls in other lands
That governments divide
They rule with an iron hand
And take the people's pride.

But the Viet Nam Memorial
Forever shall remain –
It holds the list of warriors
Who lived up to their name!

END OF LIFE ISSUES

I was sitting in the surgery lounge, sipping on coffee and donuts, waiting for my gallbladder case to start, when Herb walked in, looking somewhat disheveled and forlorn.

"You look down and out, Herb," I began. "Here, have some coffee – that'll cheer you up."

"Thanks, Dr. Truewater," Herb replied. "But I'll need more than coffee to cheer me up."

"What's the problem, Herb?" I asked.

"I'm dealing with end-of-life issues, Truewater."

"Aren't we all," I replied. "You know, the heart surgeon, Jim Hardy used to park his Lexus at the first parking spot at Holy Christian every morning, 'cause he was always the first one to get here every day. Now that he's retired, some young buck parks there every day with his new Hummer – it just doesn't seem right."

"Changing times, Dr. Truewater – nothing is static," Herb commented. "But I've got more serious problems than that. It seems that I've flunked my final exam."

"What final exam?" I asked. "I thought you were all through taking those pesky board recertification exams."

"Well, you know I've got prostate cancer, and I've had chronic pain," Herb replied.

"Yes, I'm sorry you have to go through that, Herb," I said.

"I took this tourist package they offer to Switzerland," Herb continued.

"Sounds like a fun trip," I answered, "a good way to cheer up and get a new perspective on life.

"Well, not exactly, Dr. Truewater," Herb countered. "You see, it's a one-way trip – they call it an End of Life venture. You go to Switzerland, see all the usual sites, then you tell them your end-of-life issues on your final exam, and for a mere $3,000 tour package, you get euthanized, and they spread your ashes over beautiful Lake Geneva."

"Herb, I didn't know things were so serious. I'm shocked, shocked that you would consider such a thing. We're talking death, here, and you're only 75. Besides, the hospital never threw your farewell party."

"We'll, I just took stock of everything," Herb answered forlornly. "For one thing, I'm tired of paying my life insurance premiums out of my social security income. I'd like to see that money go to my kids – I've been paying for fifteen years, but if I quit paying now, they'll cancel my insurance."

"And I'm tired of all these government threats to cut my reimbursements by 20% to help pay for national health care. That 20% represents my profit margin, once I finish paying my malpractice premiums."

"And I'm fed up with all these government audits – I just had to send them 2,000 pages of medical records so they could see if I'm coding my procedures correctly. They want to see if I've got enough 'bullet points' in my progress notes to justify a $30 visit.

"Well, I'm sorry to hear that, Herb," I sympathized. "But I'm glad you decided against euthanasia in Switzerland and came back."

"It wasn't my decision," Herb replied. "You see, I flunked my final exam."

"You flunked your final exam?" I asked.

"Herb, you always finished at the top of the class on your exams. What happened? Did they ask you a bunch of anatomy questions?"

"Well, they asked me what my end-of-life issues were, and I told them I had prostate cancer and I was having a lot of pain."

"That sounds pretty convincing to me," I said.

"They said prostate cancer wasn't serious enough," Herb replied. "They said breast cancer was more acceptable, because it was more serious."

"Then I told them I was depressed about all the changes in health care and they said, 'Welcome to socialism!' They weren't very sympathetic for a euthanasia clinic. I mean, they were turning down CEOs of large companies, politicians, department chairmen, hospital administrators, you name it."

"Well, I'm sorry to hear you were rejected, Herb," I replied. "But I'm glad to have you back among us in the doctor's lounge."

"Thanks, Dr. Truewater," Herb answered. "But you want to know the worst part?"

"What's that?" I asked.

"The End of Life tour package only includes a one way ticket to Switzerland. I had to pay $3000 for a no-discount one-way ticket back to Oklahoma City!"

MY DAD

I really love my dad –
He's given me all I have!
Through tough times where we've been –
He's there through thick and thin!

He taught the fifth-grade kids –
That's no easy shift!
He taught them discipline
And how to grow within!

He likes to ride his bike
Around the Hefner hike!
It keeps him in good shape
And helps the world to take!

He likes to play guitar –
A real musical star!
And to my daughter Sage –
He really is the rage!

When I moved out of town to medical school
I needed someone my kids to rule!
My dad moved in the house
To help the kids to roust!

He takes his insulin
Since the age of ten –
Juvenile diabetes
Can give you the heebie-jeebies!

Lately my dad's been sick –
His kidneys want to quit!
I'd like to help him out –
When trouble is about!

Transplants have helped him out
But they eventually lose their clout!
Two lasted ten years at the most
Before they begin to reject their host!

We're the same blood type
And the conditions are just right –
A kidney I can give
To help my dad to live!

It's the least that I can do
For all that we've been through!
I can give part of myself
To try and help him out!

That what love is for –
Sometimes we forget and ignore –
True love is more than emotion –
It involves complete devotion!

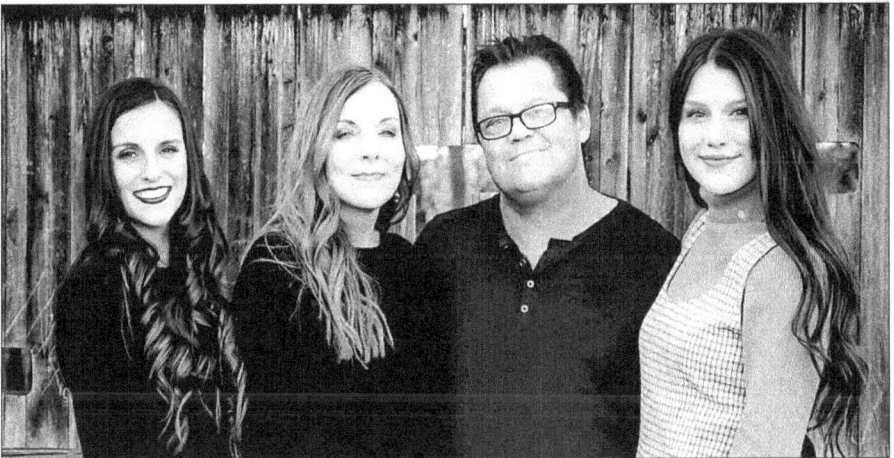

Dr. Savannah Coote (left), with her Mom, Dad, and sister.

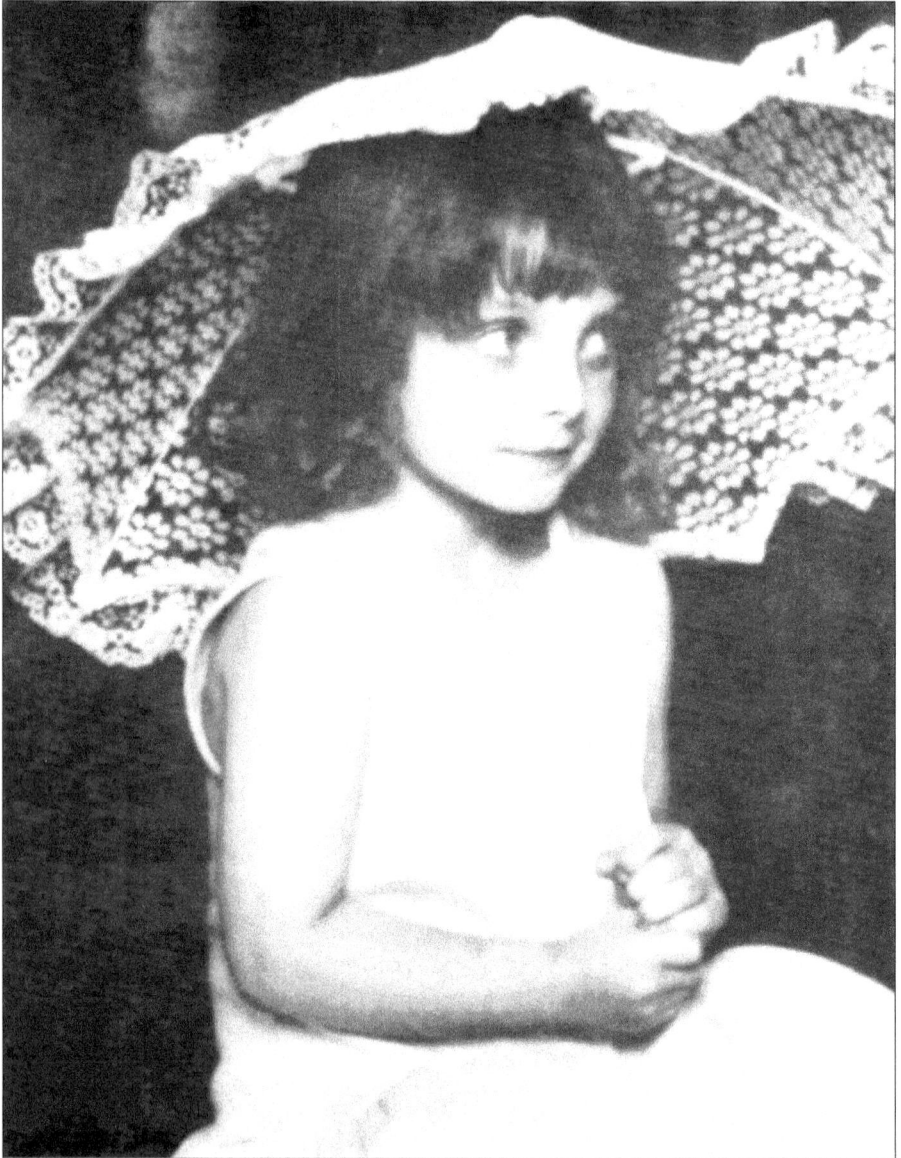

Charlotte Jones, age 4, was struck by lightning and killed while being held in her father's arms during a freak thunderstorm near Okarche, Oklahoma, on May 17, 1991. Her father, James Jones, survived with severe burns. Charlotte is also survived by her mother, Retha Jones.

TO CHARLOTTE

Did this really happen?
Is my Charlotte dead?
Or is this just a crazy dream
That rumbles through my head?

Surely I can wake you up
Your sleep seems so serene
Let me hold you in my arms
And wake you from your dream!

Looking at reality
Is such a painful task
What is real? What is true?
It's better not to ask.

I'll miss the things I used to do –
Pick up your dolls and games
I think I'll leave them on the floor
In case you come and play.

I see you with your parasol –
You loved that fancy dress
Remember how you'd bat your eyes
Whene'er you were upset?

What kind of God, what kind of fate
Would take your love from me?
Do we live a life that's real
Or is it fantasy?

I don't have all the answers
What's good, what's bad, what's true
But thank you for the memories –
I'll always think of you!

LETTERS OF REJECTION

I hate letters of rejection – you know, the kind you get when you apply for medical school. I suppose, if I had more self-confidence, I could handle rejection better. I guess it goes back to my days in high school. I always wanted to be a varsity athlete so I could wear the letter "M" on my sweater with a little picture of a baseball or soccer ball in one corner and a small Maine High School Blue Demon in another.

Not that I wasn't a success in school. I was well-liked (sort of), and I was an excellent student, but in 1963 few people gave scholars any special recognition. I thought it would be nice to have a letter sweater for top students (maybe with a small book in one corner), but the other students thought it was too corny or nerdy.

I never could understand why a top athlete in high school was more popular than a top scholar. But it was worse than that – many of the top students actually denied that they studied.

"Congratulations on your straight A's," I told one future Rhodes scholar.

"I never study," he responded gruffly. "I just hope the Blue Demons win Friday's regional game."

Thus, I went through high school in relative anonymity. That's probably why I don't handle rejection too well. You see, I always figured that, if I had been more popular, I could have handled life's ups and downs with a little more savvy – you know, turn a broken egg into an omelet. That's what a letter sweater gives you – self-confidence.

I guess I never learned how to lose – that's what rejection really is – losing. The great football coach, Vince Lombardi, once told his players, "Winning isn't everything – it's the only thing!"

Now that's very inspiring if you play football. But what happens if you lose? If winning is everything, does that mean losing is nothing? What are you supposed to do if you lose? Commit suicide?

School never really prepared me for losing – I mean, they're aren't courses on how to deal with it or anything.

I applied to seven medical schools. I was accepted at three of them, and rejected by the other four. I think I was the only medical applicant to be hurt by scoring well on his MCAT--Medical College Admission Test. The interview usually went something like this.

"Mr. Truewater," the interviewer began, "you've done exceptionally well on your admission test scores."

"Thank you, sir," I would reply humbly.

"It's just that your college grades at Northwestern aren't as high as I would expect for someone of your ability. You're a gifted student, Mr. Truewater, but you lack motivation – you're an underachiever. You know, the mind is a terrible thing to waste. How do you feel about that?"

"Oh, no sir," I would reply. "I'm a hard worker. It's just that I score better on standardized exams. And I'm well-rounded – you know, the total college experience."

Now, mind you, I didn't expect to be accepted by all seven schools. In those days, only one out of fourteen applications was accepted. It's just that I hated getting those letters of rejection.

For one thing, I hate any letter that starts out, "We are very sorry to inform you…" Right then, you know, it's all over. There's either been a death in the family, or you've been rejected from medical school. In one short sentence, your dreams and aspirations turn into hopelessness and despair.

And I wondered if they were really sorry. It was nice of them to say they're sorry, but how sorry can an admissions committee really feel for someone they've only known for fifteen minutes? Especially when all nine-hundred letters of rejection were mailed on the same day and signed by the same electronic pen!

But there was more. Each letter of rejection contained its own disclaimer. It went something like this: "Please do not feel that this refusal in any way reflects upon our opinion of your ability to succeed in medicine."

I could never understand that. I mean, how were you going to succeed in medicine if you didn't attend medical school? I could just hear myself ten years from now.

"Hello, I'm Dr. Bill Truewater. My qualifications as a surgeon are excellent, with the small reservation that I failed to attend medical school. Now, lie down and let me take out your gallbladder!"

It's now been twenty years since I applied for medical school. I survived the interviews, the examinations, the 24-hour call, and the pyramid residency programs.

I now find myself in the awkward position of selecting and evaluating medical students. With eight hundred annual applications for one hundred positions, the job is indeed difficult. How do you tell the other seven hundred applicants that they've been rejected? Someone's got to write the letter, and tell them that you're sorry.

And it's not easy to deal with rejection. Some people never learn. It's not something you learn in school – unless it be the school of Hard Knocks!

I've found that rejection, or failure, can itself be a valuable teacher. Rejection can teach you to work harder, to concentrate better, to try again, and to look for other options or opportunities that you may have overlooked.

No one likes rejection. But my experience has taught me to try to look at both sides of an issue. Maybe that's what life is all about!

THE IDEAL PATIENT

My brother Steve called me today from school. Steve teaches at Giant Cedar Middle School, and is a very good Earth Science teacher.

"I've got a hernia, Bill," Steve began. "I've decided to go ahead and have it fixed."

"That's the best thing to do," I replied. "Get it over with now before it causes problems later."

"I'm having it done at Holy Christian Memorial Hospital and, with my brother being a doctor, I'd like to make a good impression. What I need to know is, from a doctor's standpoint, what makes a good patient?"

"Look, Steve, I replied, "Don't worry about being an ideal patient. Just be yourself and everything will turn out fine."

"No, no," Steve insisted. "I want to do this right. Check with your friends, and give me a holler back tonight."

"Okay," I promised, "But you may not like what I have to say."

That afternoon, I was making rounds at Holy Christian. Danny Hoffman, the pulmonary doctor, had just finished seeing one of my patients.

"That Mrs. Lunoff is stubborn – she absolutely refuses to cough," Danny began. "Her tidal volume is only 250 ml on the spirometer. I doubt if she's ever taken a deep breath in her life – a corpse could breathe better!"

"That's interesting," I replied. "A pulmonologist can look at the chart, check the patient's tidal volume and history, and make an initial personality assessment."

"If the patient smokes two packs a day, he's already in the doghouse. If the tidal volume is low, and the patient is not breathing deeply, then the patient is lazy. If it's normal, the patient is cooperative."

"And if it's high, the patient's a blowhard!" Danny quipped.

"Each doctor tends to view his patient according to his own specialty," I concluded.

"Take the general surgeon, for example. One of the most important questions for a general surgeon is whether the patient's bowel function has returned following surgery."

"A general surgeon would walk into the patient's room and say, 'Hello, Mr. Graham. How are we doing?' Then, before the patient has a chance to respond, he asks, 'Have we passed any gas yet today?'"

Then Mr. Graham may say something sarcastic, like, "I don't know about you, doctor but I haven't passed any gas yet."

"I see what you're saying," Danny replied. "The ideal patient for a general surgeon would be someone with regular bowel habits, who wasn't too fat, and who passed gas frequently as he walked up and down the halls."

"Sort of," I replied.

Later that day, I ran into Charlie Green, the cardiologist.

"My patients are eating too much red meat!" Charlie complained. "If they would avoid greasy foods and jog a quarter mile a day or ride an exercise bike, we could cut the rate of heart attacks in half!"

The psychiatrist, Nick Ardmann, happened to overhear Charlie complaining.

"That's true, Charlie," Nick began. "But don't forget the importance of a positive mental attitude. Statistics have shown that maintaining a positive outlook can reduce stress. This in turn can reduce the mortality rate from cardiac disease and even cancer. Too many people have forgotten a very simple thing – the art of smiling," Nick frowned.

On my way out of the hospital, I stopped for a donut in the doctor's lounge. Jess Barler, the urologist, was reading the paper.

"Tell me, Jess," I asked out of curiosity, "What traits would characterize the ideal patient for a urologist?"

"That's simple," Jess replied. "There's nothing better for the kidneys than three full glasses of water a day! Keeps the kidney stones and infection away!"

"Anything else a urologist likes to see?" I asked innocently.

Jess lowered his voice before making his next response. "Well, you know, Bill, we urologists put in penile implants for a living. So, for a urologist, there's no better sign for a healthy patient than a good, firm erection. It tells me that the blood supply is good, and that my patient isn't depressed."

When I got home that night, my brother Steve called me almost before I got in the door.

"Bill," Steve said, "I'm going in the hospital in three weeks for my hernia repair. Any tips yet on the ideal patient? I want to make a good impression on all those docs!"

"You may not like this, Steve," I replied.

"Try me," Steve responded.

"Well, you'll have to give up smoking and take slow, deep breaths to keep the lung doctor happy," I began.

"No problem," Steve rebutted. "I quit smoking two days ago, because I knew what you'd say."

"And you'll have to give up red meat and French fries," I continued.

"Red meat?" Steve barked. "I was born and raised on steak and potatoes!"

"It gets worse," I added. "Do you think you could jog about a quarter mile a day to maintain your cardiovascular conditioning and maybe help you lose about twenty-five pounds?"

"I could, but I've got to have a Coke or 7-up to get me going," Steve replied, with determination in his voice.

"Caffeine and carbonated beverages aren't nearly as healthy as water," I answered sympathetically.

I had to be delicate about this next part. "The urologists also like to see firm erections – they view them as a sign of good health and happiness."

"I'll work on it," Steve mumbled.

"The most important thing, though is to maintain a positive attitude when you come in the hospital – doctors like to see patients who can smile, despite the adversity," I concluded.

There was a pause at the other end of the line. Perhaps I had said too much.

"Let me get this straight," Steve finally responded. "You want me to give up smoking, lose twenty-five pounds, jog a quarter mile a day, quit eating red meat and fried potatoes, pass plenty of gas, but give up carbonated beverages, and still maintain firm erections and a smile to boot?"

"That's it in a nutshell!" I replied.

"I've got an idea!" Steve suddenly said with enthusiasm. "Could I have this hernia fixed as an outpatient? That way I wouldn't have to worry about making a good impression on all those doctors!"

"Sounds good to me," I concluded.

I thought about all the good advice I had given my brother. No matter how well-intended, there was simply too much for one person to handle. With all the rules and regulations about eating and exercise, it's impossible to please everyone, and still maintain a smile. About the best you can hope for is to please yourself!

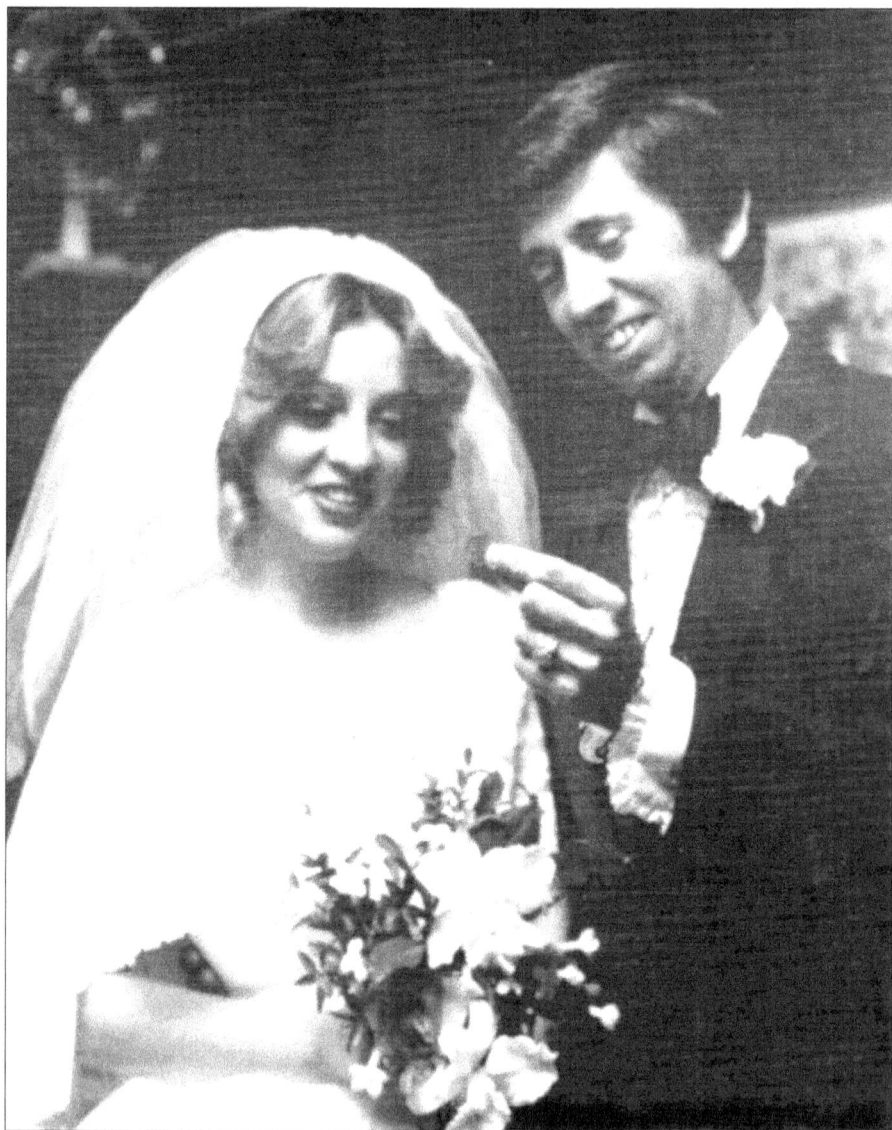

Pam and her father, Bill Montgomery

TO PAM

Oh, daughter of my creation
Where have you gone?
Struck down by a machine of iron
While in your youth
Cutting short the dreams
Of a Father's imagination.

No more shall I see you –
The curly locks of your windswept hair
Or hear your laughter
On a warm summer's night
Or give the advice
That a Father gives his daughter.

Some of my fondest memories
Will be the shortest
As if Nature is jealous
Of her greatest treasures
And must reclaim them
Before their time.

PLANNING FOR RETIREMENT

I was sitting in the doctor's lounge, munching on a diabetic donut and decaf coffee, waiting for my lap gallbladder case to start, when Herb walked in with a concerned look on his face.

"What's up, Herb?" I asked. "You look worried."

"Good morning, Dr. Truewater," Herb began. "You're right. I'm concerned. I've been trying to figure out if I've got enough money saved up in my pension plan to retire."

"Money?" I said. "Who needs money? Retirement is a state of mind – I look upon my career as a source of enjoyment and pleasure. I don't plan to retire until I'm unable to physically do the work!" I replied gleefully.

"Well, I've had enough enjoyment and pleasure being a plastic surgeon, making noses smaller and lips and breasts bigger," Herb responded. "I'm ready to retire. I just need to figure out if I can do it financially. I've got an appointment with my financial counselor."

"Financial counselor?" I quipped. "Herb, you don't need a financial counselor. You just need a simple equation that will tell you if you can retire."

"A simple equation, Truewater?" Herb asked. "I find that hard to believe."

"It's simple, Herb," I continued. "Let's say you plan to live on $30,000 a year plus your social security income."

"O.K.," Herb answered. "Then what?"

"You just take the $30,000 and multiply it by the number of years you're going to live."

"What?" Herb asked.

"Let's say you're going to live 10 more years. You just multiply $30,000 times 10 years – that's $300,000 dollars you'll need in your pension plan before you can retire. It's just that simple," I explained.

"There's just one problem with your calculations, Dr. Truewater," Herb replied. "How do you know how long you're going to live?"

"They've got tables for that," I answered. "Actuarial tables is what they call them. You just look up your life expectancy and go from there."

"What?" Herb asked again.

"Well, let's see," I continued. "I'll do the calculations for you. You're 67 years old and the average male life expectancy is 76, so I figure you've got nine years left. Women live five years longer than men – it's been speculated that male mice sacrifice longevity for bigger bodies and greater energy output required for breeding."

"Very funny. But those actuarial tables are just averages, Dr. Truewater," Herb answered angrily. "You can't use them to plan your retirement. Why, for all I know, I might be an outlier and make it to 90 – then I'd be a penniless pauper living on social security alone, if it hasn't gone bankrupt!"

"True enough, Herb," I replied. "You probably are an outlier. But you can fine-tune my equation by calculating your biologic age."

"My biologic age? Now I'm a biology specimen?" Herb queried.

"We're all biology specimens," I answered. "You should know that from medical school. We're living, breathing organisms – built of carbon, hydrogen, and oxygen. We need to eat healthy, exercise, and live a robust live style."

"Robust?" Herb asked.

"Yes," I answered. "Are you living a robust lifestyle, Herb?"

"Well, not exactly, Dr. Truewater," Herb answered. "I mean, I smoked two packs a day for 30 years, but I'm down to a half pack a day. I'm about 30 pounds overweight. And I'm not up for eating healthy – I like a good T-bone steak at least three times a week, and I love French fries and barbecue ribs at tailgate parties.

"Anything else, Herb?" I asked.

"Well, I gave my treadmill away to my daughter when she married and moved into her own house. Now, the most exercise I get is driving to the hospital and making rounds. It's not exactly what the cardiologists would call aerobic exercise."

"My advice to you, Herb, is to adopt a healthier lifestyle. Eat more vegetables, avoid fried foods, lose 30 pounds, avoid fats and sugar, stop drinking alcohol, stop smoking, take multivitamins, and walk a mile a day. That would improve your life expectancy and your biologic age. You'd be one lean fighting machine!"

"Well, I see two problems with that approach, Dr. Truewater," Herb smiled.

"What's that?" I asked.

"Well, first of all, I'm happy with my present life style – it's worked for 67 years," Herb replied.

"Secondly," Herb continued, "if I change my lifestyle, I would improve my biologic age, right?"

"That's right, Herb," I answered.

"And if I improve my biologic age, Dr. Truewater, I'll live longer according to the actuarial tables, by decreasing my risk factors, and living a robust life style."

"Exactly, Herb," I replied. "Now you're getting it."

"But that creates a new problem, Dr. Truewater," Herb said.

"What new problem?" I asked.

"Well, according to your retirement equation, if I live longer I'll need to have more money in my pension plan before I can retire. If I add another ten years to my biologic age, I'll need another $300,000 in my pension plan before I can retire!"

"True enough," I replied.

"Thanks for the financial advice, Dr. Truewater," Herb added.

"No problem, Herb," I answered, as I slipped on my mask and headed back to surgery.

As I walked back, I wondered if my advice was all that helpful. Was Herb going to adopt a life of hedonism and debauchery?

Maybe it's not wise to take financial advice from a surgeon.

RISING FROM THE DEAD

This is a true story. Have you ever heard of someone rising from the dead? Oh, to be sure, we all know it happened in Biblical times. Lazarus rose from the dead, as well as Jesus Christ Himself. No, I'm talking about modern times. And right here in Oklahoma City.

I was helping Dr. George Ruby perform a bowel resection on Mrs. Florence Kelly, a 52-year-old woman with colon cancer. A portion of the cancer was stuck to the plexus of veins along the sacrum, causing significant blood loss requiring multiple blood transfusions. Near the end of the procedure, Mrs. Kelly developed a fatal cardiac arrhythmia.

Dr. Ruby performed complete cardiac resuscitation, including electric shock paddles, cardiac drugs, and open cardiac massage. After thirty minutes, the electrocardiogram showed a straight line, indicating no electrical activity. Blood pressure and pulse were both zero.

"Why don't you close the incision, Dr. Simmons," said a heart-broken Dr. Ruby. "Dr. Truewater and I will go out and talk to the family."

I accompanied Dr. Ruby to the family waiting area, where he broke the bad news to the patient's husband, Mr. Kelly.

After about ten minutes, an obviously disturbed Dr. Simmons came rushing out to the waiting room.

"Dr. Ruby, Dr. Ruby!" an excited Dr. Simmons began.

"Dr. Simmons, don't interrupt me," Dr. Ruby snapped. "Can't you see I'm in the middle of a very painful situation? This poor man's wife has just died, and I'm trying to console him."

"But, it's about Mrs. Kelly," Dr. Simmons continued.

"Let him speak, Dr. Ruby," Mr. Kelly interrupted. "Whatever news he's got about my wife couldn't be any worse than what I've already heard."

"That's just it," Dr. Simmons continues, as he pulled Dr. Ruby and me off to one corner. "Mrs. Kelly has resurrected herself – I mean she's come back from the dead! Come see."

We ran back to the operating room, and, sure enough, Mrs. Kelly's electrocardiogram came back to normal. Her blood pressure and pulse even returned. Dr. Ruby was astounded.

"Quick, let's finish the operation and get her off the operating table before anything else happens," Dr. Ruby said.

We scrubbed our hands, and put on sterile gowns and gloves. The bleeding had stopped, so we finished closing the incision. In the recovery room, Mrs. Kelly began to awaken from the anesthetic.

We stood around her bed, anxiously awaiting her first words. Mrs. Kelly looked peacefully around the room, then looked at Dr. Ruby.

"What happened?" she asked angrily. "I feel like I've been through hell!"

"You have," Dr. Ruby began. "I mean, we had a little more trouble than we expected, but you're going to be fine now."

"Doc," Mrs. Kelly continued, "I'm not going to die, am I?"

"No, nothing quite that bad," Dr. Ruby reassured her.

Dr. Ruby took us aside and said, "Dr. Truewater, I want you to come with me. I'm going to go back and give Mr. Kelly the good news."

"I've never seen anything like this, Dr. Truewater," he confided. "I don't know if this would be classified as a miracle, but I've never seen anything like it. That woman was obviously dead when I left the operating room the first time."

"The Lord moves in mysterious ways," was all I could think to say at the time. In fact, to this day, I still haven't thought of anything better to say.

When we arrived at the waiting room, Dr. Ruby began the conversation.

"I don't know how to explain this, Mr. Kelly," Dr. Ruby said.

"Doc," Mr. Kelly interrupted, "I know you did the best you could, I don't blame you. When your number's up, and the Good Lord calls, there's no turning back. Don't blame yourself, Doc – it was just my wife's turn to die."

"That's just it," Dr. Ruby began. "You're not going to believe this, but your wife just made a complete recovery!"

"From death?" Mr. Kelly asked incredulously.

"Well, let's just say she was temporarily dead," Dr. Ruby

stammered. "I've never seen this happen before. According to all our instruments, you wife was clinically dead for twenty minutes – no heartbeat, no pulse, not even any electrical activity. I personally feel she was dead."

"She's come back from the dead?" Mr. Kelly asked, still in a state of shock. "Don't that beat all! Lord be praised. There is a God in heaven!"

"Tell me, Doc," Mr. Kelly continued, "do you think her soul actually went up to heaven and then came back again?"

"I don't think so," Dr. Ruby began. "I mean, I don't think there was enough time. The fact remains that your wife was clinically dead. Now, whether that means her soul left and then came back, I couldn't say."

To this day, I've never been able to explain what happened. With massive blood transfusions, it is possible that hypothermia played a role in her cardiac arrest, much as drowning patients can be resuscitated from cold water.

At any rate, I can only say that the line between life and death may not be as scientifically precise as we might think. And, despite our technology, the role of humility in medicine is just as appropriate today as it was fifty years ago!

WHERE DO WE GO?

Where do we go when we die?
Nobody really knows
Is there a heaven above us
Or only the north wind that blows?

If only I could remember
Long before I was born
Where did my soul arise from
At the dawn of my morn?

I hope that I'll have the answer
To where I might journey some day
For surely we go where we came from
If I could remember the way!

Too bad our life's not that simple
Lake a tapestry long ago sewn
We live in a world of mystery
Surrounded by the unknown!

GETTING IN SHAPE

"You look sick," Dr. Truewater," Herb told me as I sat in the doctor's lounge, getting ready to peel my orange.

I'm not sick, Herb," I replied. "I'm on a diet. I've lost five pounds, and I'm pretty proud of it."

"You still look sick, Truewater," Herb persisted.

"I'm not sick, Herb. I'm only eating 1,200 calories a day, so I don't have my usual strength."

"Are you sure you don't have cancer?" Herb asked.

"Don't be ridiculous," I replied. "If I had cancer, you'd be the first to know."

"How do you know you don't have cancer?" Herb continued. "Sometimes you lose weight, and you think you're on a diet, but it's really because you have cancer, and don't know it."

"I don't have cancer, Herb," I replied. "Why, just the other day, I had my prostate blood test at the annual Physician's Appreciation Day, and it came back normal."

"O.K., so you don't have prostate cancer. There still could be something else going on," Herb replied.

"You know, Herb, you're beginning to bother me," I answered angrily. "I'm afraid you're turning into a hypochondriac – and a paranoid one at that!"

"I'm just worried that you're losing weight, Truewater," Herb persisted. "Is it wrong to feel concerned about a fellow physician? You look washed out."

"I told you, Herb, I'm on a diet. I've got a low H.Q."

"You mean I.Q.? Herb asked facetiously.

"No, Herb," I answered. "H.Q. stands for Health Quotient. At the Physician's Health Fair the other day, they took my family history, weight and height, checked my blood cholesterol, glucose, and PSA level.

"Then they put it all on a computer and told me I was suffering from low H.Q."

"I was right," Herb replied. "You're sick and now you're going to die."

"I'm not going to die, Herb," I answered. "I just need to change my lifestyle. I need to eat low-fat food, lose weight, get more exercise, and live a low-stress life.

"A low-stress life – does that mean you're giving your children up for adoption, and quitting the practice of medicine?" Herb joked.

"Very funny, Herb," I answered. "I'm just not going to let things upset me so much – like the federal government or insurance companies telling me how to practice medicine. No, I'm just going to take things in stride."

"And I'm going to enjoy life," I continued, as I loosened my tie and leaned back to relax.

"That doesn't sound good, Truewater," Herb said. "You're beginning to worry me."

"What's wrong with enjoying life?" I answered.

"You're not planning to get a divorce, are you?"

"Of course not, Herb," I answered.

"Well, you know what happened to that ENT doctor in Norman, don't you? He started losing weight, just like you. Then he traded in his Cadillac sedan for a sports car, and then he bought one of those glue-on hairpieces. The next thing you know, he was filing for divorce, and ran off with one of Holy Christian Sinai Hospital's best oncology nurses."

"Herb, I'm not going through a middle-age crisis," I answered. "I'm just trying to lose a little weight."

"That's what they all say," Herb grumbled.

"Look, maybe you ought to get your H.Q. checked," I told Herb. "You don't look to be in such great shape yourself."

"I feel just fine," Herb answered. "When I was in medical school forty years ago, we were told that a blood cholesterol of 300 was normal. Now they've lowered it to 180 and tell us that half of the American adult male population is suffering from high cholesterol levels. I don't buy it."

"But most of the data from the third world countries shows cholesterol levels below 100, Herb. Those people have lower rates of coronary artery disease."

"That's because they're dying from malnutrition, Truewater," Herb answered sarcastically.

"I'm sorry, Bill, but I don't want to go around looking like some undernourished weakling with rapid stool transit times, just so I can brag to people about how healthy I look."

"Besides, what do those people die from, if they don't die from a heart attack? They die from cancer, Truewater. No, I'd rather go from a heart attack any day than die from cancer."

"By the way, Bill, you mentioned family history earlier. Do you have a positive family history?"

"Yes," I replied. "My father died at age 54 of a heart attack."

"That's not good, Dr. Truewater," Herb replied in a somber tone.

"Why not?" I asked defensively.

"You've got bad genes, Truewater. It doesn't' matter if you lose five pounds or twenty-five pounds. I don't want to sound fatalistic, but your death is pre-determined. You're a goner."

"Not so fast, Herb – my father was a heavy Lucky Strike smoker, and led a sedentary lifestyle as a draftsman."

"Besides," I added, "for all we know, you may die before me – I still haven't seen your H.Q. score."

"Of course, I'm going to die before you, Truewater," Herb said. "I'm ten years older than you. Studies show that older people tend to die sooner. And every year I sign that federal form that threatens me with imprisonment if I mis-code a diagnosis, my hair gets a little grayer."

"Look," I concluded, "the whole idea of preventive medicine is to identify the risk factors, and change the factors that can be corrected. Certain things we can't change, like death and taxes, or heredity. And even if we can't improve the length of our lives, we can at least improve the quality. And that's just as important."

"A little while ago, Herb, you asked if it was wrong to be concerned about a fellow physician. Well, I'm concerned about you too, Herb. I'd like to see you lower some of your risk factors."

"You're right, Dr. Truewater," Herb answered, as he put down his donut, and began peeling an orange from the Eli Lilly fruit basket.

"Perhaps it's time for me to change my lifestyle, too!"

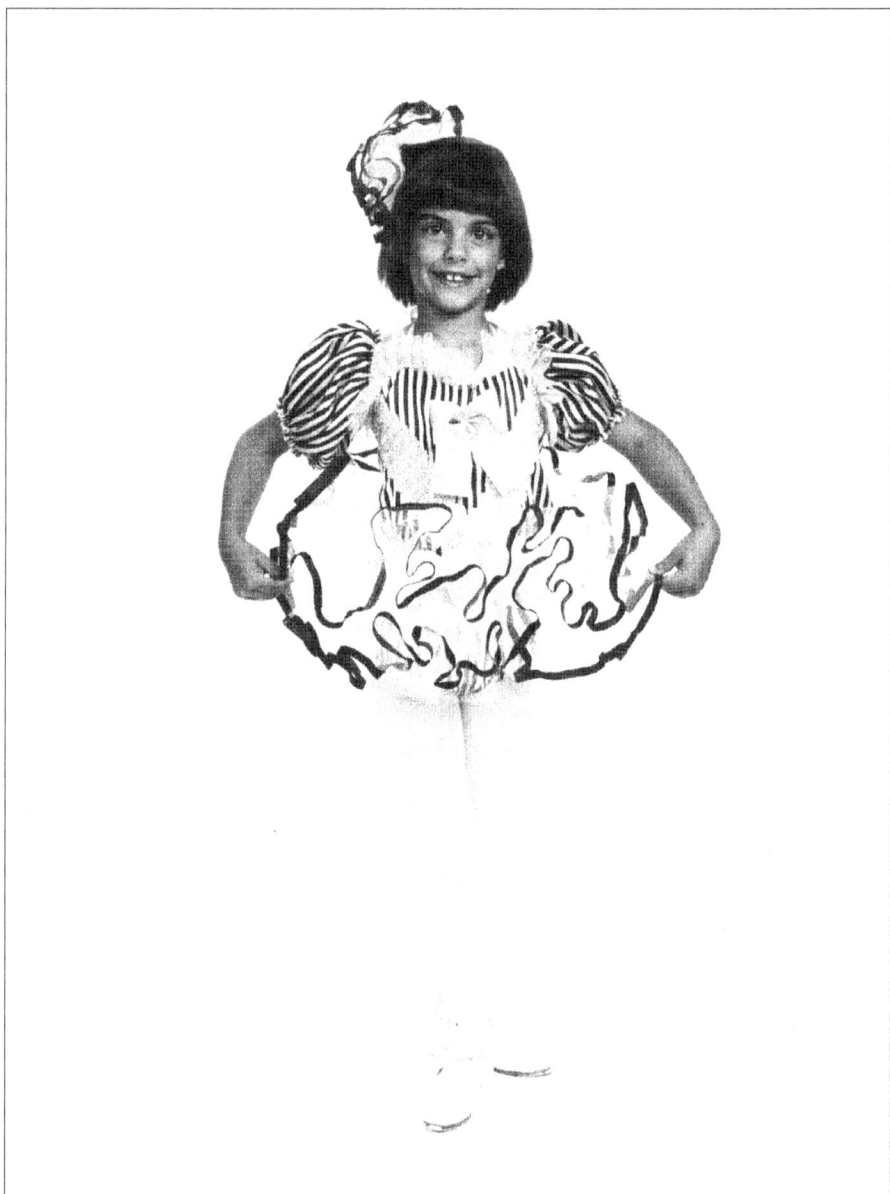

Tracy Truels

MY LITTLE GIRL

I pick you up and hold you tight
My little girl sleeps in the night
And as I hold you in my arms
I think about life's special charms.

How lucky can a Father be
To hold another just like he
With soft brown hair and eyes that shine
How could Nature be so kind?

Someday soon you'll hold your child
And cradle him the longest while
You'll think about the days gone by
And how the stars change in the sky.

Life is such a transient phase –
A pause upon the cosmic stage
Cherish each moment as you live
And question not the One who gives.

TEN SIGNS OF DEATH

I was sitting in the doctor's lounge waiting for my case to start when Herb walked in with a big smile on his face.

"Why so happy, Herb?" I asked.

"Well, Dr. Truewater, I just finished planning my grave marker," Herb grinned. "I don't want my family forced to do any last-minute planning when I pass. Martha and I have a double gravestone, with our birthdates already engraved in marble."

"Isn't that a little premature, Herb?" I asked. "I mean, you're still alive and practicing plastic surgery."

"True enough, but you never know what can happen, especially at our ages – Martha and I are in our sixties now. And a double gravestone saves money – when you kick the bucket, all they have to do is chisel in a few numbers and dump you in the ground!"

"With a double gravestone, you and your wife are permanently united in death, just as you were united in life," Herb added.

"I don't know if I want to be permanently united in death," I quipped. "I might want to run around a little after I die. I'm not ready for a land of milk and honey – I'm a diabetic with lactose intolerance!"

"Besides, Herb, 60 is the new 40. Why, what would happen if you and Martha got divorced – it's kind of hard to cut a marble gravestone in half, and move it to another plot!"

"We're not getting divorced, Dr. Truewater," Herb answered. "I'm way past my mid-life crisis. Nowadays, I'm just looking for a good death."

"A good death?" I replied. "That sounds like an oxymoron. I mean, death can't be a good thing. As doctors, we make a business out of preventing death and prolonging life."

"Why, I remember one Filipino resident during my training at Cook County who never wanted to let anyone die on his shift. You hated to follow him on duty!"

"We don't prevent death, Dr. Truewater," Herb answered. "As physicians, we can only delay death. When you're young, you're like those novice pilots, who think they're invincible. After you've been in battle for a few years, you begin to realize your own mortality!"

"True enough," I answered. "But then, what's a good death?"

"According to the hospice care team, a good death is when you make the terminally ill patient as comfortable as you can, with as little pain as possible, with your final plans in order."

"You mean, like funeral arrangements and legal documents in order?" I added.

"Yes," Herb replied. "But it also means being at peace with yourself in those final days – resolve family conflicts as best you can. Resolve personal conflicts. If possible, you want to have a chance to say good-by to those you love."

"And leave a legacy," Herb added. "Each person leaves some sort of legacy behind – something he or she wants to be remembered for."

"So, what's your legacy going to be, Herb?" I asked.

"I'd like to be remembered as a good plastic surgeon, someone who helped children overcome birth defects, like a cleft palate," Herb replied.

"But, more importantly, I'd just like to be remembered as a good person – a little argumentative and confrontational, I admit, but basically a good person."

"That's very good, Herb," I answered, "but how do you know when your time has come?"

"Easy," Herb replied. "There're ten signs that death is near."

"Ten signs of death?" I asked. "What are they?"

"The first one is loss of appetite," Herb began.

"I haven't been that hungry lately myself," I commented. "What else?"

"Secondly, excessive fatigue and sleep," Herb said.

"I've been kind of tired lately myself," I added, getting a little worried. "I slept fourteen hours last night."

"Thirdly, increased physical weakness can be a sign of impending death," Herb added.

"I've been having trouble doing more than five push-ups," I stated, getting a little nervous and quickly checking my pulse for tachycardia or any extra beats.

"Besides, my cardiologist says my aortic stenosis shouldn't be a problem for another ten years. And I've never had any symptoms – never had chest pain, dizziness, or sudden death, that I know of."

"Mental confusion or disorientation is another terminal sign," Herb added.

"I couldn't find my car in the parking lot yesterday, after shopping four hours with my wife," I commented. "I had to use my key fob to sound the horn. But I'm sharp as a tack."

"Fifthly, labored breathing can be a terminal event," Herb said.

I sighed deeply and checked my nail beds. I was showing all the signs of a dying person.

"I notice I'm getting a little short of breath climbing the stairs at Holy Christian Hospital these days," I replied. "I'm using the elevator more. But my pulmonologist says my asthma and chronic bronchitis are under control."

"Social withdrawal is the sixth sign of a dying person," Herb replied.

"I'm getting to where I don't like parties anymore," I added. "Sometimes I just want to sit in front of the TV and watch a good movie, instead of going out to a bunch of noise and commotion. My psychiatrist says that's not a problem."

"Changes in urination are the seventh sign of a terminally ill person, sometimes with urinary dribbling," Herb added.

"That's getting a little too personal, Herb," I replied angrily. "My urologist says I'm doing just fine. He says it's like you take your finger off the tip of a straw – there's always a little dribbling. What are some other signs of impending death?" I asked nervously.

"Swelling of the feet and ankles is the eighth sign of terminal illness," Herb added.

"I wear support hose to solve that problem," I answered. "My cardiologist says I have a good ejaculation fraction."

"Coolness in the tips of the fingers and toes is the ninth terminal sign," Herb replied.

"Well, it was a little cold this morning walking through the parking tunnel under the giant rotating cross at Holy Christian, and my fingers were a little numb, but they're fine now," I said confidently.

"Mottled veins with bluish mottling is the tenth and final sign of impending death," Herb added.

"Well, I've had varicose veins with mottling for years," I replied defensively. "I'm just fine."

"I find it hard to believe that I could be in the final days or hours of my life," I told Herb, even though I'm positive for all ten signs.

"But I have outlived both my Father and Mother. Maybe I'm in my final days and I just don't realize it. I know the medical students look at me like I'm some sort of historic figure, when I talk about practicing medicine in the good old days, before laparoscopic surgery, lasers, electronic medical records and socialized medicine. They think I'm a relic."

"It's later than you think, Dr. Truewater," Herb added. "I can remember when plastic surgeons didn't use any plastic!"

"Besides, you just told me you've got a cardiologist, a pulmonologist, a urologist, and a psychiatrist, in addition to your family doctor. Too many doctors is not a good sign."

"Dr. Truewater, you need to think seriously about retiring from surgery, and planning for a good death."

"You may be right, Herb," I quipped, as I put on my mask and headed back to surgery. "But I'd like to work as long as I can."

"A good death for me is when they have to pry the scalpel from my cold, dead fingers!"

THE COLORADO MODEL

Here's some good news for all those tired of hospital advertising: I came across an unusual but highly successful medical practice while on vacation. I shall call it the "Colorado Model" since I discovered it while skiing in Colorado. This clinic does absolutely no advertising, maintains a deliberately low profile, and actually discourages referrals from other patients! But I'm getting ahead of myself.

My wife and I were taking skiing lessons at a popular Colorado resort. Mike McGee, our instructor, was showing us how to snow-plow with our skis and how to side-step up a steep slope. He was an unusually patient teacher for a young man who had to deal every day with rank amateurs.

Suddenly, I noticed a snowmobile racing down the slope in the distance behind us. It was pulling an orange stretcher and the patient was all bundled up with orange nylon canvas, a portion of it even covering up his face to protect from the rather severe wind chill in the mountains. Nobody seemed to take notice, but being a physician, I was naturally curious.

"Did you see that man in the stretcher?" I asked the woman taking lessons next to me.

"No," she replied. "I'm too busy concentrating on getting up this silly slope with these confounded skis!"

Mike, our instructor, was standing at the top of the slope. Each member of the class would side-step up the practice slope, then ski down using the snow-plow or wedge maneuver.

"Stay relaxed! Don't tighten up! Don't worry! Let gravity take you down the mountain!" Mike exclaimed.

When I made it to the top, I was rather short-winded, but whispered to the instructor in a low voice, so as not to scare any of my classmates, "Mike, did you see that see that stretcher that just went by? What happened? Did someone break a bone?"

"Stretcher? No, I didn't notice one. But every once in a while they have to take someone off the mountain. It's nothing to worry about."

Not satisfied, I persisted further. "Well, what's the usual thing that goes wrong? A broken arm? Broken ribs?"

"Nope," Mike replied rather nonchalantly. "It's usually fatigue. The air up on that mountain is pretty thin, and a lot of newcomers just get wore out and have to ride down."

After we made it down the mountain, I went straight to the hot tub for about two hours, then had a light dinner with my wife. As we strolled through the lobby, Margaret said, "Bill, look at that man over there! He's got a cast on his leg."

I casually walked over and introduced myself. His name was Mac Behrens from New York and this was his first day on the slopes. Mac had been skiing for over thirty years.

"What happened to your leg?" I finally asked.

"I broke it going too fast over the moguls," Mac replied.

"Doctor Lindstrom was upbeat, Mac added. "It could have been worse, especially if it had gone through a joint or torn a ligament. He splinted it right there in the clinic."

"Tell me, Mac, were there any other patients in the clinic?"

"You better believe it!" Mac exclaimed. "During the two hours I was there, a man came in with broken ribs, another with a broken left arm, a woman with a broken thumb, and a man with a broken ankle that they had to take to town. Of course, you've got to realize there were over 5,000 people skiing that mountain today!"

Finally it dawned on me. Here was an outpatient clinic that was maintaining such a low profile, it didn't even want people to know where it was located. No advertising. No hype. Yet it was extremely successful. People knew the service was available. The staff were friendly and courteous, maintained an upbeat tone and didn't dwell on illness. Here was a man with a broken leg who felt lucky because the fracture wasn't any worse, yet his whole vacation had been ruined!

I thought to myself about the "Colorado Model." What if other hospitals were to adopt such a plan – restrict competitive advertising, maintain a low profile, and emphasize service? Should a doctor or hospital have to advertise excessively to promote their services? Must we be so enamored with our technology that we can't get back to the basics of patient care? And why should society expect hospitals and doctors to extract every last ounce of life from a patient?

Perhaps the best philosophy can be summarized from our ski instructor, "Stay relaxed! Don't tighten up! Don't worry! Let gravity take you down the mountain!"

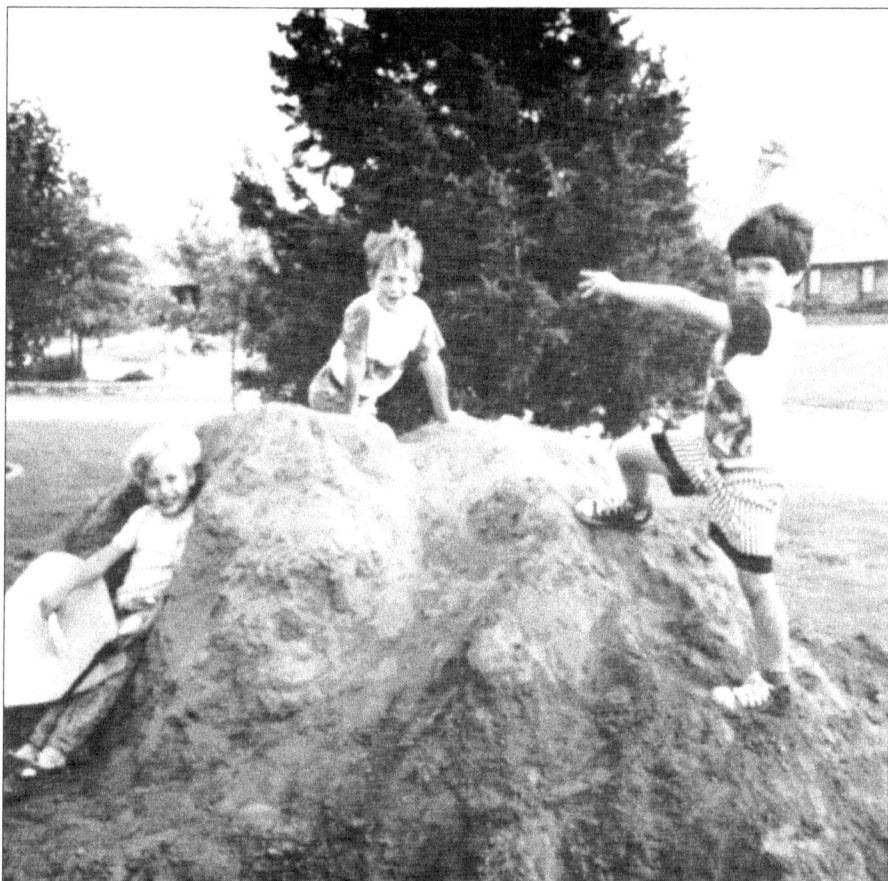

Jaime Chastain, Judd Blanscet and Michael Truels

THE SANDPILE

"This sandpile is the greatest thing!"
My son yells down to me,
"I'm the highest kid in all the world
As anyone can see!"

I shovel the sand upon the lawn
To make it soft and smooth
My little boy digs in the pile
And tries to tunnel through.

Little men in little trucks
Play beneath the sun
If only they were big like me
My work would soon be done!

All the educational toys
Are sitting in his home
A sandpile is the greatest thing
A little boy could own!

ANSWER THE CALL

I was sitting in the doctor's lounge last week, waiting for my hernia case to start, when Herb Silverstein walks in. His cleft palate reconstruction was delayed, so we had a few minutes to chat.

"I heard that Curt Winter, the orthopedic surgeon was going to quit medicine and become a preacher," Herb began.

"That's surprising," I answered. "Why, I just scrubbed with him a couple of nights ago on a trauma case. He was putting some hardware on a hip fracture while I was closing on a ruptured spleen."

"He never mentioned anything about the ministry, although he did say it was by the grace of God that our patient survived the accident – his car was rear ended by an eighteen-wheeler!"

"I guess the truck driver forgot his energy drink and fell asleep!" Herb quipped.

"But why would you forgo all that medical education and start in the ministry?" I wondered.

"Why Curt and his brother, Jerry, are two of the best orthopedic surgeons in Oklahoma City!" I added.

"They did the best Putti-Platt during my residency of anybody in town!"

"Nobody does the Putti-Platt anymore, Dr. Truewater," Herb quipped.

"Well, I guess a lot's changed since I did a rotating internship in orthopedics, as part of my general surgery residency."

"Nobody does a rotating internship anymore, Dr. Truewater," Herb replied.

"But why is Curt entering the cemetery, I mean the seminary," I corrected myself.

"That seems like a waste of all his medical training."

"It seems that Curt made a covenant with God," Herb began.

"You see, his brother, Jerry, was sick with some kind of bone marrow problem, hypoplasia or something, and wasn't making any white blood cells. Things looked bleak for a while, and Jerry was in isolation."

"So Curt talks to God and makes a covenant," Herb continued.

"I didn't think orthopedic surgeons could talk to God," I interjected.

"I know they're high and mighty and everything. But I thought only preachers could talk to God – that's the reason you went to seminary school."

"No, anybody can talk to God, Dr. Truewater. God speaks to everyone – you just have to know how to listen."

"Does he speak to general surgeons?" I asked.

"Sometimes," Herb replied. "Anyway, Curt makes a covenant with God, and says that if his brother Jerry survives, then Curt will go into the seminary."

"So, long story short, Jerry survives – I guess he had some sort of viral infection – and Curt signs up for the ministry."

"I guess this was God's way of getting Curt into the seminary," Herb added. "You see, God always has a Greater Plan for us."

"But why would God give Jerry a viral infection in order to get Curt to go into the ministry?" I asked.

"I mean, why couldn't God just talk to Curt – you said he talks to orthopedic surgeons – and just straight out tell Curt to join the ministry?"

"God moves in mysterious ways," Herb added. "Far be it from us to know the Greater Plan!"

"That reminds me of Sister Mary Rock up at Mercy," I said. "She was in a tornado in Edmond – there was this terrible noise like a freight train and, when it was over, her house was intact, but the house next to them was leveled down to the slab – thank God nobody was home!"

"Anyway, Sister Mary takes that as a sign from God. She had always thought about building a large retirement village. She felt like the tornado was God's way of telling her to get going – and that's how Epworth Villa got started – no joke!" I added.

"Well, sometimes God does things that don't make sense to us at the beginning, but look, we've got a great retirement village now!" Herb replied.

"Are you saying that God controls the tornadoes?" I asked Herb.

"God controls everything," Herb replied. "Why, God even controls your hand while you're operating in surgery!" Herb added.

"He does?" I asked. "I hope God knows his anatomy – medical students today don't learn anatomy like we did. I mean we spent a whole year on the cadaver – students today spend only a few months in the cadaver lab. I'm thinking about not even bothering to donate my body to science!"

"God doesn't need to take anatomy, Dr. Truewater! God created the anatomy – why, just from Adam's rib he created an entire woman!"

"Well, if God is guiding my hand in surgery, and He's that good, maybe I should step over to the left side of the table and let God do the surgery – kind of like an Attending Physician when the resident gets in trouble."

"Does that mean the Attending is God?" I asked.

"No, Dr. Truewater, you're getting confused," Herb replied.

"God works through us, like he worked through Curt and Sister Mary for a Greater Good."

"Humans still have to do their part," Herb added.

Just then a voice came booming over the intercom in the doctor's lounge.

"Dr. Truewater, your case is starting in room nine!"

"I've got to get going, Herb," I replied. "God is calling!"

ON REACHING FORTY

I guess I've started my decline
I'm no longer thirty-nine!
It's the autumn of my life
Though I'm feeling quite alright.

My friends who want to celebrate
Think that it is really great
"You're catching up to us," they say,
"We turned forty yesterday!"

I've got a little balding spot
That's very thin upon my top.
And if I comb a certain way,
I can cover up the gray!

I still have my lust for girls –
I still notice all their curls.
But though I know just what to do,
My body doesn't take the cue!

Oh, thank goodness for my golf
I still like to take time off.
But when I wind up for my swing,
Arthritis makes me miss that thing!

I still look at my big screen--
Those football games are really keen.
Remote control – I'm glad it's there –
It's just too hard to leave my chair!

Though this has all been one big joke
I really do sincerely hope
That when I get to forty-nine
You'll all be here to share the wine!

FALLEN HEROES

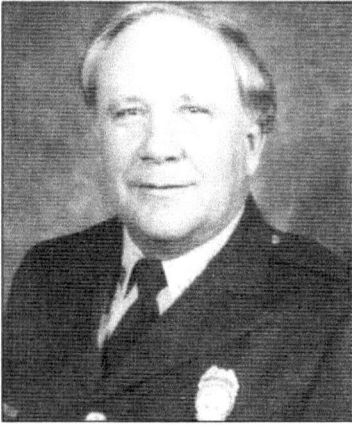

Captain Jimmy L. Ayers was a 23-year veteran of the City Of Oklahoma City Fire Department. He was Station Captain at Station #21, 3240 S.W. 29th. He is survived by his wife, Betty Lou, and three children, Curtis, Crystal, and Christopher. Jimmy L. Ayers has been nominated for the City of Oklahoma City Employees Recognition Awards.

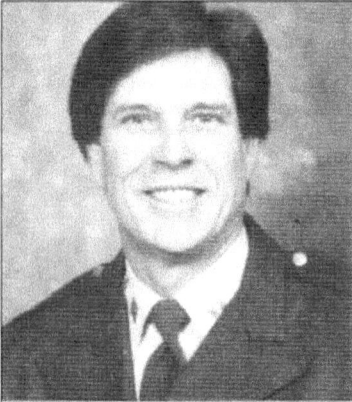

Captain Bennie D. Zellner was an 18-year veteran of the City of Oklahoma City Fire Department. He was Station Captain at Fire Station #8, 1939 West Exchange Avenue. He is survived by his wife, Sandy, who works as a nurse at the Paul Silverstein Baptist Burn Center, where all three firemen were treated. Bennie is also survived by his son, Kevin, and four step children, Patrick, Patricia, Travis, and Troy.

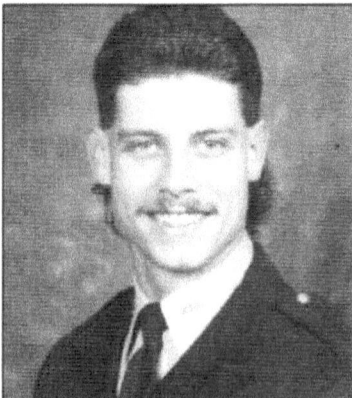

Jeffrey N. Lindsay started his career with the City of Oklahoma City Fire Department on July 12, 1985. He was a Firefighter at Fire Station #21, 3240 S.W. 29th. Jeff is a second-generation firefighter. His father, Robert Lindsay is a captain at Fire Station #7. His brother, Mike Lindsay is a Firefighter at Fire Station #31. Jeff is survived by his wife Melissa, and son, Jeffrey, born July 3, 1989.

The above three firemen died tragically in an Oklahoma City fire on March 8, 1989.

HOW WILL I REMEMBER?

How will I remember
The good times that we shared?
Why do things we cherish most
Vanish in the air?

I've gathered all your pictures –
I've got your valentine –
Remember when we had a love
That conquered space and time?

It truly is a paradox
That nature does create –
The perfect shapes and perfect forms
That soon evaporate!

They say that time will heal all wounds –
The pain soon disappears
But every time I think of you
I see you through my tears!

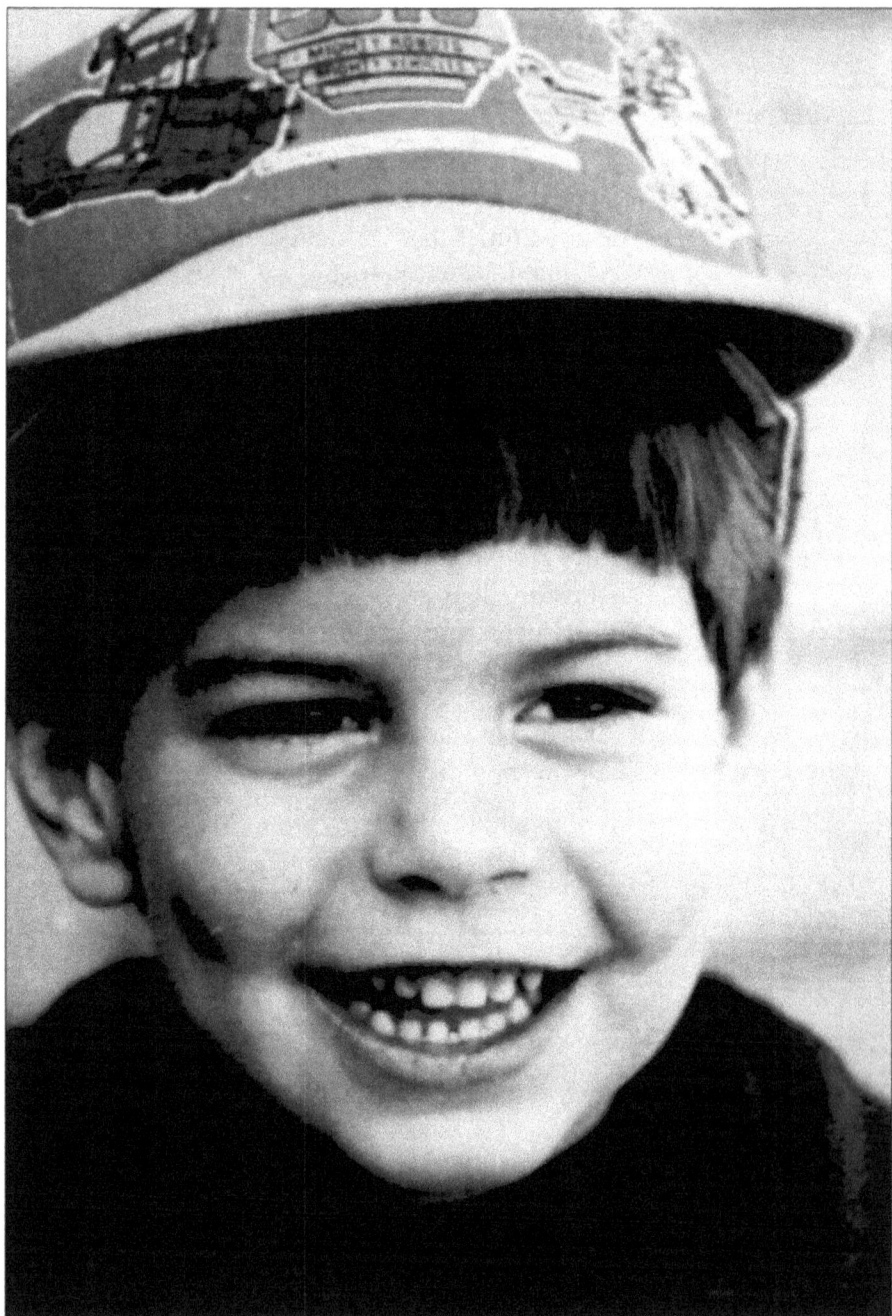

MICHAEL'S BATH

The little toys are in a row –
They form a perfect path
With soap suds flying everywhere
My boy begins his bath.

Tiny man-made submarines
Begin their slow descent
They must find golden treasure
Before their air is spent!

The Ninja man is next in line
He jumps into the sea
He must destroy the hidden mine
And set the people free!

The motorboat is next to cruise
Upon the soapy waves
But look out for the submarines
From underwater caves!

And so the little bathtub
Becomes a giant sea
Where battles rage and people fly
In dreams of fantasy.

His bath is done, I mop the floor
I try to clear my head
It's nice to settle all your scores
Before you go to bed!

JUST LIKE OLD TIMES

I'd been retired for a while, so I thought I'd visit some of the old crew at the surgery lounge, and get a free cup of coffee and some doughnuts. The combination to the lounge hadn't changed – 1-2-3-4-5 – and, sure enough, Herb was there, waiting for his case to start.

"Hello, Herb," I began. "Nice to see you again!"

"Dr. Truewater is back!" Herb exclaimed. "How's retirement treating you?"

"Great!" I exclaimed. "I thought I'd drop by for some coffee and doughnuts. Where's the coffee pot?" I asked.

"The coffee pot? Why that's obsolete, Dr. Truewater. K-cups are the rage now – each person can make their own flavor of coffee or tea – that's progress!"

"Great!" I exclaimed, as I waited for the water to heat up before popping in a Lake and Lodge K-cup.

"I'm just getting ready to do an ulnar nerve release," Herb continued.

"That requires a lot of eye-hand coordination," I stated.

"Oh, I don't' touch the patient anymore- we use robots now," Herb replied. "Everything's mechanical!"

"That's amazing!" I said, as I sipped a cup of Lake and Lodge coffee.

"The only thing new we do ahead of time is what's called a time-out," Herb added.

"A time-out? You mean, you take a short break?" I asked.

"No, Dr. Truewater. We ask the patient their name and birthday," Herb replied.

"Don't they know their name and birthday?" I asked.

"Of course," Herb added. "That's our way of making sure I'm operating on the right patient. Then we get an orange Magic Marker and have the patient write 'Yes' on the operative site."

"I suppose that's to make sure the robot doesn't operate on the left side versus the right side," I added.

"Correct!" Herb replied. "But we've got few more pitfalls to avoid than years ago."

"How's that?" I asked.

"Well, the other day, I misgendered a patient named Leslie."

"Didn't you do a physical?" I asked.

"Well, yes, I did," Herb replied. "Based on my physical exam, this man – I mean woman – was a man."

"I'm getting confused, Herb," I replied. "I know you're a plastic surgeon, but you still had to take cadaver anatomy in medical school."

"Things have changed, Dr. Truewater. People can now declare to be whatever sex they choose, regardless of their physical attributes or their genetics."

"I mean, did you ever think that way down deep you might be a woman?"

"Not lately," I replied, "although I do have my ups and downs."

"Well, it's important," Herb continued, "to use the right pronoun."

"What's grammar got to do with it?" I asked.

"Well, if a man believes that he's a woman, you must address him as 'she' or 'they', not 'he' or 'him'".

"If you use the wrong pronoun, you've committed a microaggression and you're guilty of misgendering."

"Well, at least you've got a 50 per cent chance of being right," I quipped.

"Not exactly, Dr. Truewater. You see, there are 72 genders and 78 gender pronouns and with gender fluidity this can change from day to day."

"You know, I've just had an important insight, Herb," I replied, as I sipped on my Lake and Lodge coffee.

"What's that, Dr. Truewater?"

"I'm glad I'm retired!"

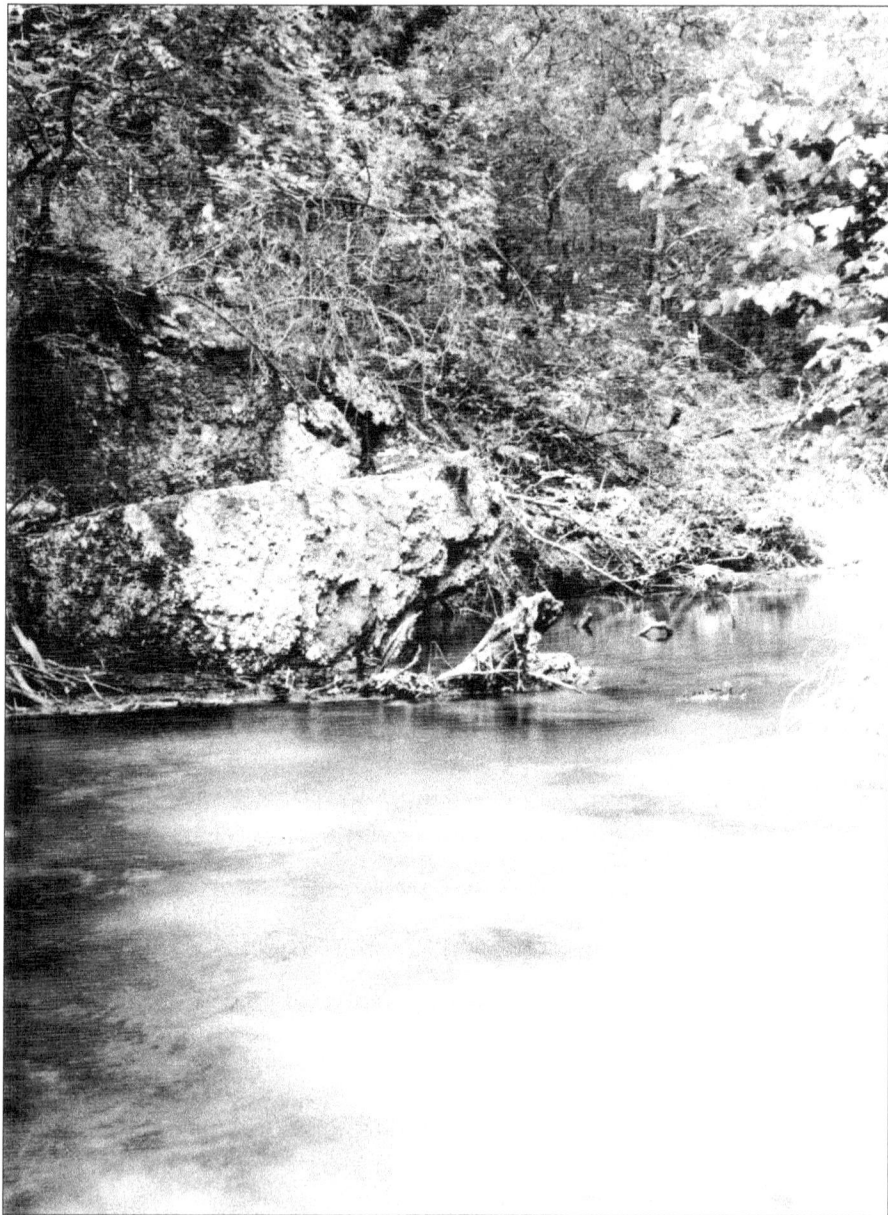

The stream at Martin Nature Park.

THE STREAM

I throw a pebble in the stream
And watch the ripples fade
It's nice to have some time alone –
I like to get away.

The water rushes round the rocks
And churns an airy foam
As I journey through this life
I've wandered far from home.

I close my eyes and float
Along the channels of my mind
I see the scenes of yesterday
The people left behind.

And as the circles widen
They share a common lore
Like all the friends that 1 have known
They touch the one before.

And though the ripples of the past
Have faded long ago
I love to sit here by this stream
And watch the water flow.

THE MOST IMPORTANT ORGAN

I was sitting in the doctor's lounge waiting for my hernia case to start when Herb Silverstein, the plastic surgeon walked in. I'd just got back from a long road trip with my wife, Maggie, and was dying to ask Herb this question.

"Tell me, Herb," I began, "What's the most important organ in the human body?"

"That's easy," Herb began. "As a plastic surgeon, I can tell you that the skin is the most important organ – you can't live without your skin. It protects you from infection, it keeps you warm, it cools you off when you sweat, and it affects your self-image – how you look is a function of how your skin feels."

"True enough," I answered, "for a plastic surgeon."

"But I think most people would say that the heart is the most important organ," I added. "It circulates the blood, responds to stress by increasing output, and some would say it's the seat of emotion. Lovers even say, 'I love you with all my heart!'"

"But the brain is the true seat of emotion – perhaps even the seat of the soul," Herb replied. "It's nature's own computer and allows us to try and comprehend the world around us- it was Einstein's brain that showed that gravity was a warping of the fabric of space-time, and that time was not constant, but varied with the relative velocity of the observer."

"But if you're a liver specialist," I countered, "You believe that the liver is the most important organ. It stores and metabolizes the food we eat and helps purify the blood. The ancient Greeks believed that the liver was the seat of human emotions. You can't live without your liver."

"Which brings us to the kidney," Herb replied. "It's the kidney that purifies the blood and maintains the all-important 20:1 bicarbonate to CO_2 ratio that keeps the ATP pump working, which keeps us alive."

"Which in turn brings us to the lungs, which oxygenate our blood and blow off carbon dioxide to preserve that 20:1 base to acid ratio, which keeps our transaminase and phosphatase enzymes working," I added.

"But, if you leave it up to the general public, they would no doubt say that the sex organs are the most important- some people say that everything revolves around sex," Herb replied. "It's nature's way of procreating the species."

"True enough," I replied. "Although after the initial attraction begins to fade, it's more important that people get along with each other to create a coherent family bond."

"I'm beginning to get your point, Dr Truewater," Herb replied. "The importance of each organ is a function of the observer. Each physician views their area of expertise to be the most important. And each patient views their illness, or their area of interest to be the most relevant."

"Exactly, Herb," I replied. "Which brings me to my next point."

"I spent the week-end on a long road trip with my wife, Maggie and our pet mongrel. We stopped every 30 minutes to let the dog out to pee, or let my wife out to pee, or to let me out to pee with my enlarged prostate."

"I concluded that the most important organ in the human body is the one most likely to trigger a divorce. I decided that the bladder is the most important organ in the human body. A well-functioning bladder is the key to a happy marriage. You can carry on your activities at a normal pace without frequent disruption, leakage, odor, or pain."

"I know that doesn't sound romantic or scientific," I concluded. "But, as a senior citizen, I'll put my money on a healthy bladder over the liver or lungs any day!"

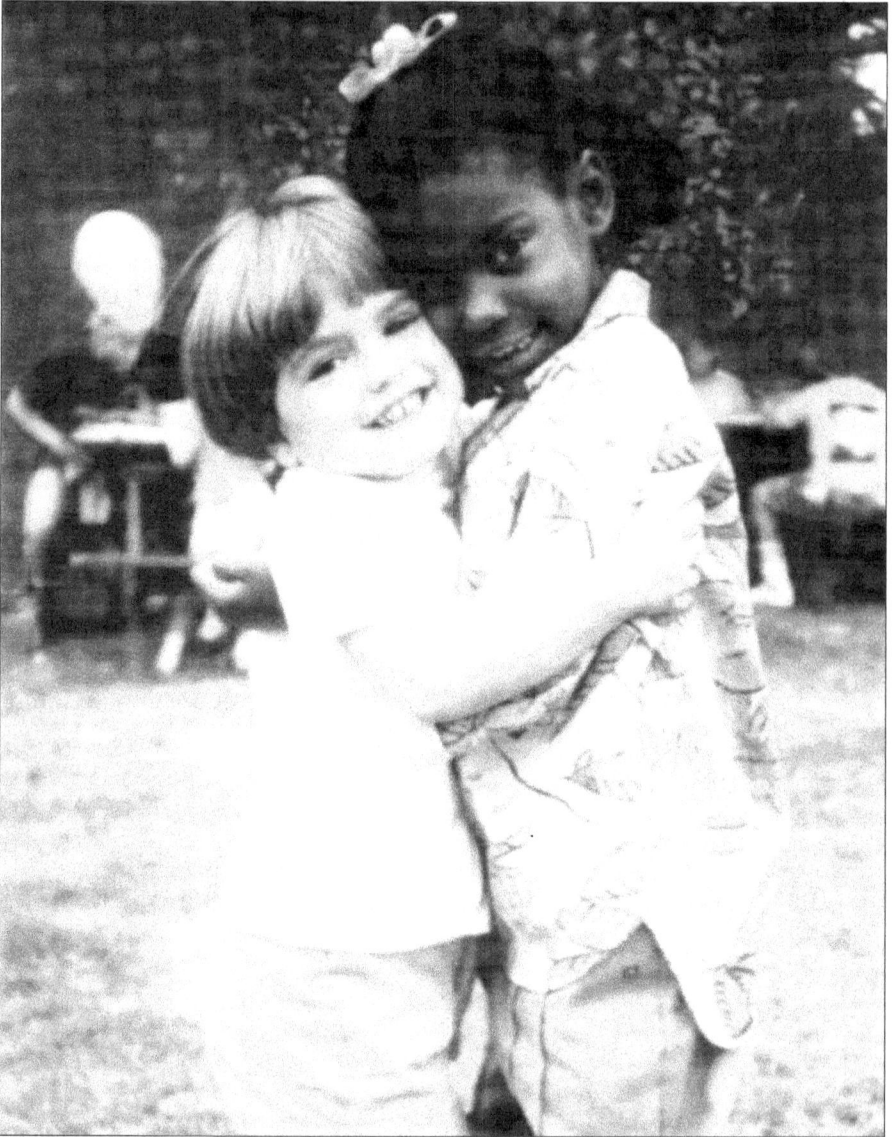

Pictured are Katie Brumbaugh (left), daughter of Peter and Marlene Brumbaugh, and Tara Williams, daughter of Darrell and Arnita Williams, playing at the Oklahoma City Zoo. Their parents both work in the Surgery Department at Baptist Medical Center in Oklahoma City.

CAN YOU PLAY?

The sun is out – it's a happy day
Can you come outside and play?
The days are long, school is out
It's time to run and dance and shout!

I've got my bike – you've got one too
I'll go to the park with you!
They've got some swings – it's not that far
They've got a slide and monkey bars!

We could spray each other with the hose
That's down by the old swimmin' hole
Or we could get a ball and bat
And play some baseball in the back.

Your skin is black and mine is white
But I think everything's alright
There's lots of things that we could do –
I'd like to have some fun with you!

A DAD REMEMBERS

Tracy,

This week marks the beginning of a new era in your career. I admire you for the courage and compassion you have shown for spending two years of your life helping to educate underprivileged children in the most crime-ridden part of Chicago, complete with muggings and drug dealers. You also put up with two years of city school politics and lived in a noisy, underprivileged neighborhood.

In the past, you dealt with the stresses of high school and college. Now, you are returning to Indiana University for graduate school, and I wish you well. Once again, we will miss you, but we wish you well in creative writing at Bloomington.

P.S. Some of the things a Dad remembers (you were easy to raise!):

1. Reading a children's book at a very early age—I would turn the page, and you would "read" it to me. (I think you might have memorized it.)

2. Swim meets at the Greens, where you had to work hard to get to the other end of the Olympic pool, but you never gave up. Playing tether ball in the back yard. Learning to ride a two-wheeler bike, without even having to practice, after we took off the training wheels.

3. Going to the Mercy ER during a life threatening asthma attack around age two, and one year later to St. John's in Tulsa in the middle of the night.

4. Dance lessons where you memorized your steps after only one or two tries.

5. Playing basketball against much bigger girls in junior high school.

6. Singing "Crazy" at the high school's talent show, making the auditorium go crazy with cheering.

7. Singing a tribute at my mother Georgia's funeral.

8. Pulling you, Lisa, and Michael on a sled after a rare Oklahoma snow storm

9. Going to a JFK assassination meeting in Dallas—Bob Groden still mentions you!

10. Shaking hands with Senator Bob Dole at Baptist Hospital.

11. Going to a Chicago Cubs game with Luke and Mike at Wrigley Field. Visiting your apartment in Chicago and eating out at the Thai restaurant and the Cuban café.

12. Pulling a mattress over your head and lying in the bathtub while you were alone in the house during a tornado alert on one of your visits back to Oklahoma.

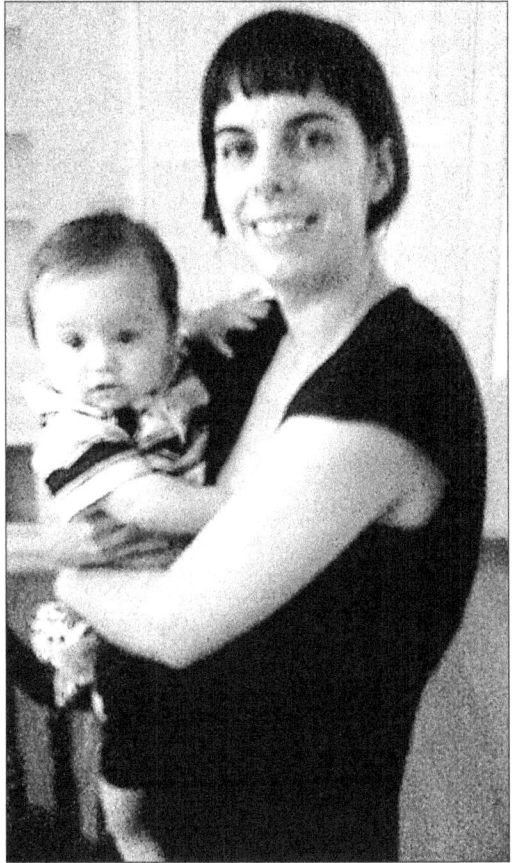

13. Making that picture calendar with all the family pics—a true collector's item for us!

15. Cheering Mike's home runs at Santa Fe baseball games.

16. Helping Lisa study for her GED.

17. How extremely important it was to try and get your driver's license on your 16th birthday.

One thing I notice is that, once you set out to do something, you do it with full commitment, like finishing the Teach for America program in Chicago, and doing the full two years, where I would probably have bailed out after one year. I think that's a good trait, and I admire your stick-to-it-iveness (if that's a word).

Anyway, good luck in the next chapter of your life, Tracy—we're all pulling for you, and we all love 'ya!

MY ENDLESS LOVE

If I should count the stars
That shine in our heavenly sky
They say I would never finish
Though I count 'til the day I die.

Like the stars my love has no limit
It is timeless, endless, and bright
Like a rose that blooms in the sunshine
Your beauty is my delight!

Some things go on forever
Though I will never know why
Yet true lovers like you and me
Are the flowers that blossom and die.

But why count the grains of sand
Or even the stars above –
Though Nature may long outlast me
It's you I always will love!

YELLING AT TORNADOES

I was sitting in the doctor's lounge waiting for my case to start when Herb Silverstein, the plastic surgeon walked in.

"You know, Dr. Truewater, there's just too much emphasis on bad weather in Oklahoma," Herb said, as took off his galoshes following a recent rain storm. "It's bad for business!"

"How's that, Herb?" I asked.

"Well, companies do research on where to expand. They look at Oklahoma- a sunshine state with lots of labor, and then they look at all these negative weather reports about Oklahoma."

"They talk about hail storms and high winds and wind shear. Then it's tornado this and tornado that. Why, in forty years in Oklahoma I've only seen two tornados, and only one came close!" Herb continued.

"You only need one tornado to come close, Herb, before you get lifted up into heaven."

"That's Wizard of Oz fairy tale kind of stuff," Herb answered. "We're not in Kansas anymore!"

"Why, it shook the doors on the storm cellar, but that's as far as it got!" Herb added. "We were all a little scared as we huddled in the underground shelter in the front yard, but that's Mother Nature for you!"

"I agree with you, Herb," I replied. "Why, you can get struck by lightning playing golf, and that could happen anywhere, although mostly on a golf course."

"In fact, the only tornado I ever saw was where I grew up in Illinois- I was in third grade and the tornado took off part of the school roof! We were all hiding under our desks, like it we were practicing for a nuclear attack or something- the teacher just wanted us to be safe! Those big old-fashioned school windows shook, but they didn't break!"

"Those were crazy times!" I added. "It turned out that the weather was a bigger threat than the Russians during the Red Scare in the sixties!"

"Speaking of crazy times, that reminded me of that crazy dermatologist, George Spears. Do you remember him, Dr. Truewater?" Herb asked.

"Wasn't he that elderly dermatologist who thought everything was a skin cancer? I mean, he missed one melanoma, along with the pathologist, and from then on, he got paranoid that everything was a skin cancer!"

"Right, well George was our next-door neighbor, and one day I was in the shelter with my wife and kids eating our rations, and I could hear George's wife next door, yelling at him to get in the shelter."

"'Get in the shelter, George!' she yelled."

"I had to open our shelter door and peek out, which you're not supposed to do, because by then the wind was blowing pretty hard, and the doors were rattling!"

"Well, it was pitch black in the middle of the afternoon on Easter Sunday, but you could still see this big tornado, kind of spindly, with a deafening roar, like some angry God, sucking up everything in its path – lawn chairs, cars – you name it – and crazy George was throwing his hands up in the air, yelling at the tornado. It was the craziest thing I've ever seen!"

"You see, George was a buttoned-down kind of guy, and he couldn't handle disorder. The tornado was messing things up."

"I yelled at George to get in the shelter. George was a good golfer, and we needed him for the upcoming *Member-Guest Spring Fling Tournament*, if we had any chance of winning."

"Lord, take me!" George yelled. "I challenge you to take me!" as the hailstones whipped against his body.

"It was a classic case of Man vs Nature – our desire to assert ourselves against all the forces that seek to destroy us. For a moment, I thought George was admiring the sheer power of the damned thing!"

"Was it suicidal? I don't know. But George was challenging the Destructive Force – he was immersing himself in the destructive element – Joseph Conrad would have been proud!"

"It reminds me of Dylan Thomas," I added. "Do not go gentle into that good night – Rage, rage against the dying of the light."

"I still can't figure out why George would yell at that tornado," Herb interjected. "Perhaps, like ancient times, he was offering himself as a human sacrifice – take me and spare my family!"

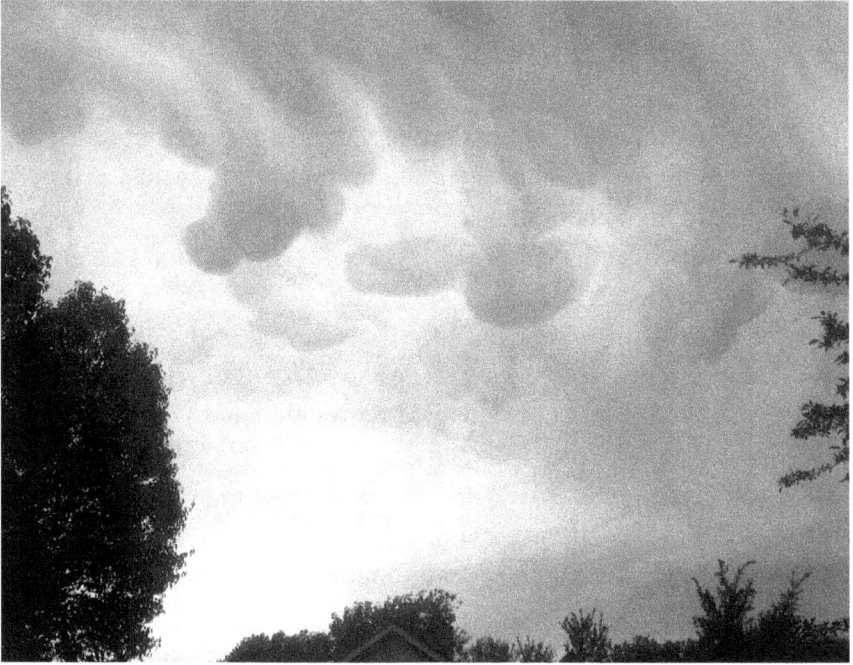

Taken from my front porch on April 24, 2020

"Well, it was foolhardy, nevertheless – and stupid," I said. "It's not good to get angry at God. Sometimes we are our own worst enemy! Be careful what you wish for!"

"Some people interpret tornadoes and natural disasters as a sign that God is punishing them for past sins," Herb replied.

"Others, like Sister Mary, who was next door to a house that was flattened, took it as a sign that God was telling her to get on with her dream of building a retirement center. That gave rise to Senior Villages, complete with walking paths and a beautiful garden."

"But why couldn't God get Sister Mary's attention by just leaving her a note to build her retirement center?" I asked.

"Wouldn't be as dramatic," Herb answered. "Flattening that house next door got her attention. And she took it as a miracle that her house was untouched."

"At any rate, George got a second chance. He pulled the wood splinters out of his skin, took some time off to heal his wounds, and then resurrected his practice."

"Perhaps it was a catharsis – I don't know. He seemed happier after that – like he had stood up and challenged the tornado and won!"

"Or perhaps he had seen the face of God!" I added.

MINI-MAE'S LAST RIDE

Mini-Mae limped up into her travel seat in our van, anxious for her daily ride. With her neck bowed down from arthritis, she could barely raise her head high enough to see out the window.

We loved Mini-Mae, now 13 years old. She started out as our granddaughter's dog, with her fluffy fur and bouncy gait. In her younger days, Mini-Mae loved to run fast, jump in the air, and land with a somersault! As she grew older and less agile, my wife and I adopted Mini-Mae and accompanied her on her many veterinarian's visits for scoliosis of the neck and arthritis in her right front leg that would sometimes cause her to fall flat on her face as she raced against our other dog, Mia--chasing a squirrel in our back yard!

I remembered one night, several months ago, when I woke up and found Mini-Mae standing alone in the bathroom panting. We rushed her to the emergency room, convinced she was having a heart attack. After a thorough exam and overnight stay, the veterinarian informed us that Mini-Mae was having chronic, severe pain and we began an around the clock pain pill regimen.

I held up Mia, our little chihuahua dog for Mini-Mae to see, as I stood in the garage. Mini-Mae held up her head, almost gloatingly, for she was going on her ride, while Mia was staying home! Mia quickly looked away, as if she sensed something was wrong. This was late in the day- not the usual time for Mini-Mae's daily ride.

Despite her age, Mini-Mae had a good memory – she would remember all the places she had been. When my wife and I drove past our old house in the Village, Mini-Mae's ears would perk up as she stuck her head out the window and stared at her first house. I'm sure the strangers who lived there now wondered why that old dog barked at them, like she was reclaiming her old territory!

We drove past the old ice cream shop that Mini-Mae enjoyed, as she looked out the window and barked. We bought Mini-Mae a small bowel of soft serve ice cream and let her lick it dry, as my wife wiped away a tear. Mini-Mae must have wondered – what was the special occasion?

We slowly drove around the old walking path in our neighborhood. Mini-Mae recognized each of the houses where her doggy friends used to live, and barked or whimpered at each one as we drove by – as if begging their spirits to come out and play! Most of Mini-Mae's friends were gone now – she had outlived most of them.

We drove by Lake Hefner where Mini-Mae liked to walk around and let her gaze at the ducks and roll in the soft, fluffy grass. She watched

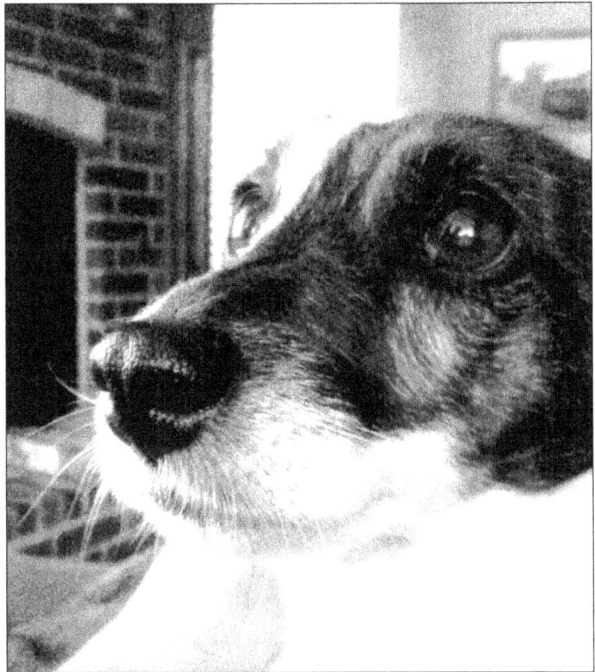

Mini-Mae

the wind surfers take off into the air and do somersaults, wondering if one day she might be able to do somersaults again!

When we arrived at the veterinarian, he put us in a small room and let Margaret and I visit with Mini-Mae. We said a quiet prayer, and Margaret wrapped Mini-Mae in her favorite blanket- gently, for all her legs were sore now from the arthritis. I was already beginning to tear up and had to step outside for a few minutes.

Mini-Mae must have wondered why the veterinarian was starting an IV in her arm. We softly stroked her white fluffy fur to reassure her. When the doctor injected the medicine, Mini-Mae suddenly looked up at me for one last time, and for one brief second our souls touched each other. It never seems like the right time to die!

The doctor carried Mini-Mae off, wrapped in her favorite Dora the Explorer blanket, as her head drooped down. Mini-Mae was in pain no more, but our pain over her loss was just beginning! Maybe she was jumping in the air and doing somersaults once again!

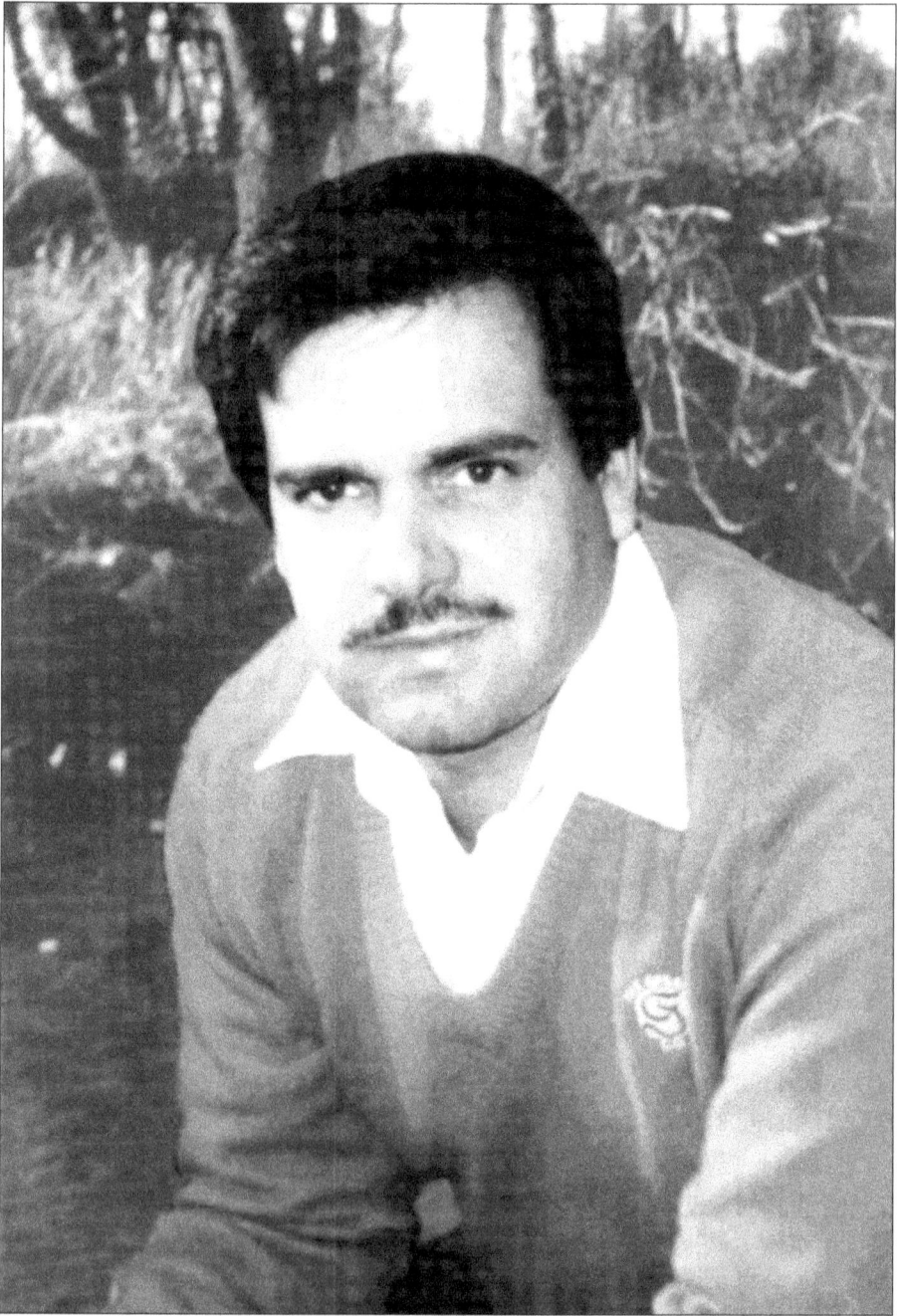

HAIKUS FOR DAD

A true Wanderer
not afraid to leave the crowd
or ask it questions

A rad Raconteur
the fly, Marilyn, and poems
each shines like a coin

A mad Scientist —
fan blades at just the right speed
looking for answers

A fierce Protector —
tires, coughs, a/c and engines
asks *how's that working?*

A Gifted healer —
listens, observes, and reflects
never in a rush

A devoted Friend —
happy just to sit in quiet
not one missed phone call

And always a Dad —
singing to our higher selves
always believing

– Tracy Truels
July 12, 2013

BACK TO THE BASICS

Little Susie sat on the old wooden exam table, waiting patiently for Dr. Hale to arrive at his south Oklahoma City clinic. Her long blond hair was neatly braided into pigtails that gently brushed against her oversized, hand-me-down sweatshirt. Her bright blue eyes stood in stark contrast to her rosy red cheeks, flushed from the fever which had overtaken her these last few days.

Being six years old wasn't easy. With Mom and Dad separated, it was hard for Mom to make ends meet. Susie wore mostly jeans, which were hand-me-downs from her older brothers. Susie looked proudly at her high-top tennis shoes with the words "Air Special" printed on the side, a gift from the Baptist Medical Mission. They were the joy of her life. For once she had gotten something brand new – even her older brothers were jealous. Susie would fly through the air at recess, just to show off her new tennis shoes.

But for the last two days, Susie was too sick to run, or even go to kindergarten. The fine, red rash that covered her body, along with her sore throat, didn't respond to Mom's usual home remedy of warm cinnamon water and toast.

"Hello, Susie!" Dr. Hale began. "How's my little girl?"

"I don't feel good," Susie said. "My throat hurts."

"Let's have a look," Dr. Hale answered, as his partially paralyzed right arm gently examined her throat. His wife, Sandy, a registered nurse, and also a victim of multiple sclerosis, passed him his stethoscope, and Dr. Hale listened to Susie's chest.

Of course, Dr. Hale had already made his diagnosis. The fine red rash, sore throat, and elevated temperature were the classic signs for scarlet fever.

"I'm glad you brought Susie to the clinic," Dr. Hale told Susie's mother. "If unchecked, this kind of infection can spread to the kidneys, causing permanent, sometimes even fatal damage."

Susie received a penicillin shot and some antibiotics to take home – at no cost, thanks to donations from concerned pharmacists, nurses, and physicians.

I decided to make my own contribution the following week, tucking my donation box under my right arm as I approached the mission door. Little Susie had made a complete recovery. As she waited in the mission lobby, her Air Special shoes flashed from room to room. I managed to talk with her for a fleeting moment, when she stopped to catch her breath.

"Susie," I began, "why do you think there are doctors?" I asked rather naively.

"To help get people well," Susie answered.

I thought about Susie's answer as I sat on the mission steps, watching the people waiting patiently in line. In my private medical practice, with all its DRG frustrations, pre-certification approvals, oversight committees, and health care rationing guidelines, I was losing sight of my original purpose. What this country needs is to get back to the basics of medical practice!

Just then, Susie's Air Special shoes flashed by, as she prepared to leave the mission with her mom.

"Susie," I began. "I'd like you to have this present."

I pulled out the brown box that was still tucked under my arm, and watched Susie's big blue eyes get even bigger as she unwrapped the present, and held up a brand new, bright red dress.

"My first dress!" Susie smiled, as her eyes welled up with tears of joy. "I will always remember you1"

"And I will never forget you, Susie," I answered, fighting back my own tears. "You see, we're all involved in some type of struggle, but by pulling together, we can help each other. That's what medicine – and life – are all about!"

Author's Note: Dr. William Hale founded the Baptist Medical Mission Clinic in Oklahoma City.

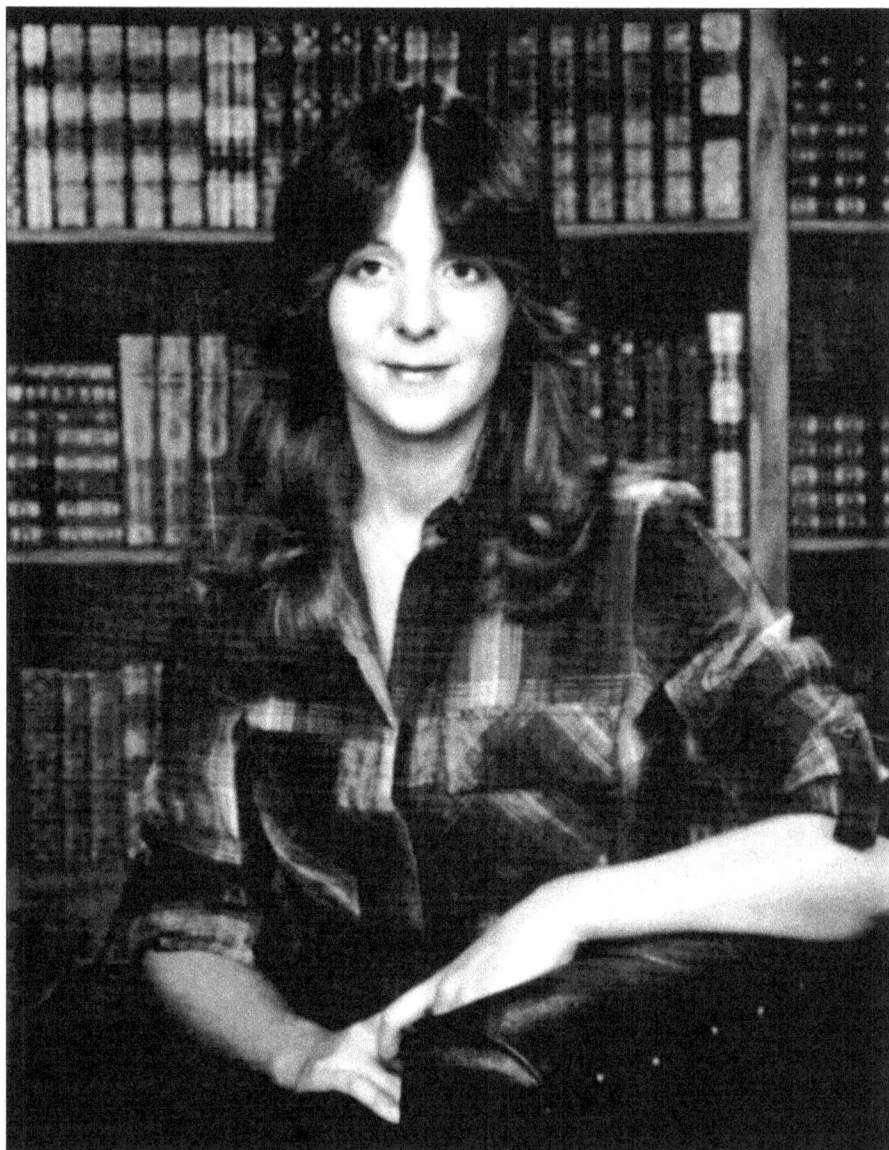

Nancy Morgan, age 34, sustained severe brain injury in a car accident on July 18, 1982, at the age of 25. She was cared for in a private home by her mother, Mary Ann Waken, and sister, Mary Pearson. Nancy has two other sisters, Jain Fair and Linda Franklin, and one brother, Dave Morgan.

TO NANCY

Each day I come to see you girl
To find if you still sleep
I know not where your soul has gone
I only wait and weep.

It doesn't seem that long ago
That fate got in the way
The accident that knocked you down
Seems only yesterday.

So I sit here by your side
And talk of days gone by
I don't know if you hear my words
Do you laugh or cry?

I dreamed the dreams that Mothers do-
Your destiny was mine
I thought that we'd together be
For the longest time.

I still hope that you'll come back
I know it's very sad
I still come to visit you
And talk of what we had.

One day when we both are gone
Our souls will upward go
Then we shall be joined as one
My girl, I miss you so!

THE GREAT PRETENDER

"Did you ever think of yourself as an imposter?" I asked Herb, as we sat in the Doctor's Lounge at Holy Christian Hospital, waiting for our cases to start.

"Not hardly," Herb replied. "It took me six years after medical school to become a plastic surgeon – I'm no imposter – I'm a real plastic surgeon!"

"Well, sure," I answered. "It took me six years after medical school to become a general surgeon. Then I had to pass a written exam, followed by an oral exam to get board certified."

"I'm not talking about credentials, Herb. What I mean is that sometimes I feel like I don't deserve all this credit and respect- I mean, I'm the same person I was in high school and college. Back then, I put on a white jacket and worked as a bus boy in a sorority. People barely noticed me!"

"And for good reason," Herb joked. "You were just a Nerd back then, who studied hard and didn't know how to enjoy college life!"

"True enough," I said. "But now people walk up to me and say, 'Doctor this' and 'Doctor that' – I mean, sometimes I think I don't deserve all this attention."

"I've done some pretty stupid things in my time – I'm lucky to be a doctor, thanks to a few people who stood up for me that I never got to thank. I mean, I was smart – I just wasn't mature. I just don't know that I deserve these accolades!"

"The important thing is that you learn from your mistakes," Herb replied.

"But, I'll just call you Mr. Truewater, if it makes you feel any better!"

"I think back to my medical school days," I continued. "I was a second-year medical student in Chicago, steeped in book learning, and short on social skills."

"I was assigned to do a patient history and physical. I put on my White Coat, told the patient that I was a student, and bravely proceeded to pretend like I was a doctor."

"Then I saw one of my colleagues – you know, the ones that are always one year ahead of you in school – you never catch up to them. He was walking in the medical ward of Holy Christian, wearing his scrubs, with his white coat and stethoscope- just like he was a real doctor!"

"I mean, isn't that what we do – we pretend – we play the role of a doctor."

"True enough, Dr. Truewater, we all have a role to play. You can be humble like a pediatrician or obnoxious like a surgeon!" Herb quipped.

"We go through a solemn, almost mystical, White Coat ceremony," I continued. "They call it a Transformation Ceremony – sort of like an anointing. But do clothes really make the man – or are they costumes that we use to masquerade?"

"Then we have a Graduation Ceremony, and we put on a robe and a fancy hat that has a tail on it, and we get a paper certificate that puts an MD or DO after our embossed name – and we keep on playing the role- we keep on pretending that we're doctors!"

"People worship us, but we're all just ordinary people!" I added.

"Trying to do extraordinary things!" Herb replied.

"But, it's not like you're some Charlatan, or some Great Pretender," Herb added. "You worked hard to get where you are today – you deserve a little respect, and society gives it to you!"

"We're not movie actors on a stage, Dr. Truewater. Movie actors pretend to be someone who they're not – and they're good at it. But we're not pretending to be doctors – we really are doctors, for God's sake!"

"I saw an interview with a rock star on TV," I interjected. "He says he adopts a Persona on stage when he's performing. Isn't that what we all do? I mean, if you're a judge in front of the jury, you put on a black robe, and you learn to play the role. We adopt a very serious doctor Persona when we're doctoring. Then we go out and have a beer at the local pub to let off steam!"

"True enough," Herb replied. "But do you think it's any easier for other professions? Take the ministry – do you think that first time preachers have a few self-doubts when they give their first sermon, preaching hellfire and brimstone to a crowded congregation, and promising eternal life to the believer?"

"We each have a role to play, Dr. Truewater. The doctor's role is to keep the patient alive and healthy. The preacher's role is to marry them and bury them!"

"That's all well and good, Herb. But we're dealing with human lives here – we're claiming to cure people of their afflictions by performing surgery and writing prescriptions. I don't know if I can promise that!"

"I mean, for the first five years, I looked too young and had some self-doubts. Then, for the next thirty years, the doubts vanished and everything was fine. Now, in the last five years, with my patients becoming senior citizens, I'm beginning to realize my shortcomings. I'm busy extolling the wonders of modern science, but my patients are dying, for God's sake – I'm calling the preacher to help!"

"Most of the time we don't cure people, Dr. Truewater- we don't prevent death- as doctors our role is to delay death and improve the quality of life."

"Besides, it's been shown that if you honestly believe that you're a doctor and you convey that self-confidence to your patient, then your patient is more likely to be healed! It's important to believe in yourself, Dr. Truewater, so that your patients can believe in you!"

"Of course, you have to be honest with your patient," Herb added. "You can't promise pie in the sky – you have to be realistic with your patient and explain the downside."

"And as a physician, it's important to give back to the community- look at those eye doctors who travel to Africa every year – or those doctors at St. Jude who treat children with cancer for free. Look at those missionary doctors who travel to far-off lands to treat disease and heal the afflicted!"

"You're right, Herb," I said. "Perhaps I'm being too critical!"

"I think to love and be secure in a profession, Dr. Truewater, is to be able to criticize it," Herb responded.

"But, you're right in a sense, Dr. Truewater," Herb added after further introspection.

"We all have self-doubts from time to time. In that sense, we're all actors – we're all role playing. You put on a White Coat and a stethoscope and you go play 'Doctor'. Then you go home and you play, 'Mommy' or 'Daddy' and 'Husband' or 'Wife'."

"Perhaps the most important thing," I concluded, as I put on my cap and mask and headed back to surgery, "is to learn to play multiple roles- don't play 'Doctor' so hard that you forget to take off your White Coat, slip into something casual, and play 'Parent' or 'Spouse' when you get back home!"

THE THRILL OF YOUR TOUCH

I want to be close
Let me put it this way –
I want to be next
To you night and day.

Physical love
Is gone in a flash
But the thrill of your touch
Has no other match!

There's all sorts of ways
To say I love you
There's all kinds of words
That say, "My love's true!"

I play all my records
The songs talk of love
I want you to know
I just need your hug!

For the one thing I like
About you the most
Is when I'm with you –
I love being close!

SOLVING THE AMELIA EARHART MYSTERY

The People wondered,
"Who were the perpetrators of this loathsome deed?"
But no one dared tell the People!
So, the Council decided, rather than share the Truth,
"Let the People live their Delusion!"
Thus, did the Myth endure!

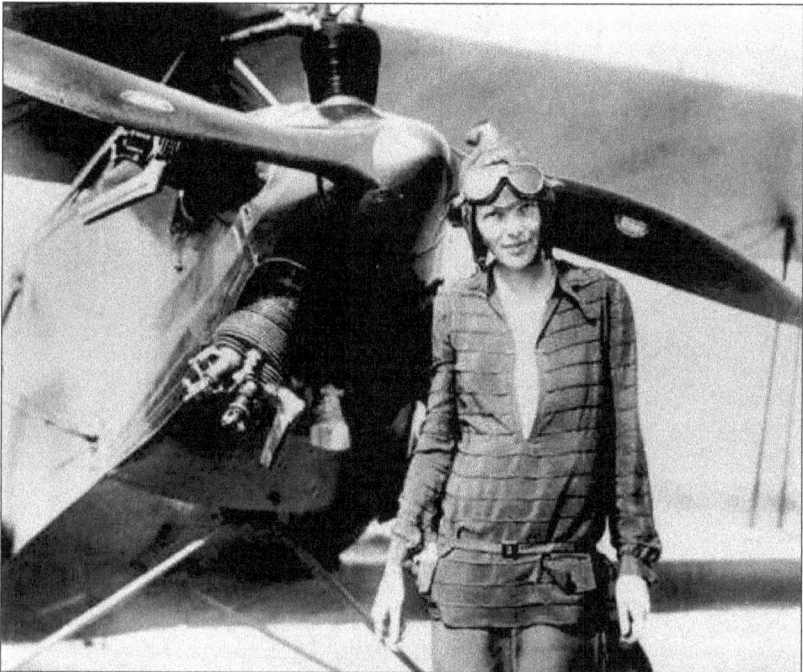

"Tell me, Dr. Truewater," Herb began, as we sat in the doctor's lounge, waiting for our cases to start.

"Oklahomans all know what happened to Will Rogers and Wiley Post, who died in a plane crash near Point Barrow, Alaska, in 1935. There's a 99s Museum of Women Pilots at Will Rogers Airport on Amelia Earhart Drive. But what happened to Amelia Earhart? You seem to be knowledgeable on these things – was Amelia and her navigator really lost at sea in her attempt to reach Howland Island?"

"There're a few things you've got to know first," I began. "Our military was very interested in knowing what the Japanese were up to in the Pacific in 1937. Now, Amelia was a commissioned officer in the U.S. Army Air Force Reserves – she actually met with FDR and Eleanor Roosevelt before her trip. Major Earhart and Merchant Mariner Fred Noonan will one day be honored with a state funeral and a military flyover!"

"Now, Amelia described her plane as a flying laboratory- it was state of the art, and souped up by what would be later known as the Kelly Johnson Lockheed Skunk Works for the extended range required to fly across the Pacific. A few days before her flight, the port engine turbo, which was also used to pressurize the cabin, actually overheated and caught on fire during a test flight and was successfully extinguished upon landing!"

"So, how was the plane brought down, if she was pressurized and could fly higher than the open-cockpit Japanese fighters?" Herb asked.

"I believe the port engine overheated and caught on fire," I replied. "There are reports that she was treated for burns to her left hand, arm, and shoulder at a hospital on Saipan."

"You mean, native islanders reported seeing Amelia Earhart?" Herb asked.

"You know, over 200 natives saw or heard of Amelia on the Mili Atoll in the Marshall Islands and Saipan in the Marianas – a white female pilot on a small Asian island with short hair, wearing long pants and boots, made quite a sensation! The American government solved that problem by calling it a mass hallucination on two islands 1,800 miles apart!"

"Using his sextant, Fred radioed a star fix to the Lexington aircraft carrier and was furious that the Americans cancelled a rescue – after all, the two countries were not at war! But the Japanese were demanding an agreement that the U.S. would stay out of the Pacific, which FDR refused!"

"In fact, FDR wanted photos of the illegal Japanese build-up on Truk island in Micronesia, as well as the Marshall Islands, that he could refer to the World Court!"

"Despite the secrecy surrounding Amelia, her presence in Saipan at the Garapan prison was common knowledge among the Chamorro natives! The little island would eventually issue commemorative stamps in 1987, with Amelia and Fred Noonan standing next to their damaged plane on the coral reef!"

"The Navy actually did a limited hangout in the movie, *Flight For Freedom* in 1943, with Rosalind Russel playing an animated, ground-breaking female aviator who was recruited by the Navy Intel boys to take reconnaissance photos and document the Japanese military build-up over the Marshall Islands!"

"When we invaded Saipan, Amelia's plane was found in a hanger with state-of-the-art Fairchild wing cameras still attached. In addition, a sailor broke into a safe and found Amelia's passport along with a Macy's receipt. Both were destroyed on orders from James Forrestal."

"If this is all true," Herb interjected, "why haven't the American people been told – I mean, this all happened over 85 years ago!"

"True enough," I replied. "But the Japanese are embarrassed because they executed Amelia and Fred for a peacetime venture in violation of international law."

"And the Americans are embarrassed because they would be forced to admit that Amelia was on a dangerous spy mission, which they had previously denied. In addition, a rescue mission had been cancelled, along with a refusal to negotiate and concede the Pacific waters to Japan. So, both sides agreed to bury the story," I concluded.

"The official story, provided by James Forrestal was that, since Japan and the United States were no longer at war, it was important to bury the Amelia Earhart story in order to limit anti-Japanese sentiment."

"That just seems hard for me to believe," Herb responded. "I mean, why would our government go to such extremes to hide the truth?"

"I call it pride – some people call it arrogance!"

I put on my mask and headed back to surgery. Sometimes the truth is just too much to handle – it's much easier to sell the deception and let sleeping dogs lie!"

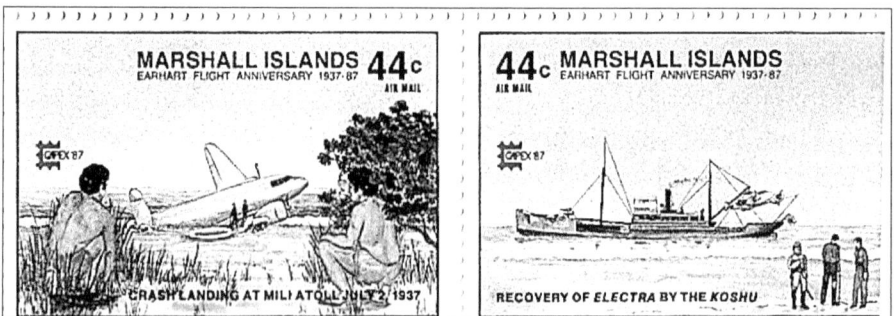

Stamps issued by the Marshall Islands in 1987, showing Amelia and Fred standing next to their damaged plane on a coral reef in the Marshall Islands.

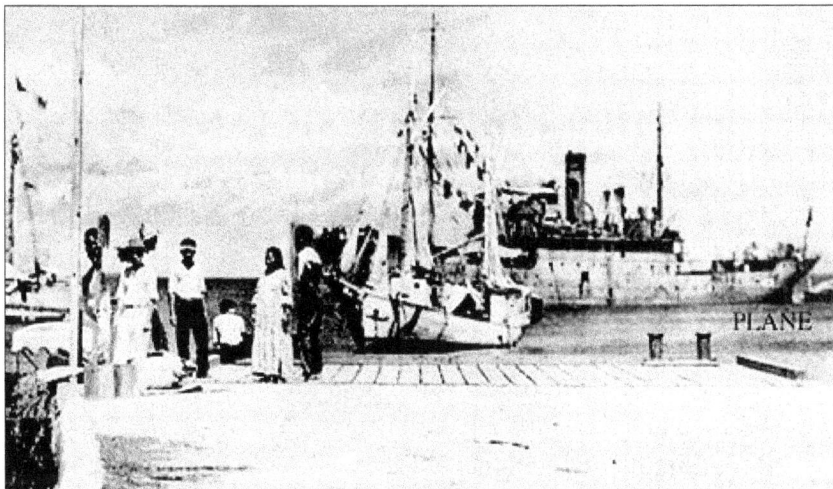

Earhart and Noonan on dock in Jaluit in the Marshall Islands with Koshu ship in background and Electra twin engine plane on rear deck.

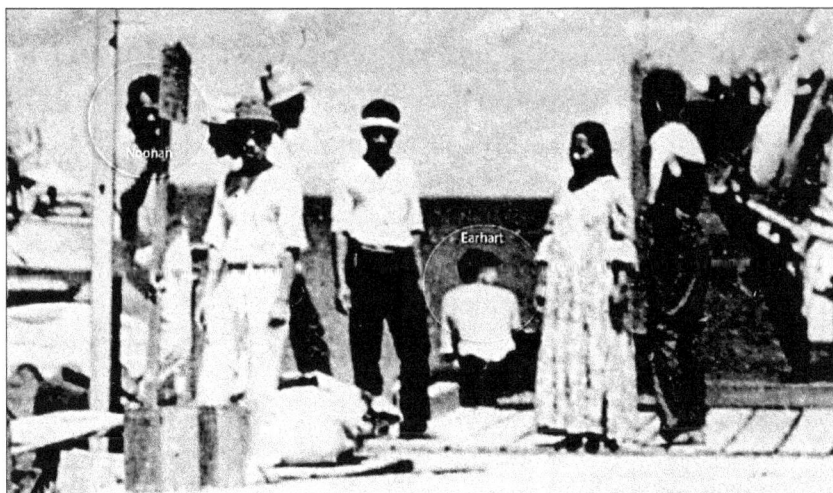

One photo analyst concluded that this photo was a "very good" match for Amelia and Fred, as well as the Electra plane. Native women did not wear short hair or slacks and the photo is also a match for Fred's hairline and thin, six-foot height.

THE ELDER PHYSICIAN

I look upon the Elder Physician
Like a wizened sailor
Who has traveled near and far
And seen the open ocean with all its fury
And the quiet sea like a placid lake
Beguiling its true nature.

The Elder Physician is quiet and smiling
As he views his younger compatriots,
With brand new medical degrees and credentials,
Scurrying by with a quick hello,
To an old man with a black bag and a dark suit,
As they scamper around the hospital
With a full sense of mission and purpose,
Imbued with new powers and tributes –
Healing the sick, birthing the children,
Prescribing cures with the latest scientific remedies –
Much better now than they used to be, mind you,
And surgically mending worn arteries and weakened tissues
With man-made devices.

The Elder Physician has done all that
And more
He is no longer mesmerized
By the wonders of science.

With his thick skin
He brushes off the angry arrows of the afflicted
And with his soft heart,
He understands with sympathy the human condition.

He treats the soul now
And his patients revere him
With all the wonder of an elder parent
Who has stood the test of time.

The Elder Physician
Has weathered the storm of all life's indignities
And tragedies and shortcomings
Joining with his declining census of elderly patients
Who by now are senior friends
Having shared the births and deaths
Of Mothers and Fathers and children and grandchildren,
And seen the ravages of time which science cannot avail.

The Elder Physician, with one quiet statement,
Proves the bond that joins us all,
As he turns his weathered, time worn face
To his awe-struck patient, and smiles, and says,
"How are we today?

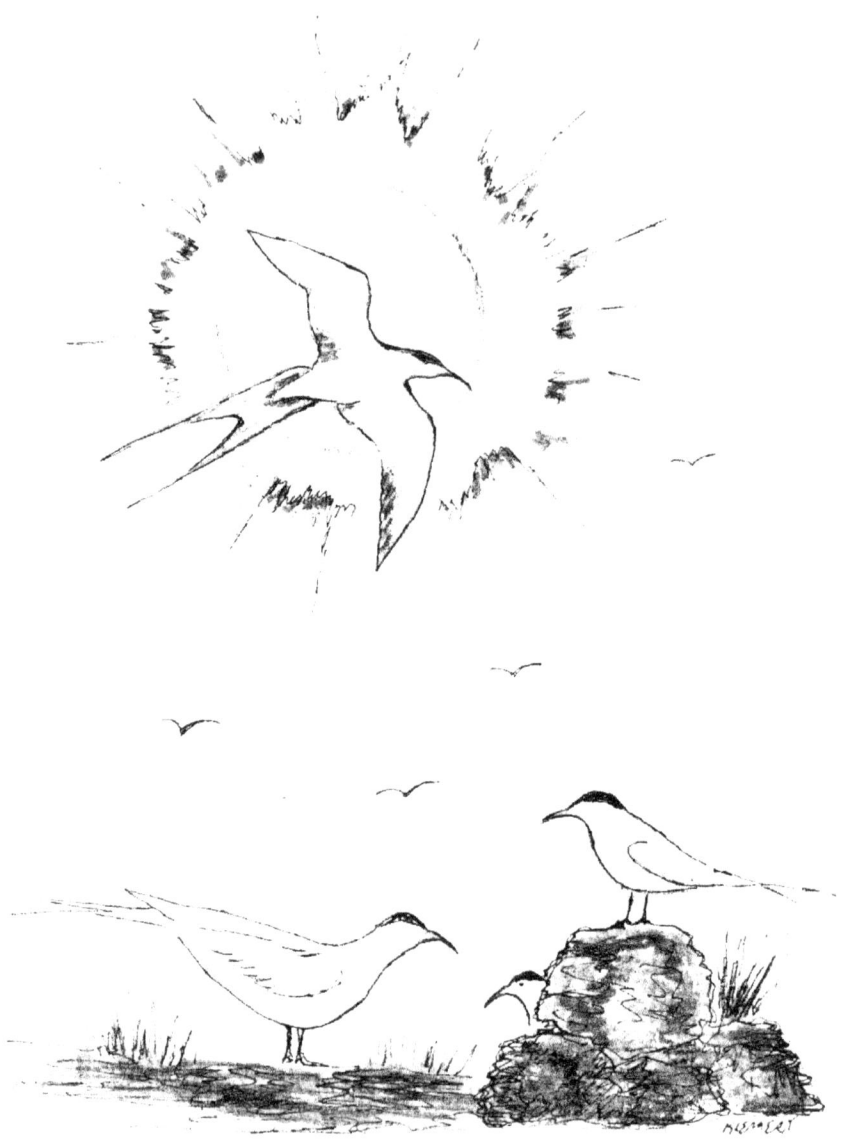

THE ARCTIC TERN

I am an Arctic tern
I seek the summer sun
In my heart I always yearn
To go where the spring is young.

I fly 'round the world each year
From Northern to Southern Pole
I stay when the weather is warm
And leave when the cold wind blows.

I sail down the Western Coast
Then 'round the Cape of Good Hope
And when my days start to shorten
I head for the Northern Slope.

And though I must travel far
In my quest to follow the sun
I may not find all the answers
But the journey is half the fun!

THE ANOINTED

I never considered myself to be "anointed." True, I'm a physician, but I had to fight to be a physician. It wasn't handed to me. And I had to fight to be a surgeon. Nobody gave me that, either. But I was never the "anointed one" – I always struggled to achieve my goals.

I also had few illusions about myself or the world about me. I never viewed the universe as a friendly place. Sure, I had people helping me, and I'm eternally grateful for them – my parents, my sister, my extremely valuable friends, my professors, and my wife.

But when bad things happened, I never tried to find anything good about it – I figured things were bad because they were bad. I wasn't bitter about it – I just accepted it as best I could and went on.

I know it's possible to be awed by the natural beauty of birds chirping in the trees. I think that's important. But I'm also aware that those birds are chirping because they are fighting over territory, competing for a mate, or warning of danger.

Even the tree is involved in a struggle for existence, reaching down with its roots to gather water, and spreading its leaves to gather the all-important sunlight necessary for survival.

While I'm not a skeptic, I never really believed in the power of positive thinking, either. Somehow, positive thinking reminded me too much of the door-to-door salesman – there was always some part of reality that you were denying. Why should broken eggs always be turned into omelets? Maybe they weren't meant to be omelets. Maybe they were just meant to be broken eggs.

I believe in God. I think there is an Almighty Being that guides our actions. But I'm not sure that God punishes us for our actions. I think we do that to ourselves. In many ways, we create our own heaven and our own hell. John Kennedy once said, "In this world, God's work must truly be our own," and I believe that. However, I still give God the glory, for God is the one who makes it all possible in the first place.

When I was in medical school at the University of Illinois, there were always a few students who considered themselves "special" or even "anointed." They felt they were born to be doctors, that being a doctor was part of their destiny. Often, one of their parents was a doctor or some famous person. They were often gifted, and didn't have to work hard for their grades. They viewed the universe as basically friendly, and the world as a nice place to live.

The professors liked "the anointed ones", because they scored well on their exams, and always had a positive attitude. In fact, they acted like they were already doctors – even though they hadn't yet seen a patient. I was friendly with my professors, but I never had a religious experience with any of them – they just seemed like regular people to me.

During my surgery residency, there were always one or two residents who felt they were "anointed." They quoted Halsted's principles of surgery like the Ten Commandments. I sometimes worried about them because they would walk the hospital halls at night muttering things like, "maintain meticulous hemostasis", and "avoid tissue injury by gentle handling of the tissues." They hung onto every word of their attending physician, as if he or she were dropping pearls of gold – which would sometimes be fashioned into bullets for unsuspecting medical students.

I always wondered how some surgery residents could maintain such an adoration for their attending physicians and, at the same time, such complete disdain for the medical students. Didn't they realize that, once upon a time, attending physicians were medical students too?

As I look back twenty years later, I'd have to say it's all a matter of personal perspective. The "anointed" people start out with a positive view of the world, and, after the usual round of divorces, bankruptcy, war, and personal tragedies, decide it's not such a friendly universe after all. The "unanointed" people start out with a slightly more negative view of the world and, with a little success, become slightly more optimistic.

There is one important difference, however. The "anointed" feel that, in the end, God will protect us from our misdeeds and shortcomings – that our lives, and even our existence, will have a positive, happy ending. The "unanointed" feel that man will reap his just desserts – that man is ultimately responsible for shaping his own destiny, and that what you sow is what you reap.

The world becomes less certain, and life becomes more tenuous. That is why I will always remain "unanointed."

THE ROBERT KENNEDY ASSASSINATION

The year was 1968
Filled with war rallies and political hate!
During a time of great turmoil –
Our country was about to boil!

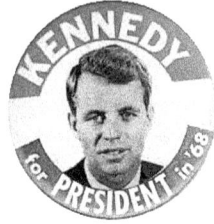

"Dr. Truewater," Herb began as we sat in the surgery lounge waiting for our cases to start, "I'm not a conspiracy theorist, but is there one piece of evidence you can tell me that would convince me that Sirhan Sirhan was not a lone gunman in the Robert Kennedy assassination?"

"Robert Maheu," I replied.

"Wasn't he personal assistant to Howard Hughes?" Herb asked.

"More than that," I replied. "Robert Maheu acted as a liaison between the CIA and the Mafia. He testified that he was contacted by CIA "wet works" manager, William Harvey, in the late fifties to organize an assassination team in the ill-fated attempt to take out Fidel Castro. Allen Dulles, CIA director, was later fired by JFK."

"Maheu recruits Johnny Roselli in the Mafia to organize a hit team. Roselli in turn contacts Sam Giancana in Chicago and Carlos Marcello in New Orleans to form an anti-Castro hit team."

"But what does this have to do with Senator Robert Kennedy?" Herb asked.

"Fast forward to 1967," I replied. "I was a graduate student in biochemistry at Indiana University one cold morning in October, 1967, when anti-Viet Nam protestors booed Secretary of State Dean Rusk. Indiana University made national news!"

"Later, Robert Kennedy decides to run for President and gets a standing ovation at Indiana University in April, 1968, promising to end the Viet Nam War. I couldn't get into the auditorium due to the large crowd, so I waited outside. I was less than ten feet away from RFK, cheering him on, as he got into his open-air convertible in front of the auditorium and left the campus."

"Needless to say, the CIA was not too happy about Robert Kennedy's anti-war stance. He seemed to be following in the

THE ROBERT KENNEDY ASSASSINATION

footsteps of brother John, who had threatened to break the CIA into a thousand pieces. The last thing the Deep State wanted was another Kennedy President!"

"But what does this have to do with Robert Maheu?" Herb asked.

"Fast forward again to June, 4, 1968 at the mafia-run Ambassador Hotel. It's midnight, and Senator Robert Kennedy has just won the California primary and finishes his victory speech. There was no Secret Service protection. And there was a last-minute replacement in RFK's hotel security. His security guard, Thane Eugene Cesar, is a newly added member of the Ace detective agency, which is also a new hire for the Ambassador Hotel. RFK was routed through the kitchen by multiple unknown individuals, which was not the planned route. Cesar is directly behind and to the right of RFK as he walks through the crowded kitchen and Sirhan Sirhan opens fire. Author Lisa Pease, who wrote *A Lie Too Big to Fail* about the RFK assassination, found two databases that listed a man named Thane Cesar as a CIA hitman. Cesar then states that he 'retired' from his new job one week later."

"Sirhan worked as a trainer at the race track and was an inveterate gambler with a large gambling debt, according to Giancana. Let's just say they made him an offer he couldn't refuse."

"Witnesses report Cesar, the security guard, pulling out his gun and firing some shots. Robert Kennedy is shot and pulls off Cesar's clip-on tie as he falls to the ground and makes the sign of the crucifix. Forensic pathologist Dr Cyril Wecht analyzes the powder burns to RFK's head wound and determines that one fatal shot was fired from behind within one inch of RFK's right ear. Dr. Noguchi determined that all of RFK's wounds were fired from behind, and RFK also has powder burns on the back of his jacket."

"From Sirhan Sirhan?" Herb asks.

"According to Roosevelt Greer, Sirhan remained in front of RFK and, according to 70 witnesses, never got closer than three feet to RFK because of a steam table while Greer held him. Sirhan, firing multiple shots, makes an excellent decoy, wounds several bystanders, and even puts a bullet in the door frame, which is later removed and disappears. One student takes multiple pictures in the kitchen, which establishes everyone's position, but police chief Daryl Gates and the Los Angeles police classify the photos for 20 years and then manage to lose them."

"And Robert Maheu?" Herb asks. "I'm still waiting."

"It turns out that Robert Maheu created the Ace Detective Agency, and that this is Cesar's first and last assignment. An audio recording relates two double sounds that are too close together to be fired from the same gun. And thirteen recorded shots means that two guns were involved."

"So, the same man, Robert Maheu, who the CIA hires to organize a Mafia hit team to take out Fidel Castro, later creates the Ace Detective Agency that is hired by the Ambassador Hotel to protect Robert Kennedy!"

I'm not a conspiracy theorist," Herb replied, as he put on his mask and headed back to start his cleft palate surgery. "But if this Robert Maheu involvement is not a coincidence, then my lone gunman view of the world is beginning to crumble!"

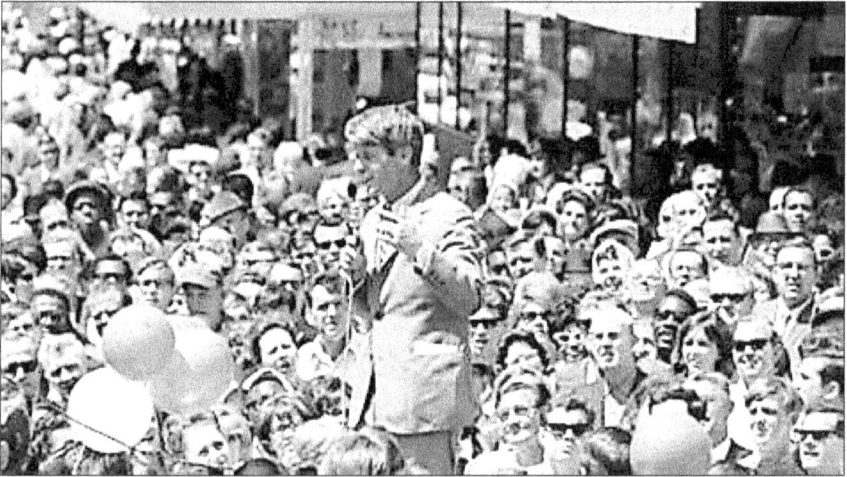

Senator Robert Kennedy, 1968

Thus, the murder of Robert Kennedy
Would go down in history
As the random act of a crazy man
Who was never part of a conspiracy plan!

MAXIMUM BOB

Every once in a while, you meet someone you never forget. Such was the case with Bob Macintire. Bob was one of the most well-rounded surgery residents in Oklahoma history. Standing 6 ft 6 in and weighing in excess of 250 pounds, few people, not even chief residents, argued with Maximum Bob. I'm not sure how he earned his nickname – some said because of his size. Others said because of his forceful personality.

Bob started out as a preacher for one of those churches where you didn't have to go to seminary school. His photographic memory for Biblical scripture, coupled with his story-telling ability, made Bob the most popular and knowledgeable Sunday School teacher in Hominy, Oklahoma. Later, Bob moved to Piedmont, where he started his own congregation in the auditorium of the Will Rogers Elementary School. The church was half-way between Mustang and Yukon, so he called it MY Church. Rumor has it that Bob performed a little faith-healing on Sunday nights, when the "Voice of God" spoke to him.

After about five years, with a successful congregation of over 100 families, Reverend Macintire decided to become a doctor. I'm not sure exactly why, though Bob made numerous references to Christ the Physician, and turned his church over to his assistant Pastor.

Being a naturally gifted student, the University of Oklahoma Medical School Admissions Committee had only one stipulation: no faith healing – Bob had to adhere strictly to the principles of human physiology for his diagnosis and treatment of the human condition.

After medical school, Bob enrolled in the general surgery program, where he was my junior resident. With his slow, lumbering walk, you could literally feel Maximum Bob approaching, as the old wooden floor of the Main South surgery ward began to tremble.

"I've got a problem, Bob," I began.

"What's that, Truewater?" Bob asked. Bob always called his fellow surgery residents by their last name, sort of like basic training.

"I've got a little seven-year-old boy with a hot appendix," I replied.

"Fix it, Truewater," Maximum Bob barked.

"But there's a problem," I answered. "The parents don't want it fixed. They say that God is testing them, and if they pray hard enough, their son will heal without surgery."

"Then they went into this story about Abraham and Isaac, and how God tested Abraham to see if —"

"I know the story," Bob interrupted, "but that has nothing to do with faith healing. We'll have to get a court order."

"I threatened to get a court order, but the parents say their religious beliefs are protected by the Constitution."

"Let me talk to them," Bob offered.

I went back to the emergency room and explained to little Franklin's parents that I was calling in a consultant. I had no idea what Maximum Bob was planning. I had heard of such cases making headlines in the national newspapers, and I was not about to become a celebrity. Worse yet, I feared for little Franklin's life – he was now beginning to double over with pain.

"We believe in the power of God Almighty to heal our son," Franklin's father said.

"But sometimes God expects us to handle our own problems," I tried to reason. "I believe that God acts through us, in order to help us solve our problems."

"By now, little Franklin was beginning to cry with pain, and I was about to lose my temper.

"Nothing can change our minds," Franklin's father replied resolutely, as the floor began to vibrate with Maximum Bob's impending arrival. The bewildered couple turned toward the door to face the source of the disturbance.

"I'm Dr. Bob Macintire," he began.

"We're Mr. and Mrs. Hempstead," Franklin's father replied. "We believe in the power of God to cure Franklin's malady."

"Then, why did you bring Franklin to the emergency room?" Maximum Bob asked.

"I wanted to make sure what was wrong," Franklin's father answered, somewhat flustered. "Besides, I can't stand to see the sight of little Franklin in pain. I'm sure that God will act to help Franklin."

What happened next absolutely boggled my imagination. Maximum Bob fell to his knees with a giant thump that shook the picture of St. Luke the Physician off the south wall of the Holy Christian Hospital emergency room. He broke out in a sweat that drenched his forehead, and began talking in a language that I couldn't recognize. After about five minutes, Maximum Bob slowly got up, with a smile that made his entire face glow.

"Are you alright?" Franklin's Mother asked, as they came out of the corner. "For a moment, we worried about your sanity!"

Maximum Bob spoke not a word, but slowly looked about the room, as if to make some magnificent revelation. He looked carefully at Franklin, then slowly turned to Franklin's parents.

Maximum Bob lumbered over to the beleaguered parents. The shadow from his massive 250-pound frame easily dwarfed them like a pair of shivering toothpicks. The couple slipped back to the wall, and wrapped their arms around each other, as if preparing for the wrath of God.

Maximum Bob looked them slowly in the eye, then whispered softly, as a lone tear rolled down each cheek.

"God spoke to me," Bob began. "It was the most wonderful experience of my entire life!"

"What did he say?" Franklin's mother asked, as she drew even closer to her husband.

"He told me, 'Fix Franklin's appendix!'" Maximum Bob somberly replied. "He told me, sometimes God's work must truly be our own!"

Just then, little Franklin, who had been silent during the entire interview, decided to speak.

"I want Big Bob to take out my appendix!" Franklin demanded.

And that was that. The bewildered parents readily signed the operative permit, and we took out Franklin's ruptured appendix that night. Little Franklin went home five days later.

As the happy couple prepared to leave the hospital with their beloved son, I overheard Franklin talking to his parents.

"Did God really talk to Dr. Macintire?" Franklin asked his father.

"I believe in divine intervention," Franklin's father replied. "And it was absolutely divine that Dr. Macintire intervened!"

DON'T ROCK THE BOAT!

Gladys Schmidt called me today. Gladys has been a patient of mine for fifteen years. She is 89 years old and amazingly healthy.

"Dr. Truewater, I have a bone to pick with you!" Gladys exclaimed irately.

"What's the problems, Gladys?" I asked somewhat defensively.

"I went to the Pheasant Springs Shopping Mall Senior Health Fair today as part of their 'Respect Your Elders' celebration."

"Good!" I exclaimed. "Did they find anything wrong, Gladys?"

"Everything was normal except for my cholesterol. They told me to contact my doctor right away. You never told me I had a cholesterol problem, Dr. Truewater!"

"How high was your cholesterol on the screening exam?" I asked.

"It says my serum cholesterol is 220!" Gladys sobbed.

"That's about what you normally run," I explained, trying to allay her anxiety.

"You mean, I've had a cholesterol problem all these years and you never told me?" Gladys screamed.

"Well, not exactly, Gladys," I replied. "I mean, yes, you've always run a serum cholesterol around 220. But, for the last fourteen years, that's been considered normal."

"I don't understand," Gladys interrupted. "How can a serum cholesterol be considered normal for fourteen years, and the same value become abnormal on the fifteenth year? That doesn't make sense!"

"Well, Gladys," I began, "what they've done is change the definition for what's normal. The upper limit of normal for serum cholesterol used to be 300. Then the National Heart, Lung, and Blood Institute lowered it to 240, and most recently, they lowered it again to 200. With your total cholesterol value of 220, you've now got a cholesterol problem," I explained.

"I'm getting confused!" Gladys exclaimed.

"I wouldn't worry too much about it, Gladys," I stated, trying to console her. "Besides, total serum cholesterol isn't all that important, anyway. What's really important is the ratio of high density to low density lipoproteins."

"I'm getting more confused!" Gladys exclaimed. "I can't figure out how a cholesterol value can be normal for fourteen years and be abnormal on the fifteenth year!"

"Well, what they did, Gladys, was compare serum cholesterol with people living in other parts of the world, like Africa, where people eat a lot more roughage and have lower rates of heart disease. They also have a lower stool transit time and a lower risk of colon cancer."

"Stool transit time?" Gladys queried. "You mean, somebody actually measures how long it takes for the poop to travel?"

"Yes," I responded, "we in the medical profession like to see large, bulky stools! It's a sign of good health! It means you're eating lots of fiber. Eating more roughage and less fat also helps lower your serum cholesterol," I explained.

"First, you measure serum cholesterol and after fifteen years they change the values for normal! Now, you tell me you're measuring stool transit times. I suppose the next thing you'll tell me is that doctors walk around the hospital eating apples and bananas!" Gladys exclaimed.

"As a matter of fact, they do," I responded, "though I must admit the cookie tray disappears first!"

"Let me say this, Dr. Truewater," Gladys concluded. "I respect the efforts of the Pheasant Springs Mall Senior Health Fair and the concern they show for my well-being. But whatever I've been doing for the last eighty-nine years is working just fine for me, and I'm not about to buy a stopwatch and worry about my stool transit time or my newly discovered cholesterol problem! Thank you very much1"

What patients sometimes don't understand is that medicine is not an exact science. Due to genetic and geographic differences, a normal lab value for one person may be abnormal for another. And certainly, if someone has been healthy for eighty-nine years, my advice would be, "Don't rock the boat!"

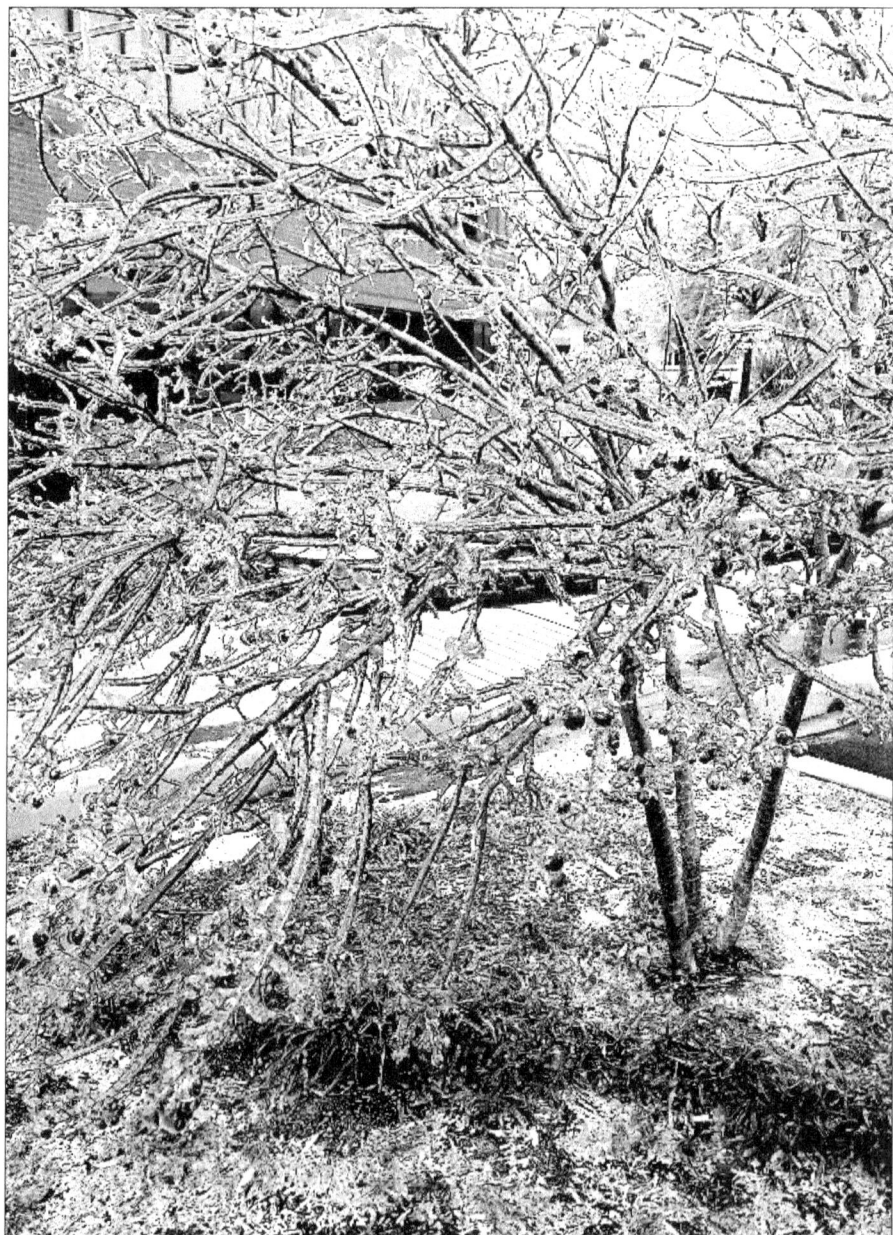

THE FLAME OF PEACE

One night as I meditate
I pretend to levitate
I float above the frozen ground –
I can see for miles around!

The ice storm petrifies the leaves
The little birds hide from the breeze
The nights are cold as winter drones
And people huddle in their homes.

And as I leave the city's light
The stars above shine oh so bright!
I look upon the virgin earth
And think about our planet's birth.

I see no boundaries down below
All the earth is one big globe!
If man could somehow stop his fight
Perhaps the world would then unite!

As I come down from the air
I see small steeples everywhere
People there inside do pray
And hope that peace will come some day!

I wake up – the room is cold
I put a log upon the stove
If I could a spark ignite,
The flame of peace would burn so bright!

GETTING SLEEP

The most difficult part about being a physician is getting enough sleep. In fact, as a medical student, I had a hard time getting any sleep at all. One emergency phone call would usually ruin my whole night, as I found it difficult to forget about my patient and go back to sleep.

After a middle-of-the-night phone call, I would toss and turn for about thirty minutes, wondering how my patient was doing, half-expecting another call. If it didn't come, I would pick up the phone and call back myself, just to make sure everything was alright. Besides, my chief resident, Alex Knockbutten, never let me get any sleep.

"Always cover your rear, Truewater," Alex would say. "Remember Murphy's Law – if something can go wrong, it will!"

As a result, I spent most of my residency worrying about Murphy's Law and covering my rear. Every time I did a procedure, I explained it thoroughly to the family, as well as the potential complications, documented it carefully in the progress notes, then dictated my operative procedure. Not that any of this was bad – being paranoid, I was much better prepared to meet the unexpected. It's just that my sleep suffered as a result.

As the years have gone by, however, I have gradually adapted to my profession. After all, with the exception of medical students and residents, a person cannot live forever without sleep. Sooner or later, your performance suffers. I am proud to say that after ten years of private practice, I am now capable of sleeping the whole night, even if a few midnight calls for sleeping pills or even admitting orders should chance to wake me up. Perhaps, with my years of experience, I have gained a certain security that has given me peace of mind, to say nothing of a restful night.

Oh, occasionally, I'll have a worrisome dream or two, wondering how my patients are doing, but at least I'm able to sleep. Take last night, for example. I dreamed that a patient of mine, Ralph Greer, was admitted with early symptoms of appendicitis. Then I dreamed that I had criticized the charge nurse, Mary Atwater, for waking me up in the middle of the night. I told the nurse to place Mr. Greer under observation and give him intravenous fluids. When I work up the following morning, I wondered what in the world made me dream about Ralph Greer, since I hadn't seen Ralph in several years.

"The subconscious mind is an amazing thing," I said to myself, as I walked into the hospital. I resolved to call Ralph that day, just to put my mind at ease.

I made leisurely rounds with Mary Atwater that morning on Three West Quad.

"It's so nice to make rounds after a full night's sleep without interruptions," I told Mary. "I also think the patients appreciate having a surgeon who's well-rested."

"No doubt about it," Mary replied. "I could use a little rest myself – I started work at 11 pm last night and won't finish the back half of this double shift until 3 pm today."

"You nurses need to get more rest," I answered sympathetically, knowing that Mary was the sole supporter of her three children."

"You're right, Dr. Truewater," Mary replied. "There's nothing worse than a crabby nurse except maybe a crabby doctor," Mary added with a half-smile on her face.

"I agree completely," I added.

As I left the floor to start my office, I saw Mary waving her arms to come back.

"Dr. Truewater!" Mary exclaimed. "There's one more patient you forgot to check!"

"Are you sure" I asked. I carefully rechecked my list as I walked back toward the floor.

"Don't you remember?" Mary asked.

"I've seen everybody on this list," I replied confidently.

"But what about Ralph Greer?" Mary asked.

"How do you know about Ralph Greer?" I asked suspiciously. Up until now, my supposed dream had been the object of my own private thoughts.

"You admitted him last night at 3 am with possible appendicitis," Mary said. "I apologized for waking you up, and you placed him under observation and gave him IV fluids. I'm surprised you don't remember."

I'm at the age where very few things make me blush any more. But this time I was genuinely embarrassed. This must be what old age is all about.

"Why, yes, of course," I mumbled. "I thought he was on a different floor," I added lamely, as I scribbled Mr. Greer's name on my patient list.

I took out Ralph Greer's acutely inflamed appendix that afternoon. The following morning, I was again making rounds when I noticed Nurse Atwater.

"Oh, Mary," I said. "I want to thank you for reminding me about Mr. Greer yesterday morning. I must have made a Freudian slip or something."

Suddenly, I remembered that I had been rude to Nurse Atwater in my dream.

"I'm sorry if I was rude to you on the phone yesterday," I said. "It was late at night and I was tired. You're not going to believe this, but I actually thought I was dreaming when I talked to you about Ralph Greer."

"I accept your apology, Dr. Truewater," Mary replied.

"You see," I explained, "when I started medical school, I never got enough sleep. Now it seems, I'm sleeping too well!"

LEARNING TO COMPENSATE

They say that one sure sign of old age is loss of memory. I've always been a little forgetful, but I never really worried about it too much. In fact, I think that sometimes people expect their doctor to be a little absent-minded – take, for example, the well revered absent-minded professor, who is adored by everybody.

After many years of denial, I've decided to accept my forgetfulness. I've even learned ways to compensate for it. Take, for example, the halls at Our Lady of The Saints Hospital. I've been taking care of patients at this hospital for ten years now, and I still get lost! Part of the problem is that the hospital was built in four stages, with each stage being tacked onto the one adjacent to it. Needless to say, there was never any thought given to central planning. I've actually seen visitors try to walk into the morgue after making a wrong turn on the way to the cafeteria!

There are two banks of elevators at Our Lady Hospital that face each other. If you get off the west bank, you must turn left to get to the doctor's parking lot. If you get off the east bank, you must turn right. Unfortunately, the two banks look identical when you step off the elevator. Most visitors do a double or even triple take before they get their bearings.

This, however, does not look very professional. Instead, what I now do is always turn left when I get off the elevators, doing so in a rather positive, confident fashion. Half, the time, this turns out to be correct, and I'm on my way to the parking lot. The other half of the time, I realize that I'm going the wrong way. At this time, I have several options. I can stop and get a Coke, as the canteen is in this direction. Or I can stop and talk to the volunteer at the desk before changing directions.

I've also learned the art of triggering my beeper with a flick of the wrist (especially handy when I want to leave breakfast meetings early). If I realize that I'm going the wrong way, I set my beeper ringing, suddenly stop to silence it, and then reverse my direction, as if heading to answer a page. The last thing anyone suspects is that I'm lost.

My resourcefulness knows no bounds. One day, I walked out to my car to go home for the evening. I was carrying a dozen long-stem roses – a surprise gift from one of my patients for removing her gallbladder. My mind was also preoccupied with the care of a patient who wasn't doing well.

Needless to say, when I got to the parking lot, I had completely forgotten where my car was parked. Not to panic. Instead of wandering aimlessly through the parking lot, looking this way and that for my car, I resorted back to my days of military training. This involved systematically "sweeping" the parking lot by walking up and down each of the rows in a purposeful fashion.

This particular day, however, the new parking lot attendant noticed my behavior and began looking at me rather suspiciously, like I was about to hot wire someone's car and drive away, roses and all.

"Do you belong in this parking lot?" he asked rather gruffly, not realizing that I was one of the doctors.

"I'm Dr. Truewater," I replied. "I'm just trying to get a little exercise," I added, too flustered to tell him that I couldn't find my car.

"Oh, sorry doctor," the embarrassed guard replied before driving off in his golf cart.

At this point, I was getting desperate. Suddenly, I had a flash of inspiration. I triggered my beeper, then pulled my cellular phone out of my coat pocket, as if answering a page. I put in a quick call to my office.

"Hello, Dr. Truewater," Lola answered. "I didn't expect to hear from you so soon after leaving the office."

"I need you to do me a favor," I told Lola, as I continued my authoritative walk through the parking lot, trying not to look lost.

"Sure, Dr. Truewater. How can I help?"

"I want you to look out the south window of the office and see if you can spot my car with the binoculars. I seem to have misplaced it," I whispered into the phone.

"I don't see your car, Dr. Truewater," Lola replied after a few minutes. "However, I do see someone who looks like a security guard walking in circles. He's holding a walkie talkie, and he's in the third row to the south. You might ask him for help."

"That's me," I responded. "I'm using my cell phone."

"Oh, sorry, Dr. Truewater," Lola replied. "Come to think of it, didn't you tell me you parked on the covered north side of the building today because of the hailstorm warning this morning?"

"Very good, Lola, "I said, turning toward the north parking lot.

When I arrived home that evening, roses in hand, Margaret greeted me at the door.

"A dozen long-stem roses – I don't believe it!" she shrieked, as she jubilantly accepted my patient's roses. "For the first time in ten years, you actually remembered our anniversary!"

Somewhat flushed, and momentarily at a loss for words, I smiled and replied, "Happy Anniversary, my love!"

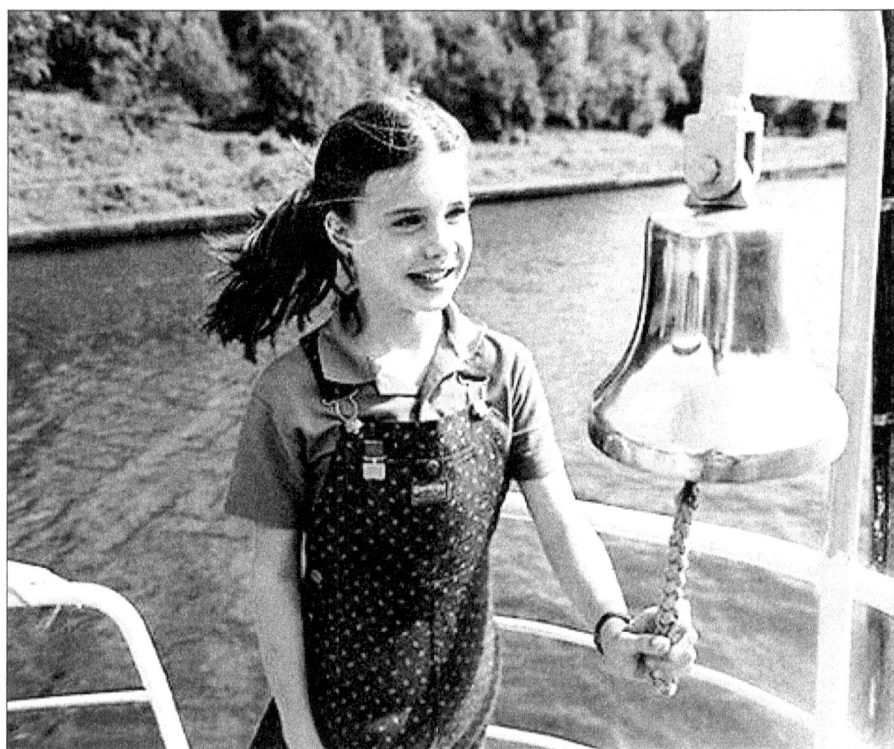

Samantha Smith

SAMANTHA'S PRAYER

Let me tell you the story of Samantha
She was a gift from God above
She wrote a letter to Russia
And went on a mission of love.

She went to the tomb of Lenin
And walked past the Kremlin walls
They talked of a time not forgotten
With soldiers and cannonballs.

She made friends at the youth camp
And wore a white bow in her hair
They asked about clothing and music
And what was it like over there?

Then all of the kids started dancing
They danced where the night never ends
She hoped with her friend named Natasha
That they would ever be friends!

Then each made a wish for the future
And tossed it upon the sea
Samantha wished something quite special –
She prayed for friendship and peace.

And though this young girl has now left us
I think of Samantha's prayer
What a wonderful seed she has planted
That there might be peace everywhere!

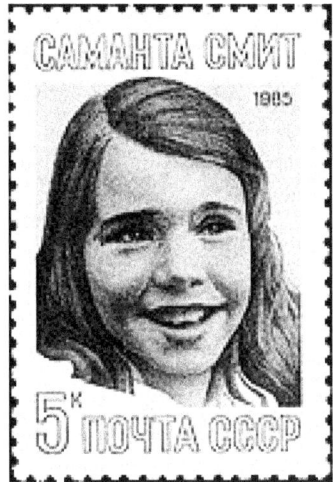

Samantha Smith and her parents, Jane and Arthur Smith, visited Russia on a mission of peace after she wrote a letter to the Russian government promoting peace and an end to the cold war.
Samantha spent time in a youth camp that summer, when she met her friend, Natasha. Tragically, Samantha and her father were killed in a plane crash in Auburn, Maine in 1985 at the age of 13 shortly after returning from Russia.

THE COMPUTER CRAZIES

I am told that computers are one of the great advances of our decade, if not the entire century – a veritable tribute to the wonders of modern science. But computers are starting to drive me crazy.

On the way home from work yesterday, my wife asked me to pick up a pizza with sausage, bacon bits, and extra cheese. I walked into Sam's Sooner Pizza and the conversation went something like this.

"I'd like to order a sausage pizza," I said. "How much are the extra ingredients?"

"Two dollars for each extra ingredient, sir," the boy politely responded.

"Then I'd like to order sausage, bacon bits, and extra cheese," I replied.

"Can't do that sir," the pizza boy politely replied. "You can only order two ingredients."

"How come?" I asked.

"Something's wrong with the pizza computer," the boy replied. "The computer charges $24 for the third ingredient. They're trying to fix it down at the main office."

"Well, what if I just pay you two dollars for the third ingredient, and you don't enter it in the computer?" I pleaded.

"Can't do that, sir," the boy replied. "Internal Revenue and all that tax stuff, you know."

I settled for a pizza with sausage and bacon bits and figured my computer problems were over. Or so I thought.

The following morning, my office girl, Anne, informed me that Andrew Kyle had just been approved by vocational rehabilitation for repair of his inguinal hernia. But someone at their office had entered the wrong code number for the procedure – 59520 instead of 49520. I called Jenny at the vocational rehabilitation office in an attempt to rectify the matter. The conversation went something like this.

"Hello. My name is Dr. Truewater. My patient, Andrew Kyle, is scheduled to undergo repair of his recurrent inguinal hernia in three days. He's already been approved for the procedure, but someone entered the wrong procedure code number in your computer," I politely explained.

"Let me look that up in our computer, Dr. Truewater," Jenny began.

After a few moments, she replied, "Yes, Dr. Truewater. I'm happy to inform you that your patient has been approved for a Caesarian section, to be performed in three days on June 20 at Holy Christian Sinai Hospital. Is that a problem?" Jenny asked.

"Yes," I replied patiently. "My patient doesn't need a Caesarian section. In fact, he's not even pregnant. He needs to have his hernia repaired. Somebody entered the wrong code number. Could you just change that procedure code number, and make the first digit a four instead of a five?" I pleaded.

I can't do that," Jenny replied sympathetically. "We'll have to repeat the application process. It's too late to approve your patient for a hernia in just three days. At the present time, you're only approval is for a C-section."

"I can assure you that this patient was never approved for a C-section," I replied angrily. "His approval was for repair of an inguinal hernia, which would allow him to go back to his job as a roofer."

"Trust me, Jenny," I pleaded. "A C-section would not help this man, even if I could figure out some way to do one."

"I understand what you're telling me, Dr. Truewater," Jenny replied. "But I can't change the listing in the computer. If you can't do the scheduled procedure as described, then you'll have to reapply for approval."

"But that could take several weeks," I pleaded. "This man needs to get his surgery and get back to work!"

"I'm sorry, Dr. Truewater," Jenny replied. "You'll have to go by the book."

Undaunted, I went ahead and fixed Andrew's hernia, and he was back to work in three weeks as a roofer. On his post-operative visit, Andy had only one question.

"Dr. Truewater," Andy began, "the hernia repair went well. But, how come my bill says 'C-section' on it?"

"Oh, that," I casually replied. "C-section – that also stands for a special kind of hernia repair. These days, with computers and everything, you've got to go by the book!"

And with the rise of gender dysphoria, no one suspected a thing!

* Author's Note: This article was written in jest –
Please correct any procedure approval codes before doing surgery!

MEDICAL SLANG

TV sports commentators, by the nature of their occupation, are not highly versed in medical matters. Hence, a complete set of slang terms has arisen to describe sports injuries.

I was watching my favorite football team, the Chicago Bears, on television. I saw one poor soul, Charlie Waters, running full speed at the ball carrier when his heavier opponent, running full speed in the opposite direction, ran directly into him, smashing him to the ground. How did the announcer describe this vicious assault?

"Charlie Waters was taken out nicely on the play," the announcer stated, almost casually. "Let's take another look on the video replay."

In this context, "taken out" means slamming into one's opponent at full speed, causing massive blunt injury, leaving him sprawled helplessly on the ground.

I switched the channel for a few minutes to see how my favorite boxing match was going. Sugar Ray Leonard had just smashed his fist into Roberto Duran, leaving him dazed and momentarily senseless. How did the announcer describe this tragic event?

"Roberto's going to be O.K.," the announcer assured the listeners. "He's just had his bell rung!"

Now, I've spent nine years in medical school and residency, and I've never heard the phrase "having your bell rung" to describe a head injury. What really happened is that Roberto's brain went bouncing around inside his skull, causing a cerebral contusion, with transient loss of memory, which would ultimately result in the death of millions of Roberto's brain cells. In a few minutes, Roberto is back boxing again!

I flipped the station again to catch my favorite basketball game. Larry Bird was leading the Boston Celtics in a blitzing scoring attack against the Los Angeles Lakers. As Larry goes up to shoot, he is crushed between two defenders and falls to the floor, gasping for breath.

But the announcer is quick to reassure us, lest we quit watching and lower the ratings. "He's going to be O.K. folks," we are told. "He's just had the wind knocked out of him."

In medical terms, Larry Bird has just sustained massive blunt chest trauma, possible fractured ribs or traumatic pneumothorax with pulmonary contusion, and even a possible cardiac contusion. Larry hobbles over to the bench, sits out for a few minutes, and then returns for more punishment.

While doctors may have a more sophisticated vocabulary to describe human trauma, I decided that surgeons and TV announcers really have a lot in common. They both sometimes downplay the seriousness of the situation.

The following Monday in surgery, I sliced a patient open, separated her rectus muscles, dissected out her gall bladder, cauterized her bleeding liver, then sewed her muscles and skin back together again.

"Your wife's going to be alright," I reassured her husband. "It was a fairly routine gall bladder surgery."

Despite years spent in medical school learning the proper medical terminology, doctors would do well to learn medical slang. Last week, little Bobby Duncan was injured in a car accident. I could have gone out and explained to his mother that Bobby suffered blunt trauma to his chest and abdomen, with severe contusions to both legs.

When I went to the waiting room, Bobby's mother was sobbing uncontrollably. I put my arm around her to reassure her.

After she quieted down, I simply said, "Bobby's going to be alright. He was shaken up a little from the accident, but I expect he'll be back to normal in a few days."

Bobby's mother understood the situation immediately, better than any long-winded technical explanation.

Sometimes, though, the sports announcers can fool you. When I got home that evening, I was watching the Chicago Cubs playing the Philadelphia Phillies. Rick Sutcliffe was pitching for the Cubs when he suddenly developed a sore arm. The TV commentator, instead of using medical slang, surprised me with a detailed medical explanation.

"I suspect Rick Sutcliffe may have a rotator cuff injury," the announcer stated in a rather serious tone of voice.

"What does that mean?" my daughter asked, obviously quite worried.

"I suspect he's pulled his shoulder," I replied.

"Why didn't he just say that?" she asked.

"He's trying to be more precise," I answered. "Sometimes, when we try to explain things too well, we end up not explaining them at all!"

THE MURDER OF MARILYN MONROE

"Hello, Dr. Truewater," Herb exclaimed as I walked into the surgery lounge.

"How's it going, Herb?" I asked.

"Both our cases are delayed," Herb informed me, "which gives me a chance to ask you something I've been meaning to ask. Rhonda, the scrub nurse, told me you wrote a chapter on Marilyn Monroe."

"That's right," I replied, "also known as Norma Jean Baker."

"I personally believe she committed suicide," Herb began, "what with her past history of depression and drug abuse. Keeping it simple, is there one fact you can tell me that would prove she was murdered, and turn me into a conspiracy theorist?"

"Of course, Herb," I replied. "My extended Greek family is from Chicago, where I was raised. There was a young lady named Eugenia 'Becca' Pappas that my relatives talked about. She was an 18-year-old manicurist and walked a little on the wild side. She befriended a 32-year-old man named Frank 'the German' Schweihs who actually lived for a while with Sam Giancana, the boss in the Chicago Outfit."

"People told her to stay away from Frank, who she met in Greektown, but Becca was in love with Frank, who even gave her a new car, and Becca loved the life style. It turns out that Frank was a Mafia hit man, but Becca didn't know that."

"Now, Becca gets invited to a party in California. So, she takes off from Palwaukee Airport outside Chicago in a private plane with Frank and some of his friends on August 4, 1962. They all go to a party, but midway through the party, Frank and his friends leave. Becca is told to stay behind."

"The next day, when they land back at Palwaukee Airport, Becca finds out that Marilyn Monroe died the previous night. Becca later hears scuttlebutt that Frank was involved. She confronts Frank but he denies any involvement."

"The two later part ways, but months later, Frank invites Becca on a double date on a riverboat on the Chicago River. Her friends tell her not to go, but Becca decides to go anyway. The double date later splits up. Becca disappears that night and her body months later is found floating in the Chicago River near Riverview Park."

"The scuttlebutt was that if Frank didn't kill Becca, then Frank would also be killed. There were ongoing questions in the press about Marilyn's death, and Becca knew too much."

"Becca's story actually made it to the Chicago Tribune, but charges were never filed."

"But why would the Mafia want to kill Marilyn Monroe?" Herb asked.

"The Mafia didn't like Attorney General Robert Kennedy and his War on Crime. But the Mafia often did domestic favors for the Deep State, who also despised Robert Kennedy."

"President John Kennedy famously said that he wanted to break the CIA into a thousand pieces, firing CIA director, Allen Dulles, after the failed 1961 Bay of Pigs invasion of Cuba. Robert Kennedy, who aspired someday to be President, shared his brother's beliefs."

"The FBI had wiretapped Marilyn's house during the renovation and knew that Robert Kennedy was planning to visit that night. Marilyn's presumed suicide could easily have ended Robert's political career, if JFK hadn't pleaded with J. Edgar Hoover to intervene and cover up Bobby's visit – thus guaranteeing Hoover's perpetual job as FBI director."

"Robert Kennedy and Peter Lawford even returned that night and said a prayer in the ambulance, as Marilyn was rushed to the hospital. She'd been given a Nembutal/Chloral hydrate suppository according to Chuck Giancana, which explains why her stomach lacked any pill residue, despite the high drug levels- something the coroner had never seen – he called it a 'presumed suicide.'"

"Sounds pretty complicated," Herb concluded, as he put on his mask and headed off to surgery. "I'm willing to believe that Marilyn was murdered, based on your extended family's account. But I would blame the Mafia over the Deep State."

"Take your pick," I answered. "Either way you look at it, Marilyn's reputation needs to be restored – she was an innocent pawn who was sacrificed in an unsuccessful effort to end Robert Kennedy's political career."

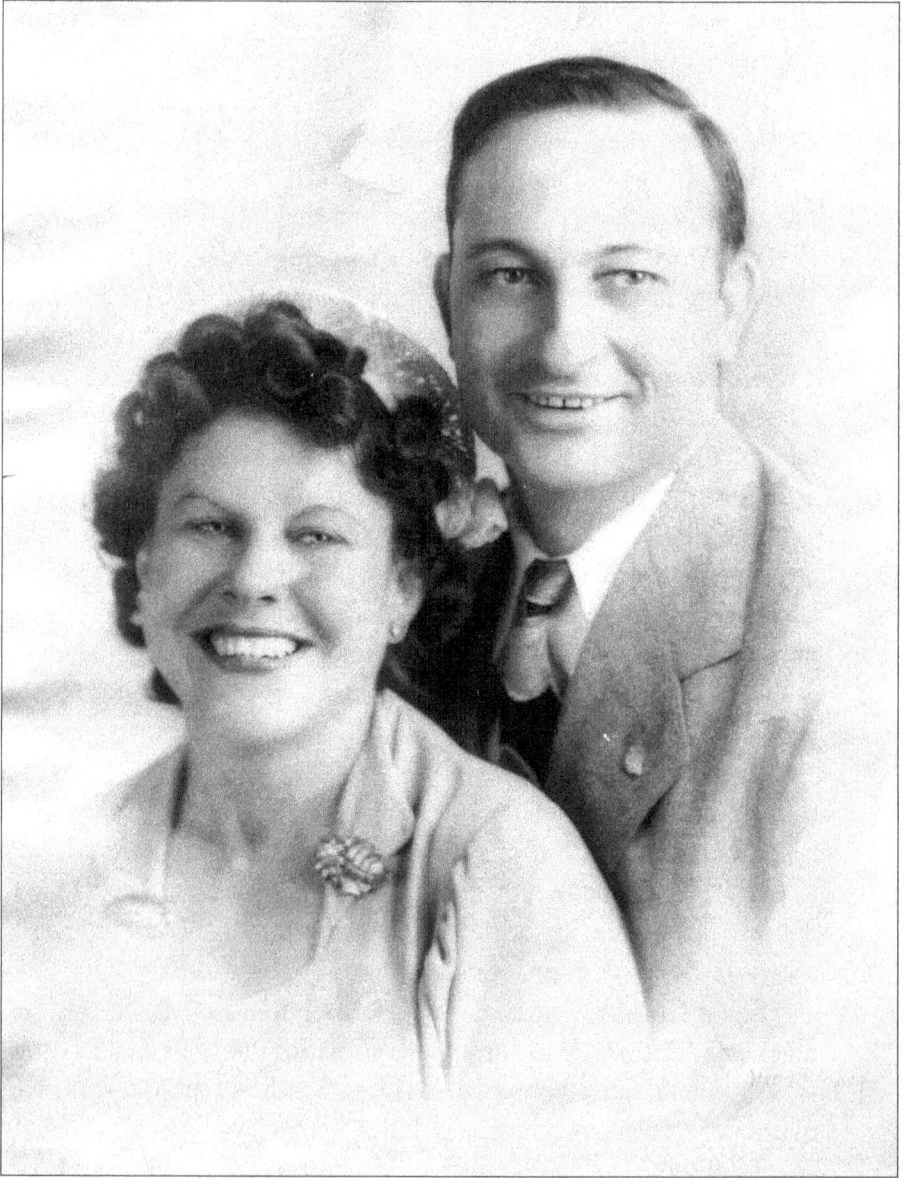

Willis and Marguerite Bettis

TRIBUTE TO WILLIS BETTIS
OCTOBER 16, 2003

Today, we gather together to honor the memory of my father-in-law, Willis Bettis. I want to thank you all for coming. I think that Willis would be especially honored to see the large gathering of friends and relatives who have come together for a final tribute.

Willis was born April 8, 1913 in Wellston, Oklahoma; He died October 11, 2003 of congestive heart failure.

Father: John Thomas Bettis from Arkansas
Mother: Julia Elizabeth Wilkerson Bettis from Texas

Brother Clyde died at an early age in 1914 and sister Mamie died in 1915 of typhoid fever; both had red hair like their sister Lillian
Burl, Charles, Lillian, John now deceased

Children: Myrtle Lillian – died at age 2 ½ of childhood illness
Thomas Willis Bettis died at age 16 of drowning
James William Bettis died in Viet Nam 1968
Ronnie Wayne Bettis died 1998 of lung cancer
Norma Joanne Bettis Montgomery of Houston, Texas
Margaret Sue Bettis Truels of Oklahoma City (wife of William Truels)

During his childhood, Willis' family lived mostly in western Oklahoma; the family did travel to Arizona for a brief period. He picked cotton as a child. When he was only four, he was sent on errands, riding a horse to the neighbors to deliver goods. Willis worked as a paper boy in Oklahoma City. He sold insurance for a while in Oklahoma City.

Willis fought for a while as an amateur boxer. As a diversion, he would sometimes ride the boxcars to Dallas or points even farther west. Once, he said, he met the Hobo Queen, an annual award, but he said she didn't have much to offer.

Willis entered the Army January 31, 1944 as a cook during World War II., and was discharged October 25, 1945. Willis had his first four children with Myrtle Faubus. He was then divorced and married Marguerite Theodora Campbell in 1946. They met on an elevator in Tulsa. (That's what I call going up in the world.)

Willis later took a course in refrigeration and became a licensed operating engineer. He subsequently worked at the Tulsa Club, from 1946 until 1978, where many of the city's wealthiest citizens dined, including the Kerr and McGee oil magnates. Willis was the chief operating engineer for the last 20 years in charge of operating the club. He believed strongly in the union, and fought to raise the wages of the everyday worker.

While lacking a formal education, Willis was a self-educated man. He enjoyed reading about history. And he loved to philosophize about anything and everything.

In his earlier days, Willis loved to play pool, and would sometimes get an angry call from Marguerite to come home for supper.

Willis loved to fish at the Keystone Dam. He would take whoever would go with, including my son Michael. We still have the picture of Michael holding a large fish—a ten-pound Drum--he caught with his grandfather.

Willis loved to go on long drives through Western Oklahoma with his wife Marguerite. He once found a dinosaur tooth in Western Oklahoma, and gave it to his grandson Scott – I believe it was a Tyrannosaurus tooth.

Willis loved to pitch horseshoes. He had a horseshoe pit in the backyard and would practice every night after work. He traveled to horseshoe tournaments with Marguerite, sometimes going out of state with friends like the Belden brothers, Bob and Al.

And Willis loved to play dominoes. He would sometimes spend hours playing dominoes with his friends as a sort of mental recreation. Willis loved to talk about OU football and professional tennis, and was well-read on both subjects.

Willis loved animals, especially cats, and would try to help stray animals. Most recently, an entire litter of cats was born under his house, and he and my wife worked to get them to the *Free to Live* pet center.

Willis was a good friend to his friends. He could be counted on to help those in need. He would sometimes help people he didn't even know.

But most of all, I loved to hear Willis tell his personal tales of his experiences in Oklahoma – which included hunting squirrels and preparing squirrel stew!

Willis pondered a lot about religion. He did believe in God and in a higher power, a Creator. Willis studied the Bible extensively, and formulated his own opinions about the hereafter.

Let us bow our heads in prayer. Our Heavenly Father, bless Willis Bettis and those of us gathered together to honor his memory. Guide us in our grief over the loss of this compassionate man. Let Willis be an example to all of us – an example of how we can overcome the hardships in life, of picking cotton 14 hours a day for $2 a week, of dealing with the loss of our loved ones – Willis lost four of his children at an early age, as well as his wife Marguerite after a marriage that lasted nearly fifty years.

In his later years, Willis suffered from diabetes and heart failure. As he got older, he saw his friends die, one by one. Yet, he carried on.

Willis would occasionally talk to me about what he called the cycles of life. He lived through the roaring twenties and the depression that followed. He was old enough to remember the influenza epidemic of 1918, when bodies were stacked like cordwood on the front porches. He remembered the good times and the bad times.

And Willis talked about the cycles of life. He would laugh about his checked coat, the one he's wearing now, which would go in and out of style every twenty years or so – right now, it's back in style again!

And so, Lord, let us remember Willis's lesson about the cycles of life – the cycles of life and death that include all of us. Let us make the most of the time we have, and say the things that we meant to say before it's too late to say them.

And let us remember, Lord, Willis' compassion for his fellow man, and use that compassion as a guide for our own lives.

In closing, Lord, thank you for giving us Willis Bettis. Today, we honor his memory. Tomorrow, we can only hope to follow his example.

In thy Holy Name we pray, Amen.

GRAVESIDE PRAYER

Lord, we are gathered today at the final resting place for Willis Bettis. I can remember many a time that we walked with Willis at this very site. I remember he was upset about that old tree, and was worried that it would fall down on the gravestones. At least I've been assured by the management that all the dead trees will be taken down in the next six months.

But, more seriously, Lord, thank you for the opportunity of knowing Willis Bettis. I know that he truly missed Marguerite and at least now they can be together again. And I know he truly grieved over all his deceased children, and now he can be together with them too.

And Lord, bless all the people – relatives, friends and acquaintances who have taken time out this morning, many of them coming from hundreds of miles away, to share our experiences and memories of Willis Bettis.

And bless Willis now Lord as we commit his mortal remains back to the ground from whence all life started, finishing the cycle of life which began 90 years ago on April 8, 1913 in Wellston, Oklahoma. May you rest in peace, Willis, and may we all live by your example of compassion for your fellow man.

In Thy Holy Name we pray. Amen

SLEEP, MY CHILD

Tell me what you see, my child
As you lie asleep
Do the stars shine in your sky
Or do they watch and weep?

I see you breathe so quietly
Your world seems so serene
Does the wind blow softly now
Or is it raw and mean?

There's a smile upon your face
As you stretch and turn
Your world must be a nicer place
Than what I've come to learn.

I often sit and wonder
When times are hard and lean –
Do we live a life that's real
Or is it all a dream?

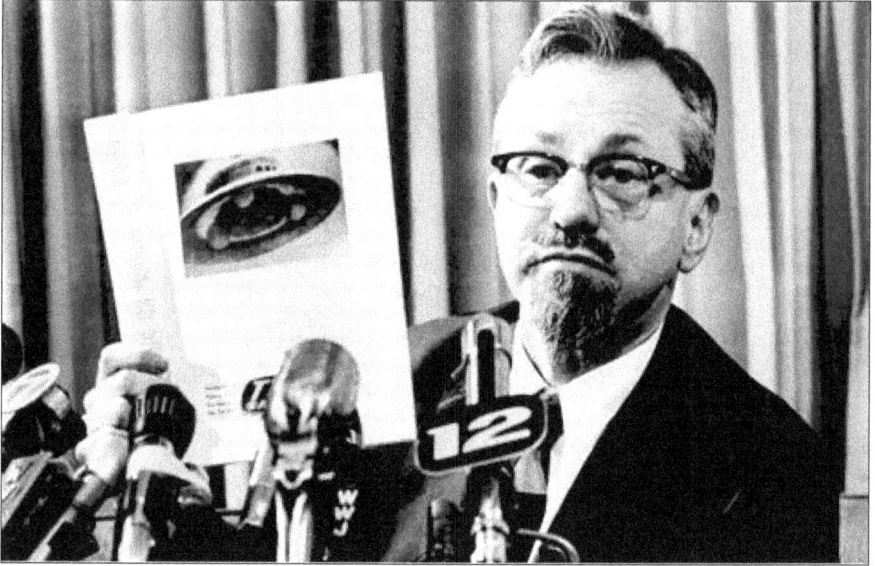

Dr. J. Allen Hynek

WHAT'S TRUE?

What's true is what I'll say to you –
It's just that nothing else will do!
History's victors will tell the story
And brag about their fictitious glory!

A fact's a fact—I don't doubt that –
Let's not create an artifact!
But the one who lives to tell the tale
Will be the one who you regale!

The Keepers of the Secret don't want you to know
About the truths that linger deep below!
Laws of Physics you cannot trust –
And off-world Beings that don't look like us!

Time is not linear when gravity departs
And history unfolds in confusing parts!
Time, it seems, is just an illusion –
When Past and Future meet in confusion!

ASTRONOMY 101 WITH DR. HYNEK

It was the spring of 1967 – three months before graduation from Northwestern University and I needed an extra class to fill out my curriculum. I decided on Astronomy 101 with Dr. J. Allen Hynek.

Dr. Hynek was the civilian head of Project Bluebook – the Air Force project that investigated flying saucers. During World War II., Dr. Hynek helped develop the top-secret proximity fuse, which would trigger an anti-aircraft shell to explode as it approached a Japanese Zero. It was so successful that the Japanese were forced to resort to kamikaze attacks!

Ten minutes before the end of a standard astronomy lecture, Dr. Hynek would read excerpts from portions of the Bluebook files which had been declassified.

Dr. Hynek had been a debunker, but to my surprise he would read tape-recorded conversations of, for example, police officers chasing a flying object as it traveled from precinct to precinct and from town to town. At the time, Jacques Vallee, the future UFO researcher, visited with Dr. Hynek at his Evanston home and later enrolled in the Northwestern graduate computer program.

Officially, the government claimed these objects didn't exist – you could literally lose your commercial pilot's license in 1967 if you reported these objects. Individuals who reported seeing flying saucers were publicly ridiculed by the government and news media!

Dr. Hynek read tape recordings from airport towers as fighter jets were scrambled to chase these objects. I was shocked to hear that some of the jets had orders to try to shoot them down! One jet lost all power as the pilot prepared to fire a missile!

Toward the end of the semester, Dr. Hynek started talking about four types of aliens that inhabited the UFOs. One Insectoid type resembled a praying mantis. Another was a Reptilian with scaly skin. Then there were the short and tall Grays.

But the group that the government was most concerned about from the standpoint of national security were the Nordics that looked just like us! They could actually be walking in the halls of the Pentagon without being discovered!

I literally had to pinch myself! Could this be true? I leaned over to the student sitting next to me in the Tech auditorium on Sheridan Road – but he was more concerned about the Viet Nam anti-war rally in Dearing Meadow that afternoon!

Questions about flying saucers and types of aliens were even included on our final exam. Characteristics of aliens, such as polydactyly and arachnodactyly (like the extraterrestrial in the movie *E.T.* where Dr. Hynek consulted) were correct answers on the multiple-choice portion of the final exam!

It struck me that a whole new field of Physics was yet to be revealed. Traveling from one star to another involved a folding of space-time. Activities portrayed on Star Trek, such as teleportation and quantum entanglement weren't just science fiction, as creator Gene Roddenberry was later found to have intelligence connections!

Albert Einstein described time as an illusion, although a persistent one. Author William Tompkins describes a weapon that, when fired at an opposing ship, causes it to crumple in a space-time warp, sort of like the Philadelphia Experiment.

Dr. Hynek talked about how we were retro-engineering captured alien craft, like the one at Roswell in 1947, which used anti-gravity and electrogravitic propulsion to go into outer space. I later learned that one of these Gray alien survivors, named Ebe, lived for five years at Los Alamos!

In the spring of 1967 the space race to the moon against the Russians was in full swing. Why were we using conventional rockets – was the moon race just a cover for these secret antigravity and electrogravitic projects?

The existence of extraterrestrial Beings that walk among us has to be the most important piece of information for all of humankind! It will change our view of the world, it will change our philosophy, perhaps even our religion.

I thank Dr. Hynek for having the courage of his convictions to report what he knew to be true. But why has the government refused full disclosure, as proposed by President Kennedy, after over 50 years? Why not publish all of Ebe's redacted revelations?

I look forward to the day when we will finally walk hand in hand with our extraterrestrial brothers and sisters!

THROUGH THE LOOKING GLASS

Our laws of physics are obsolete –
A special case is all they treat!
Tesla told the truth, you see
Now hidden from our destiny!

Antigravity is the new reality
Some would call it a duality!
What goes up does not come down
When antigravity does abound!

I'll tell you stuff you won't believe
I've no intention to deceive!
But living Beings are all around –
Some don't even touch the ground!

You can travel faster than light –
I know that causes Einstein fright!
But when you're folding space and time
Einstein's laws do not align!

I know the University
Prides itself on diversity –
But talk about changing Einstein's laws
And all the Professors give you pause!

Zero point energy is all around –
No need to burn the fossils down!
And though it may cause confusion
Future vehicles will use cold fusion!

Med-beds heal with frequency
And look at the DNA sequencing –
Damaged limbs can be restored
But the health industry is abhorred!

There's a group of oligarchs
Who like to do things in the dark!
"Human Beings must never know
About the secrets that we hold!"

Alien Beings from Outer Space
Are trying to help the human race –
But there's a real competition
To keep all this technology hidden!

You can travel back in time
And watch our history as it unwinds
But don't dare to alter history's course
Or a parallel world will be enforced!

Those who preach original sin
Are shocked to find what's pure within!
No need to bow down in remorse –
We're all fractals of one true Source!

I know you'll think of me as crazy
Or maybe just a little hazy!
Someday the people will get Disclosure
And find a world that's so much older!

EMPTY SPACES

We fill the empty spaces
That tragedy embraces –
Looking for a way
To keep the hurt at bay!

The logic of a trusted politician
Steeped in knowledge and erudition
Can easily refute a simple observation
If it can't provide the proper explanation!

Those who live in the quiet suffering of a grievous loss
Carry a burden which can never be lost –
You toil in the present and smile at the last –
As flashes of memory break through from the past!

THE JFK ASSASSINATION
NOVEMBER 22, 1963

I was sitting in the surgery lounge when Herb Silverstein, the plastic surgeon, had a question for me.

"I'm not a conspiracy theorist," Herb began, "but I know you've studied the JFK assassination. Keeping it short and simple, is there one established fact you can share with me that would convince me of a conspiracy?"

"Why, yes, Herb," I began. "I personally talked with the general surgeon, Dr. Charles Crenshaw at Parkland Hospital at one of the JFK Lancer assassination meetings in Dallas. He described a small entry wound in the right temple and a 'baseball-sized hole' in the right rear of JFK's head. James Hosty, the Secret Service Agent, who was no more than 10 feet away from JFK when the head shot occurred, publicly stated that 'the back of the head was gone.'"

"On the Zapruder film, you can see that JFK's head moves dramatically back in frame 313, when the head shot occurred. Jerrol Custer, Bethesda X-ray technician, personally told me that most of the brain was gone. Neurosurgeon Dr. Kemp Clark examined JFK in the Parkland Emergency Room, observed that cerebellum was falling out of a large hole in the back of the head, and gave orders to stop any further attempts at resuscitation."

"Jacqueline Kennedy crawled onto the back of the Presidential limousine to retrieve a portion of the President's rear skull that had been blasted off."

"The motorcycle policeman, Bobby Hargis, riding behind and to the left of JFK, was sprayed in the face and helmet with blood, brain tissue, and bone fragments that stuck in his protective vest. Large finger-sized chunks of brain tissue were also inside the limousine."

"William Neuman, an eyewitness at the Grassy Knoll with military experience, was closest to JFK when the head shot occurred. He personally told me, as seen in photographs, that he and his family fell to the ground from a shot that came from behind them at the picket fence on the Grassy Knoll. He was never called by the Warren Commission."

"Acoustics analysis from a police Dictaphone tape recorded a very loud shot which was localized, using echo location, as originating from the corner of the picket fence at the Grassy Knoll. Witnesses at the Grassy Knoll heard a large sound, smelled gunpowder and saw smoke."

"James Files, a Mafia-CIA shooter, out of Chicago, claims he fired a frangible or exploding bullet from the corner of the picket fence at the Grassy Knoll."

"The problem with a large baseball-sized hole in the back of the head is that this argues for an exit wound from a shot fired from the Grassy Knoll, to the right and front of JFK."

"The existence of a large exit wound in the back of the skull forced LBJ to preempt a Congressional investigation and create the Warren Commission, which officially denied the existence of a large exit wound in the back of the skull. All of the above witnesses were officially discredited or never called. Only one Warren Commission member, forensic pathologist Dr. Cyril Wecht, had the courage to challenge the official result and publicly disagree."

"In order to avoid being labeled conspiracy theorists, the 1976 House Select Committee on Assassinations actually suggested that there may have been two shooters coincidentally firing at JFK in Dealey Plaza at the same time!"

"Thank you, Dr. Truewater," Herb concluded, as he stood up and headed off to surgery. I think I just became a conspiracy theorist!"

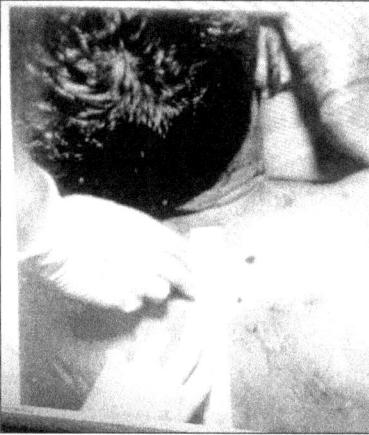

Official photo of the back of JFK's head – notice the "darkened area" at the right rear that appears to have been shaded.	A pictorial representation of President Kennedy's head wound, as described by Dr. Robert N. McClelland of Parkland Hospital.

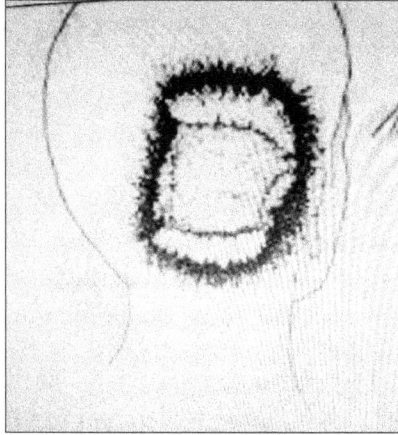

Dr. Kemp Clark was a neurosurgeon
Of one thing he was very certain –
He noted a large hole in the right occipital –
An observation that proved quite pivotal!

But the Warren Report that finally came out
Placed a small hole in the back – there is no doubt!
A shot from the rear – it had to be –
From the Dallas Book Depository!

CONTEMPLATIONS

Like the Wizard of Oz in the Emerald City
Do we live in a world of passion and pity?
Where one man rules, and controls all the force –
And occasional lone gunmen change history's course?

Or do we live in a Casablanca world?
Where all different forces rotate and swirl –
And the destiny of millions who hope to prevail
Is determined by dark forces yet to unveil?

Is all that happens part of God's divine plan –
That we must accept, however we can?
Is man able to control his fate –
Or can we only contemplate?

We all get shot one way or another –
But we always hope to recover!
You pray that you will jump right back –
But sometimes you just get laid out flat!

I'd like to think that by our actions
We can control our disparate factions!
If we could only find the truth
Then treachery we might one day uproot!

What if you knew the day of your death –
The moment you'd take your final breath?
Would you be kinder to the people you see –
And help them with their infirmity?

THE DOCTOR'S CAR

My Buick LeSabre was getting a little old, so I decided it was time to look for a new car. Whenever I enter a new car dealership, I always try to conceal the fact that I'm a doctor, hoping I can get a better deal. But inevitably, something happens that gives away my true identity.

I drove into the Sooner Red car dealership, parking in the back and walking up to the showroom. I had been careful to take my beeper off my belt and stick it in my front pocket, in order to conceal it from the salesman. I had also placed it on the "silent" mode, so as not to give away my identity.

"Hello!" I beamed, walking up to the salesman.

He quickly looked me over, as most car salesmen do, trying to determine if I was a "looker" or a "buyer", no doubt noticing my faded Bermuda shorts, old running shoes, and T-shirt that said, "Ski Oklahoma!". I was determined not to look too well-off for the occasion.

"How do you do, sir!" he beamed. "I'm Larry Johnson. How may I help you?"

This salesman was not to be deterred by my casual appearance. No doubt he had been to the Car Salesmen's School of Positive Thinking.

"I'm Bill Truewater," I replied. "Just thought I'd take a look at this year's models."

Just then my beeper started to vibrate. Being in my front pocket, I was suddenly embarrassed to find myself jabbing my right hand into my front pocket to shut the silly thing off.

I was not faced with a tough decision – either leave my right hand in my front pocket and let the salesman think funny thoughts about me, or pull out my beeper and reveal my identity. I decided to pull out my beeper.

"Oh, a doctor!" Larry exclaimed when he saw my beeper. Without missing a beat, he adds, "You don't know how lucky you are. This is Doctor's Day at Sooner Red! We're running a Doctor's Special all day today!"

"Doctor's Day?" I replied skeptically. "I don't see any signs. Besides, I never heard of a doctor's special!"

"Two thousand dollars off any doctor's car in the lot!" Larry exclaimed. "Doctors perform such a valuable service to society that it's Sooner Red's policy to give them a break on Doctor's Day!

"What exactly do you mean by two thousand dollars off any doctor's car" I asked. "What's a doctor's car, anyway?"

"Step right over here!" Larry bellowed. "A doctor's car is the kind of car other people wish they could drive. Take this coupe," Larry continued. "It's got four-way stereo speakers, a big V-8 engine, and leather bucket seats. Girls see this car and start tinging all over. Doctor, you drive down the Broadway Extension in this car, and you can pick up any girl you want! No joke."

"Well, I really wasn't interested in picking up any girls," I replied. "I'm a married man, you know, although I must admit the car is quite attractive."

In the twinkling of an eye, Larry had already moved over to the next car, a four-door BMW. The car was bright red with silver wire wheels.

"Then, what you want, Doctor, is this brand-new BMW. It's got that German craftsmanship, a German-engineered sound system, four-wheel independent suspension, and, if you buy today, we'll knock two thousand dollars off the MSRP," Larry concluded.

"Looks awfully nice," I replied. "But I don't like German cars. Some of them are too expensive to repair."

"But look at that speedometer, Doctor!" Larry cooed. "This car has a turbo and can go 120 miles an hour! This is the car you need when you've got that emergency and have to get to the hospital fast! Why, with this car, you can drive from Oklahoma City to Tulsa in one hour!"

"That's nice to know," I answered. "But I never go over 65 miles an hour, even in emergencies. Going any faster kind of makes me nervous, what with all the idiots on the road these days!"

"Then, I've got just the car for you! Larry replied, undaunted by his previous failures. "This Jaguar is the finest engineered car money can buy. It's got four-wheel independent suspension, automatic load leveling, anti-lock brakes, and the quietest ride in town. Why, it even pays for itself!" Larry jubilantly proclaimed.

"Pays for itself?" I asked. "How can a luxury car pay for itself?"

"Doctor, this car oozes professionalism," Larry explained. "Why, when your fellow doctors see you pull up in this car, you're guaranteed more business. This car gives you the professional image that a man of your stature deserves," Larry added, convinced that he had made a sale.

"Look," I began, getting somewhat frustrated. "I don't want to pick up girls on the Broadway extension. I don't want to go 120 miles an hour."

"And I don't want a car that oozes professionalism. I've got a wife and three kids, I go to six baseball, soccer, and swimming lessons a week, I like to go camping, and I like to go on long vacations in the mountain!" I explained.

"Whoa, Doctor!" Larry replied. "This is your lucky day. What you want is a four-wheel drive Rover Ranger! This car does it all. You can take the kids to school, go on vacations in the mountains, and take it to the office. It's even got a sort of Yuppie image that says 'I've made it!'"

"It's a good-looking car," I responded, "but what about that van you've got over in the corner?"

"That clunky thing?" Larry queried. "That's just a box on wheels. No sex appeal. No professional image. No charisma. It's not even a car – it's a truck. All that truck says is, 'I'm a family man.' Period. No hype. Nothing more."

"That's all I want!" I replied. "A box on wheels – no hype, nothing more – I'll take it!" I added jubilantly.

As I drove off in my new van, I could hear Larry grumbling to his boss about how hard it was to please doctors these days.

"Doctors are just like everybody else," his boss replied. "Some are flamboyant, some are trendy, and others – just plain practical!"

LOSING WEIGHT

I was sitting in the surgery lounge waiting for my case to start. Herb Silverstein, the plastic surgeon, was munching on one of the doughnuts provided by Bayer that morning.

"I just can't seem to lose weight," Herb complained.

"That doughnut isn't helping," I quipped.

"Well, I need doughnut therapy and a cup of coffee every morning to get the day started," Herb replied. "These cleft palate cases take several hours and I need the energy."

"True enough," I replied. "But if you want to lose weight, I like to follow Gary Player's advice."

"Isn't Gary Player a golfer?" Herb asked.

"An excellent PGA golfer and Master's winner," I said. "But he's also a physical fitness guru – at age 80, he does 25 pushups a day to keep in shape."

"I'm not going to start doing pushups at my age, Dr. Truewater," Herb quipped. "I'd probably give myself a hernia."

"True enough," I replied. "But Gary's got excellent dietary advice. He says that in the morning, you should eat like a king – you know, a complete, well-rounded meal."

"I'll go along with that," Herb replied. "A good breakfast helps get the day started."

"Then, for lunch, Gary says to eat like a queen."

"How does a queen eat?" Herb asked.

"Well, I presume a queen doesn't eat as much as a king-- you can't have a fat queen in the kingdom – you know, eat more delicately, more sparingly," I explained.

"I'll go along with that," Herb added. "A delicate lunch, as you put it, doesn't leave you a heavy feeling."

"But, what about dinner?" Herb asked.

"Gary Player says that for dinner you should eat like a pauper."

"A pauper?" Herb asked. "How does a pauper eat?"

"Well, you see, paupers don't have a lot of resources, so they eat sparingly."

"Right," Herb replied. "Paupers don't have a lot of money to spend on food – so they eat fast food burgers and fries and maybe a milk shake to wash it all down. Sounds pretty good to me!"

"No, I don't think that's what Gary Player meant," I replied. "You want to eat healthy for dinner – you know, fresh broccoli, asparagus, soybeans."

"Well, I'll go along with eating like a king for breakfast and a queen for lunch, but you can forget about the pauper diet for dinner."

"Besides, I'm not a pauper – I'm a doctor and I worked hard to get this far in life – I deserve better than a pauper's diet for dinner! I'll take a fresh steak every time!"

"Of course, there's always fasting, Herb--known technically as autophagy. It helps get rid of the body's waste products. Fasting goes back to our tribal history, when food wasn't always available. It even has religious significance – you know, Moses and Jesus both fasted in the desert – the rites of ablution."

"Well, I'm out of the tribe, and we're not in the desert anymore, Dr. Truewater!"

"True enough," I replied. "But the problem with being successful is that you feel like you deserve more. But more isn't always better. Aristotle taught the golden mean –nothing to excess – moderation is one of the four cardinal virtues."

"The key here, Herb, is to practice what they call sustainabilism. Our society involves too much stress, too much information, too much food, for that matter. We need to learn how to get along with less."

"You may be on to something, Dr. Truewater," Herb replied. "I scrubbed on a heart bypass with Allen Greer last week, and he told me that the enemy of good was better – we're such perfectionists that when you try to do something so perfectly right, you can actually get a poorer result."

"Maybe, instead of going for a great meal at dinner, I should settle for a good meal and lose a little weight!"

THE ONE-HOSS SHAY

You see, of course, if you 're not a dunce,
How it went to pieces all at once,
All at once, and nothing first,
Just as bubbles do when they burst.

I was sitting in the surgery waiting room at Holy Christian Hospital one day last week when I heard the most interesting conversation. The surgery waiting room is immediately adjacent to the Intensive Care waiting room and from my seat near the door, I could easily overhear the conversation in the hall.

It seems that an elderly patient, who the family affectionately called 'Grandma Nellie', had undergone surgery for a gangrenous gallbladder. She died four days after surgery, and I could hear each of the doctors involved in the case talking to Grandma Nellie's family.

The surgeon, Tim Atwater, was the first to talk to the family.

"Your Grandma Nellie put up quite a fight," Dr. Atwater began. "For a while there, I thought we could pull her through, but her heart just couldn't take the stress. I'm sorry."

Next to console the family was the cardiologist, John Blakely. Dr. Blakely knew Grandma Nellie's son, Mark, and spent most of the time talking to him.

"Nellie was quite some lady," Dr. Blakely began. "Not many people make it to be one hundred years old. I admire that lady."

"What finally did her in, Doc?" Mark asked.

"Her lungs just couldn't take the shock of the surgery," Dr. Blakely replied. "We never could get her off the ventilator."

The third doctor to console the family was the pulmonary physician, Frank McWhirter.

"Grandma Nellie gave her best shot," Dr. McWhirter told the family. "I admire anybody with that kind of spunk. I just hope when I'm one hundred years old, I'll be as healthy as your Grandma Nellie!"

"And, you know, it's a funny thing," Dr. McWhirter continued. "If it wasn't for the peritonitis and gangrene, I think Grandma Nellie might have made it!"

By now, I had quit reading my daily paper, and was concentrating intently on Grandma Nellie's demise. The family practitioner, Dr. Robert Evans, was the last to visit the family.

"Hello, Mark," he began. "I've known Grandma Nellie for over thirty years. I'm sure gonna miss her. She was quite a gal!"

"Thank you, Dr. Evans," Mark replied. "I just have one question. The surgeon says she died from her heart problems. The cardiologist says Grandma died from her lung problems. The lung doctor says she died from her abdominal problems."

"We all sort of expected she wouldn't make it," Mark continued, "what with her being one hundred years old and all. But what I'd really like to know is, what did Grandma Nellie finally die from?"

The general practitioner paused for a minute, then replied slowly, "Well, Mark, you've got to understand something about specialists. No specialist likes to admit that the patient died from a problem in their field of expertise. I guess you'd call it a matter of pride – a point of honor."

"Besides," Dr. Evans continued, "elderly patients often die of what we call 'Multiple Systems Failure.' That's where more than one system fails at the same time."

"Kind of like the one-hoss shay?" Mark asked.

"The one-hoss shay?" Dr. Evans asked.

"You've probably read about it, Doc," Mark responded. "It's a poem about a horse-drawn buggy by Oliver Wendell Holmes that was so perfectly built that each part lasted exactly one-hundred years.

"That's a very good analogy," Dr. Evans responded. "The Good Lord made Grandma Nellie so perfectly that each of her organ systems would last one hundred years. Then, when she got to be one-hundred years old, everything went kaput!"

"Thank you for the explanation," Mark replied. "And on behalf of my family, I want to thank you for the excellent job you've done these last thirty years in taking care of all of us. We wouldn't have made it without you!"

"It's been my pleasure to take care of you and your family, Mark," Dr. Evans proudly responded.

"It's nice to have all of these specialists," Mark concluded. "But it's also nice to have someone who can put it all together!"

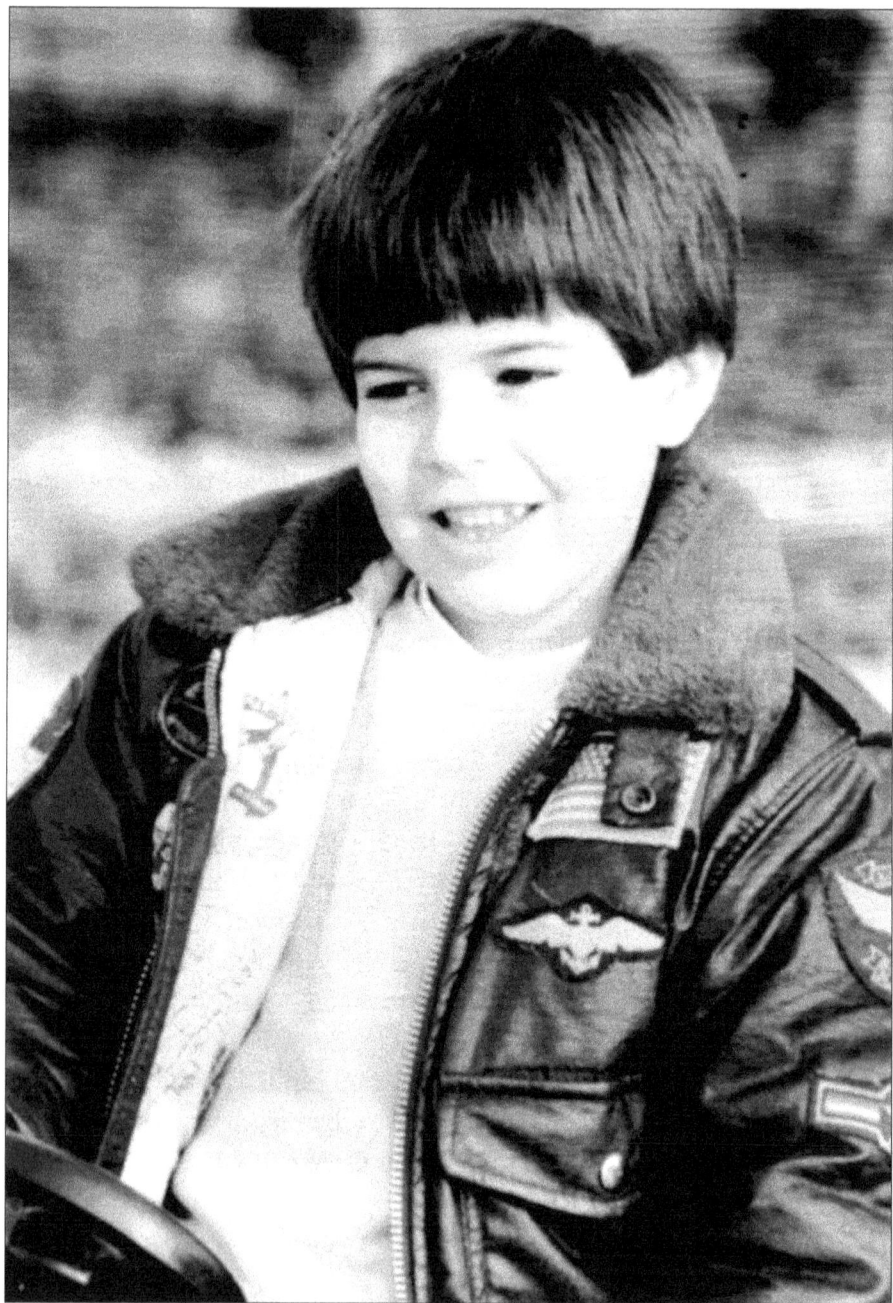

THE WOODEN SOLDIER

I pass his room
Without a noise
My little boy
Plays with his toys.

It seems so strange
My house to hear
The sound of cannon
Far and near!

Whish! Whoosh!
Splat! Boom!
The battle rages
In his room!

Laser guns
And magic beams
The air is filled
With battle screams!

The good guys must
The battle face
In order to
Preserve the race!

One laser beam
Strikes in thc head
The wooden soldier
Falls down dead.

But in a minute
He'll arise
For wooden soldiers
Never die.

The battle rages
In the park
Then moves within
The castle dark.

Transformer trucks
And magic swords
Soon defeat
The evil hoards!

"Did you win?"
I ask for fun
"Of course I have –
The battle's won!"

I only hope
When he's a man
Peace will finally
Be at hand.

Wooden soldiers
Never cry
But real people
Live and die.

If we could only
Settle scores
Without the need
To go to war.

Then I know
The world would be
A better place
For you and me!

TAKING BOARD EXAMS

Perhaps the most terrifying experience of my entire life was taking my oral exam for board certification in general surgery. Now, mind you, I'm a grown man, and very few things make me cry. But the oral exams in surgery are a distinct exception. It's not that the oral examiners consciously set out to inflict pain and suffering on the fledgling surgeons – it's just that things often turn out that way.

Part of the problem is that everything depends on passing your boards in surgery. It's possible to spend your entire life preparing to be a surgeon, but if you can't pass your examinations, it's all for naught, a big zero. Wherever you go to practice, people will ask if you're board certified. If you're not, you might not get to practice surgery in that area – it's just that simple.

To make matters worse, there're two parts to becoming board certified. The first part is an eight-hour grueling written exam, which only about two thirds of the surgeons pass – of course, they're allowed to take it again the following year. But that's not the bad part.

No, the really bad part is when you go to take your oral exams. What they do is rent a large amount of space in this giant hotel in New Orleans that has a huge atrium that overlooks the sandwich bar fourteen floors below. Then they make each candidate stand outside one of the rooms, waiting to take his or her oral exam from two qualified oral examiners.

Now, imagine standing outside this room waiting for your oral exam to start. Your whole life passes before you. Your whole future lies in that room. Who will your examiners be? Will they be fair?

Will I freeze up? Should I give the answer that I think the examiner wants to hear, based on, say his personal research, or should I give the answer that most surgeons in private practice would give?

And all the time these thoughts are going through your head, your palms are sweating, and you can feel your own heart beating. You look at the door of the room – the Inquisition Room. You look at the atrium ceiling ten floors over your head. You look down past the atrium railing to the sandwich bar fourteen floors below, and listen to the muted echoes of the people eating lunch. It's then that your mind starts playing tricks.

You think to yourself – what would happen if I vomited? If you vomited on the floor, the examiners might notice it when they stepped out to greet you. No way you could pass then. No, you'd have to vomit over the railing – the poor people fourteen floors below would never know who did it!

You wonder, how much longer can I wait before they open the door? By now your shirt is wet with perspiration and your feet are throbbing like they're going to explode out of their shoes. Your head starts to ache and you get a little dizzy. You look over the railing, but this time with a different thought. You look to your colleagues standing quietly outside their exam door, and you notice they're looking back at you, too nervous to say what's on their mind.

You think, what if I were to jump? That would solve my problems – no more anxiety, no more sweating – just a loud scream, a few brief seconds, and I'd go crashing into a sandwich table down below.

But then you think. This is just what the examiners want – they figure if you can go through the stress of this exam, then you're qualified to go through the stress of taking out someone's gallbladder or fixing their hernia.

Yes, this is all part of the game. It would be much too easy if they rented a Happy Days Motor Lodge that had only one floor, and all you had to do was stand outside with your coat on, waiting for one of those stuffy examiners to open the door.

Suddenly, the door opens. A man with a dark suit and a stern look on his face, greets you.

"Dr. Truewater, I presume?"

"Yes sir," you reply.

"I'm Steve Schwarz and this is Erwin Thomas. Would you like some coffee?"

"I decide to play it cool and take some coffee, trying not to spill it. Suddenly, it occurs to me that Steve Schwarz is the author of one of the two giant general surgery textbooks. Unfortunately, I read the other book! I carefully brush the coffee off my pants and sit down.

"Dr. Truewater, pick one of Halsted's principles and elaborate on it, please."

I looked down for a moment. Looking down has the advantage of making one appear not only humble, but deep in thought.

"Dr. William Halsted believed in the principle of meticulous hemostasis," I began confidently, looking the examiner in the eye. "This involves carefully clamping each bleeder, and tying it with a suture in order to avoid tissue trauma."

"Very good, Dr. Truewater," he replied.

Of course, nowadays everybody uses the cautery – it's much faster, and the rate of healing is identical. But this is the kind of thing you never mention on the historical part of the oral exam.

The theme of the oral exam that year was the subject of APUD tumors – unusual endocrine tumors. There was special emphasis on the Zollinger-Ellison syndrome – I must confess that, after four years of medical school, one year on a rotating internship, and five years of general surgery residency, I had never seen a single case. But I was well-prepared, and after the usual six-week waiting period, was notified that I had passed the exam.

Please don't get me wrong. The board examinations were fair, and they do perform a necessary function – maintaining quality control among a multitude of surgery programs. Furthermore, learning to develop one's oral skills is very important for a surgeon who deals with patients on a daily basis.

Nevertheless, despite their worth, the oral exams remain a stressful political and intellectual hurdle for the aspiring general surgeon. About the best advice I can give is: be humble, stay cool, and be prepared!

LIFE CAN BE DIFFICULT

Life can be difficult
That's what the experts say
But when I walk with you
I go the easy way!

Each morning when I awake
The world seems so brand new
Everything is warm and bright
And there's so much to do!

We spend each day together
I put your hand in mine
I look into those soft brown eyes
And life is so divine!

I know that there are hardships
I've already known a few
But the biggest one of all
Is when I'm not with you!

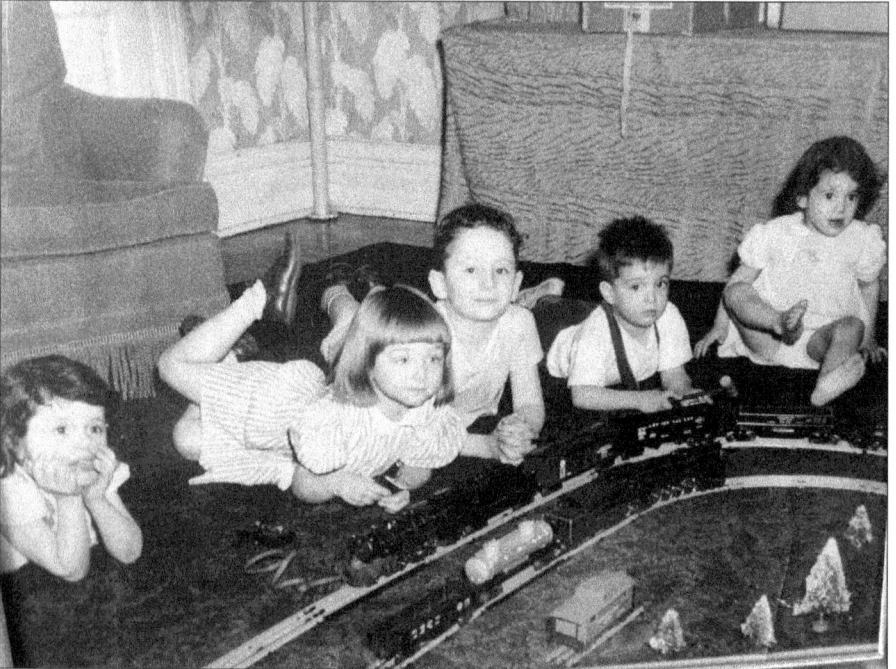

The Old Gang:
Roula, Karen, John, Bill, and Margaret Mary

MY LIFE

I might not wake up tomorrow
Sometimes that fills me with sorrow
I cherish each and every day,
As I travel on my way.

I look back upon my years –
Some with joy and some with tears
Life can be a bumpy show –
Never sure which way to go!

My friends assure me all is good
Back home in the neighborhood
These treatments sometimes make me weak –
Sometimes it's even hard to speak!

Tell my dog I'll be home soon
Sometimes I think I hear him swoon!
He wonders where I could have gone
To be away from home so long!

It's nice to see you, Mom and Dad –
I'm grateful for the days we had!
Say hello to brother Jim –
Tell him that I think of him!

When you leave, turn out the light
I'm looking for a restful night
I'll dream of when I run and play –
Praying for another day!

THE FRUIT JAR

"Dr. Truewater, if I had put my money in a fruit jar, and buried it in the backyard, I'd be better off than I am today," Dr. Lyons said as we sat in the doctor's lounge.

Dr. Fred Lyons was one of the premier gynecologists in the country. I marveled at why such an intelligent man would expound on the virtues of a backyard investment strategy.

"But what about interest?" I asked. "If you'd put your money in a checking account, at least you could collect interest."

"At the risk of repeating myself, Dr. Truewater, I would have been better off putting my money in a fruit jar and burying it in the backyard. I could probably retire today."

"I don't get it, Fred," I said. "What about that oil investment club you joined in the early '80's?"

Fred looked at me with a blank stare.

"Don't you remember that investment party with Barry Switzer and Phyllis Diller?" I continued.

"Yes, I remember, Dr. Truewater," Fred winced. "Those were the good old days. Everybody kicked in $35,000 for a piece of the action. I got to rub shoulders with the University of Oklahoma football coach, Barry Switzer. I even game him some advice – I told him he needed to pass the football more often if the Sooners were going to repeat as national champions. I knew it all in those days."

"What happened?" I asked.

"We hit a dry hole in the Anadarko basin," Fred admitted painfully. "That party cost me $35,000. And they didn't even serve dinner."

"So, I took the rest of my money and put it back in the bank," Fred replied coolly.

"Sounds like a good idea," I added. "Play it safe for a while and collect some interest."

"That's what I thought," Fred replied. "I put my money in the Penn Square Bank, and got ready to enjoy a nice Fourth of July weekend. I wondered about all those fancy investors wearing pin-striped suits. They turned out to be regulators. That's when the bank failed."

"I never could understand why they let the Penn Square Bank fail," I added.

"I mean, the Bank of New England is ten times bigger, and the government steps in and bails 'em out."

"The Bank of New England is too big to fail," Fred explained. "If a big bank fails, people might panic. But if a little bank in Oklahoma like Penn Square fails, nobody seems to care."

"Now, figure that one out," Fred Lamented. "I lose $50,000 in Penn Square Bank, but don't panic – everything's cool – it's just a small bank."

"I don't understand it either, Fred," I replied. "There's something wrong with a regulatory system that says the banks in Oklahoma and Texas are too small to save and the Bank of New England is too big to fail. I mean, why should our tax money leave Oklahoma in order to bail out the Bank of New England?"

"The fruit jar's looking better all the time," I added. "I'm almost afraid to ask what happened next."

"I got an inside tip on a good movie deal," Fred continued. "I bought stock in a movie called, The Godfather."

"For once, you did the right thing, Fred," I replied enthusiastically.

"That's what I thought, Truewater," Fred answered. "The movie grossed over $100 million dollars, but to this day Mario Puzo claims he lost money. I was lucky to break even on that deal."

"What'd you do next?" I asked with trepidation.

"I decided it was time to indulge myself," Fred answered. "You know, when you go through college and medical school, you put off spending any money. Yep, I lost a lot of girlfriends because I couldn't buy that sports car of my dreams. I decided it was my turn for a slice of the American dream. I had waited long enough."

"What'd you buy, Fred?" I asked.

"I spent $25,000 and bought me a brand-new DeLorean," Fred beamed. "You know, Truewater, the car with the gull-wing doors."

"Quite a nice car," I replied.

"The only trouble was that the company went bankrupt the following year," Fred continued. "I couldn't get spare parts, and had to sell the car for $10,000. Besides, I kept hitting my head on the gull-wing door!"

"I'm afraid to ask what happened next," I said.

"I decided to seek professional advice," Fred replied.

"You saw a psychiatrist?" I asked.

"No, an investment counselor," Fred answered. "I put $25,000 in the Fidelity Magellan Mutual Fund, the most popular and successful mutual fund of the day. Then I left for the fall meeting of the American College of Surgeons."

"That must have been October, 1987," I said.

"You guessed it," Fred answered. "Two days before Black Monday – the stock market fell 22% in one day!"

"Whenever I lose a lot of money, I vomit – don't ask me why – I guess it's just a nervous habit. Anyway, I've been vomiting a lot lately."

"You mean, it gets worse?" I asked in disbelief.

"You better believe it, Truewater," Fred replied. "Have you seen the new Medicare fee schedules lately?"

"I'm afraid to check the mail," I replied.

"Medicare's cutting us gynecologists 20% on our reimbursements – no cost-of-living adjustments, no nothing. Everything I do, except go to the toilet, is considered an 'overvalued procedure'. And instead of giving that 20% to the internists, like they promised, the government decided to keep it for themselves!"

"Dr. Truewater, where are you going?" Fred asked, as I rose to leave. "I'm not finished yet – you haven't heard about my Las Vegas Casino sports gambling trip – Oklahoma's favored to win the national championship!"

"I just remembered I've got to go to the store," I replied.

"What for?" Fred asked.

"I think I'll buy me a fruit jar," I replied. "Maybe burying my money in the backyard isn't such a bad idea!"

THE TEACHER

Do you have a minute?
I could use a little help –
Graduation's come and gone –
I can't seem to find myself!

My friends have all gone off to school
Or started off to work –
They seem so sure of what they want
I feel just like a jerk!

My counselor tells me life's a bluff –
You live your fantasy
Imagine what you want to do
Then shape reality!

I see you with your briefcase
Waiting for the train
Do you live the life you want
Or is it all a pain?

"I'm not much at philosophy
I'd like to help you out –
There's not a single move you make
That doesn't have some doubt!"

"You've got to live the life you feel
There is no other way –
Question all the moves you make
But go and join the fray!"

The man stepped up upon the train
And tipped his hat goodbye –
Sometimes the greatest wisdom
Comes from a passerby!

GRADUATION DAY

I was cleaning out my closet when I came across an old graduation picture. It showed me standing proudly between my two parents. On the back side, my mother had written, "University of Illinois Medical School, Graduation Day, June 1, 1973." I thought back to that beautiful spring day. The ceremony was held outdoors next to Lake Michigan, complete with wind and waves. It was a day of mixed emotions.

I remember my father saying, "Congratulations, Bill! You're a physician now!"

But I didn't feel any different. I had always figured that, when I graduated from medical school, some mystical presence would descend upon me, and I would know once and for all that I was finally a physician.

I must confess I even imagined I would be a wiser person, that I would finally understand the ways of the world, perhaps even the mystery of life and death.

No, this was more like a birthday. I didn't feel any older, but people would always be congratulating me for being older and wiser. I wondered if this was how ministers felt on the day they were ordained—maybe a little disappointed that the spirit of God didn't imbue them with all-knowing wisdom at the moment of ordination—or maybe He did and they just didn't always realize it.

As I looked across the waters of Lake Michigan, I thought about my first patient interview two years earlier. My professor, Dr. Mary Salkin, sensed my uneasiness.

"Just go in there, Dr. Truewater, and interview your patient," she said.

"But I'm not a doctor," I responded. "I'm just a second-year medical student."

"Dr. Truewater," Mary answered firmly, "just go in there and pretend you're a doctor. You'll get used to it. Besides, part of being a doctor is playing the role. After a while, you won't even realize you're pretending."

I slipped on my white coat, wrapped my stethoscope around my neck, stuck a flashlight and some tongue blades into my shirt pocket, and marched into the examining room.

"In my most professional tone of voice, I said, "Hello, Mr. Jackson. I'm Dr. Bill Truewater. How can I help you?"

"Pleased to meet you, Dr. Truewater," he said with a wink, realizing that I looked much too young to be a real doctor.

"I'm Jerry Jackson, and I've been having some problems with my blood pressure."

To my surprise, everything went well. Subsequent patients continued to be supportive of my pretensions to be a physician and, after several weeks, I was playing the role of physician very well.

By the time I became a senior in medical school, my confidence was at an all-time high. I had all the answers to all the questions. I even looked down at first-year medical students for being naïve and uninitiated. I was at the top of the world.

Then, something funny began to happen. As graduation approached, I knew I would soon be facing the world on my own. There would be no attending physician to supervise my actions. If something went wrong, I would be totally and completely responsible.

There was just a hint of self-doubt as I prepared to face the unknown. Maybe all this pretending was nothing more than a façade I had created—perhaps I really wasn't a physician after all! I picked up a pebble and watched it skip across the lake.

Just then, my first clinical professor, Dr. Mary Salkin, happened to notice me, diploma in hand, and stopped by for a chat.

"Something wrong, Bill?" Mary asked, as I looked over the churning waves of Lake Michigan.

"I suppose I could boil it down to one question, Dr. Salkin," I responded. "You remember my first day of clinicals, when you told me that if I pretended to be a physician long enough, that one day I would eventually become a physician."

"I would like to know when you stop pretending to be a physician and actually become one," I blurted out. "And don't tell me that holding this medical school diploma in my hand grants me the key to the kingdom."

Dr. Salkin seemed surprised at my seriousness on such a festive graduation day.

"I'm sorry to disappoint you," Mary replied after a moment's reflection. "There is no 'key to the kingdom' as you put it. Graduation Day is nothing more than the end of the beginning."

"And being a physician," Mary continued, "is nothing more than a continuation of your role-playing. Oh, to be sure, you'll get better at it. You may someday be the wisest physician in the country. But you'll never have all the answers. There will always be some pretending."

"That's not very encouraging," I replied.

"In a way it is, Bill" Mary countered. "That is why a good physician will always have some humility. As an instructor, I can tell you that the most dangerous physician is the one who thinks he knows it all, for he is least prepared to deal with the unexpected. As physicians, we will never have all the answers or solve all the problems. That keeps us humble, and that humility keeps us closer to our patients."

"Would do me a big favor, Mary?" I asked as my parents approached.

"Sure," Mary replied.

"Would take a picture of me standing with my parents?" I asked, as I posed in the center between Mom and Dad.

"Any special reason?" Mary asked.

"I'd like to remember myself on Graduation Day, and the two people who made it all possible," I beamed, "now that I've finally become a physician."

Twenty years later, as I stared at the dusty, old black and white photograph, showing me standing between my two proud parents with diploma in hand, I had only one regret—that I didn't include Dr. Mary Salkin in my picture.

Author's note: the above article was read to the graduation class of the Tulane Medical School by Dr. Ronald Lee Nichols, William Henderson Professor of Surgery, on June 2, 1992.

HAS ANYONE SEEN GOD TODAY

I went to look for God today
And learned some things along the way
I walked through fields of golden grain
Asking for His Holy Name.

The scarecrow startled me and said,
"I do believe that God is dead!
I've been here for many years
And never has His Grace appeared!"

I climbed the mountains to the sky
Looking for a reason why
I traveled in the caverns deep
Wondering if He was asleep.

I asked the sick man, "Can you tell?
Is there heaven or is there hell?"
I asked the soldier in the dirt,
"Is God alive or is He hurt?"

I dreamed that God came down to me
And asked me what I'd like to see,
"A world at peace – no need for war
Who could ever ask for more?"

Then He turned and slowly smiled –
God has been here all the while
The beauty in the swaying tree
The baby on her Mama's knee!

All these are part of God's creation –
The miracle of procreation
If only man will do his part,
How soon he could reveal God's art!

To make a world that's not at war
Man must learn to quit the sword
For God's work truly is our own –
We pay the price for what we've sown!

THE MISSION DOCTOR

One of my most rewarding medical experiences was working as a mission doctor in Nicaragua. I was a fourth-year medical student in 1972 at the University of Illinois Medical School and had an optional three-month alternate quarter. The Moravian church had a medical mission in eastern Nicaragua for the Miskito Indians, arranged through a Doctor Ned Wallace at the University of Wisconsin Medical School. You paid for your own transportation, but once you arrived in Bilwaskarma, Nicaragua, near the Rio Coco River, the mission provided your room and board – and all the beans and rice you can eat!

I traveled first by jet, then C-47 twin engine transport to Tegucigalpa, Honduras and finally by Piper Cub, flown by a missionary pilot, to land on a grass field in Bilwaskarma, Nicaragua.

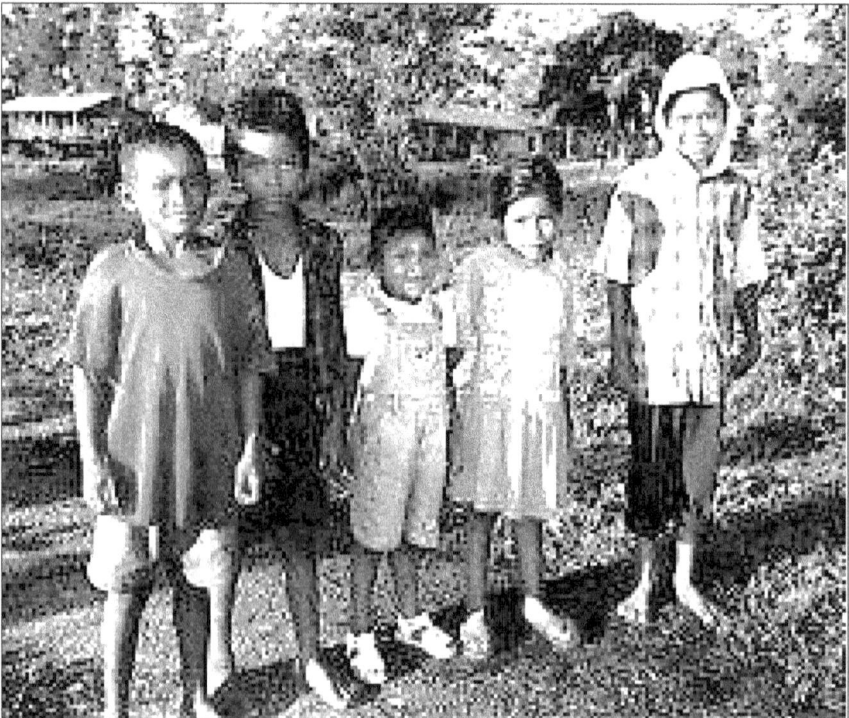

The mission doctor had two years training in general surgery and was a member of the Moravian Church. There were several wooden structures, built on stilts, that provided housing for the Nicaraguan nurses and medical students, who were required to spend a year working in a remote village.

The village had an electrical generator that provided electricity during the day, and was shut off at night. The only air conditioning was for the one-room operating suite. The tin roof on the dorms was elevated one foot off the houses to provide for through-and-through air flow, but did little for mosquito prevention.

You could ride for four hours in the bed of a Toyota pick-up traveling 20 miles an hour over the bumpy dirt roads and rickety bridges to visit Puerto Cabezas for a two dollar all-you-can-eat lobster dinner and a swim in the Caribbean Ocean with pelicans circling overhead.

A few days after I arrived, a pregnant Miskito Indian woman, who I knew as Mrs. Green, was carried in by stretcher to the hospital from the hinterland. Her right foot had been bitten by a snake while she worked in the fields and the bush doctor was unable to stop the spread of the poison. Four men had carried her by stretcher on their backs for three days to get her to the Thaeler Moravian mission hospital. By then, her right leg was grossly swollen and mottled, and she was unconscious, in septic shock.

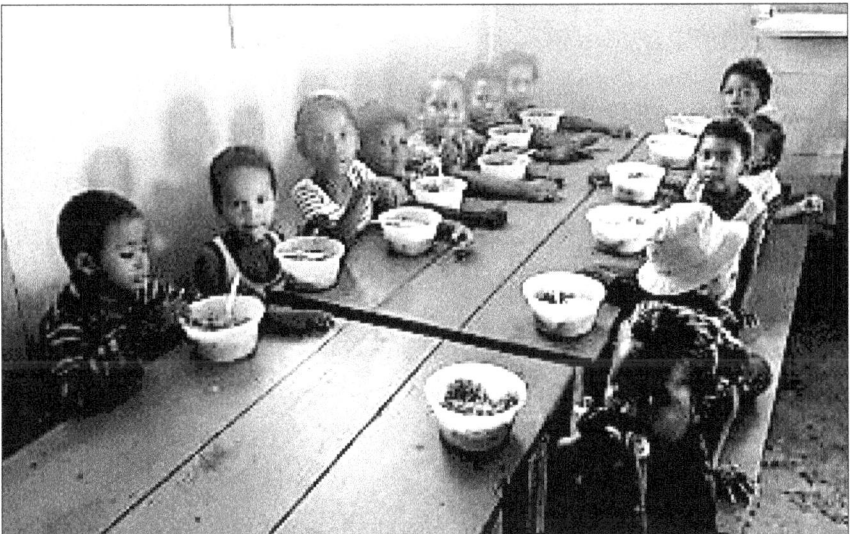

With limited oxygen, no recordable blood pressure, and only penicillin available, the mission doctor said that she had only hours to live, and that it was too late to save this unfortunate woman. I had just finished rotating through the Cook County Burn Unit in Chicago, and had done a few fasciotomies on burn victims.

I asked Dr. Peter Haupert to let me give it a try. He agreed, so we started an IV and began giving normal saline fluids and penicillin. With no anesthesia for this unconscious, hypotensive woman, and with the help of the nurses, I performed an extensive right leg medial and lateral fasciotomy from the upper thigh to the ankle, with several pints of creamy white pus pouring out. We irrigated with saline and then packed both wounds.

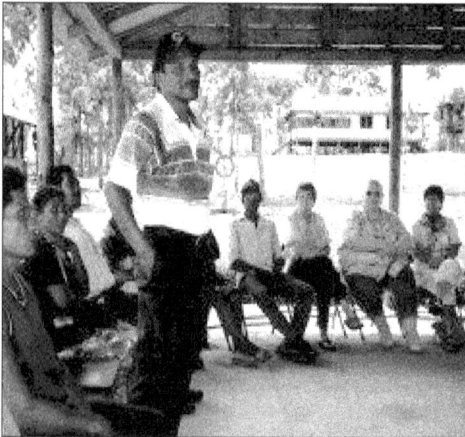

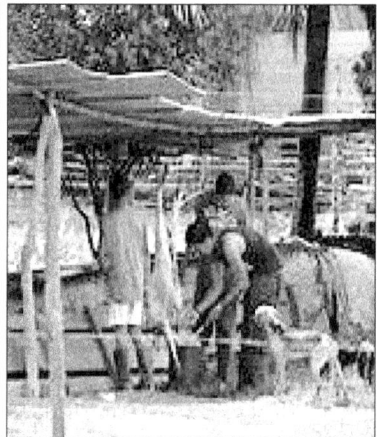

We continued packing the wounds daily with wet saline dressings, continued the penicillin and IV fluid resuscitation, and, to everyone's surprise, including my own, this lady survived. She returned to the bush country and, seven months later, gave birth to a healthy baby Brian. I even got word that the bush doctor, who practiced a totally different brand of medicine, was grateful to me for her survival and began sending some of his patients to the Moravian clinic.

After three months, I returned to the states, took a general surgery residency, and practiced forty years as a general surgeon in Oklahoma City. The entire Moravian village, including the Thaeler Hospital, and other Miskito villages, were later burned down by the Sandinistas, but the hospital and many of the Miskito villages have since been rebuilt.

Through the years, certain events occurred that reminded me of those three months in the boonies in Nicaragua. I'm always turning off light switches to save electricity. When we run out of something at the hospital, I don't get upset, because I know it will only take a few days, instead of a few months to re-supply. When it's too hot and muggy outside, I'm grateful for my air-conditioned house – without mosquitos!

But for all the surgeries I've done, I periodically think about Brian Green and where he might be today. What if I hadn't gone to Nicaragua? My third world alternate quarter rotation was one of my most rewarding, life-shaping medical experiences – and I wasn't yet a doctor!

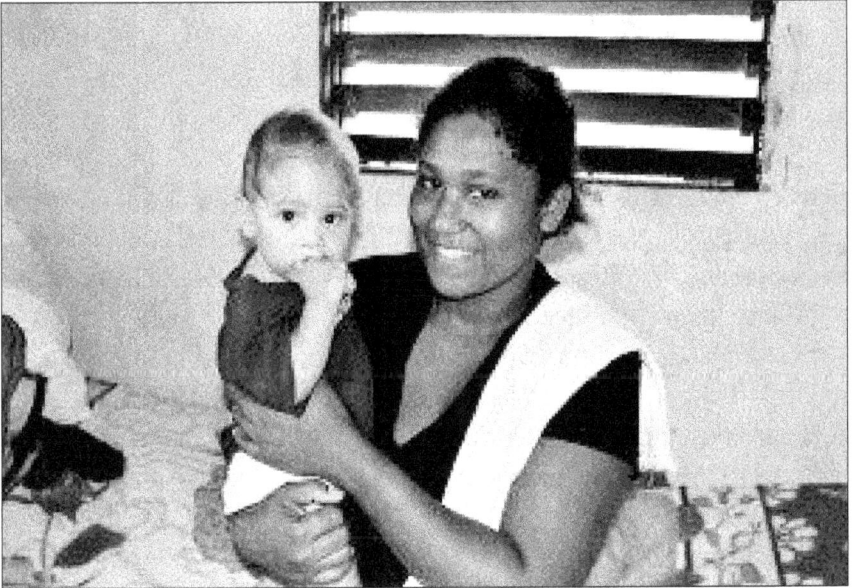

THE INDIAN NICKEL

One thing that separates medicine from most other professions is dealing with death and separation. Of course, this is a part of life, but in the medical profession, it happens on a more regular basis. One surprising source of comfort has been my own patients. If a doctor takes the time to listen, one's own patients can provide valuable insight.

I met Jack Raincloud when he was in a leukemic crisis. I was not his regular physician, but was called by Nurse Mary Adkins to insert a central venous catheter for purposes of giving blood and platelets. Jack was a pleasant man, sixty-one years old, and had retired three years earlier because of his leukemia.

"How important are these platelets?" Jack asked, as I prepared to insert the catheter. "Can I live without them?"

"You can't live without platelets, Jack," Nurse Adkins answered sympathetically. "Right now, you've only got 20,00, and you need 50,000 to keep from bleeding internally."

Nurse Adkins gently massaged Jack's forehead to help relieve his anxiety. Oncology nurses like Mary were a hospital's greatest, and perhaps most unappreciated asset. They provided invaluable moral support to the patients and doctors, in addition to their usual nursing activities.

"One thing I don't understand," Jack replied. "If my body needs the platelets, why does it destroy them?"

"That's part of the leukemic process," I said. "We really don't have all the answers, but these platelet transfusions are a temporary substitute."

I inserted the transfusion catheter and left. The following day I stopped by to check on Jack. Nurse Adkins informed me that his platelet count had dropped again. It seemed Jack's body was destroying the platelets as fast as they could be given. When I entered his room, Jack was calmly looking out the window at the expressway traffic below.

"Tell me, Dr. Truewater," Jack began. "Do all these people really know where they're going?"

"How do you mean?" I asked.

"Well, it just seems that everyone's so busy going back and forth, here and there. What do they really accomplish? Carpools, dance classes, soccer games, baseball, and football games, swimming lessons…"

"That's part of the American system," I replied. "These activities help kids in the socialization process – it's part of being well-rounded and well-adjusted."

"I guess that's what I'm getting at," Jack replied. "When your platelet count gets down to 1,500 and you know you're probably not long for this world, it makes you take stock of what's important."

"You mean, things like religion?" I asked.

"Not only that, Dr. Truewater," Jack said. "I've been blessed with three wonderful children. Two of them, Jason and Alicia, were what you would call well-rounded. I mean, they did all the right things – good students, active in extra-curricular functions in school, and highly competitive. They were both self-starters."

"And where are they now?" I asked.

"Jason transferred out of Oklahoma City two years ago. He's a successful executive for General Mills in Minneapolis," Jack replied. "And Alicia's a successful New York stockbroker."

"You should be proud of both of them," I beamed. "What about your third child?"

"Leon was our third child," Jack answered. "For a while, we thought he was the black sheep of the family. The teachers all told us he was an underachiever, and we could never get him motivated. For some reason, he never bought the go-for-the-gold psychology that pervades our society."

"What's Leon doing now?" I asked.

"He's got his own auto repair shop in South Oklahoma City," Jack said. "But that's not the interesting part. You see, of all the three kids, Leon's the one who checks on us now. After my wife's stroke three years ago, Leon made a point of stopping by every day to check on his parents."

"That means more to us," Jack continued, "than all the wealth in the world. I actually think that loyalty is more important than success."

Jack held up an old Indian nickel that he kept for a keep-sake.

"Good friends, Dr. Truewater, are like this Indian nickel. I've had it for over forty years. It's tarnished and beat up and been through a lot of abuse, but it's never left me."

"It's people who take time out of their busy schedule, like you're doing now, Dr. Truewater, that give life meaning."

"Thank you, Jack," I replied.

Jack smiled peacefully as he looked out his hospital window at the traffic below. As I stood next to him, I suddenly shared his frustration. In our herky-jerky, upwardly mobile society, we may be losing our most important values – the family bonds that tie us together and connect us to our roots.

Leon, the black sheep of the family, was providing something to his parents that neither of his more successful children could accomplish – something that didn't show up in test scores or earned income. Leon, the lost son, was now the glue that held the family together, simply because he was available – he could be counted on to tend to his ailing mother if something should happen to his father.

He wasn't smart, and he wasn't gifted, and he wasn't even highly motivated, but Leon cared enough to spend time with his parents on a regular basis.

It was getting late, and I excused myself to go to surgery.

"See you tomorrow, Dr. Truewater," Jack said. "Thanks for stopping by!"

"See you tomorrow, Jack," I answered.

Jack Raincloud died the following morning as a result of his leukemic crisis and low platelet count.

"That's the one thing I don't like about medicine," I said to myself. "One day you see somebody and have a normal conversation, and the next day their room is empty."

"One day you're among the living, and then next day your soul joins the billions who have preceded you. All we have left are the memories."

I stood in Jack's old room and gazed at the traffic below.

"How would I remember Jack?" I asked myself. Perhaps by remembering his words. The most important values are the relations we form with our loved ones – not the money, not the success, but the loyalty.

"May I help you, Dr. Truewater?" Nurse Adkins asked, as she gently placed a hand on my shoulder, fully aware that I was standing in Jack's old room.

"Thanks, Mary," I replied, brushing a tear from my cheek.

"I think I've got things under control. Some patients affect you more than others. And some patients are capable of teaching their own physician. I learned a lot from Jack."

"Jack wanted you to have this, Dr. Truewater," Mary added.

In Mary's hand was Jack's old, beat-up Indian nickel. A sliver of light reflected off the old Indian's face, and for the briefest moment, I thought I saw Jack smiling peacefully.

"Thanks, Mary," I replied, as I put the nickel in my pocket.

"I'll always cherish this."

"You're most welcome," Mary responded. "See you tomorrow, Dr. Truewater."

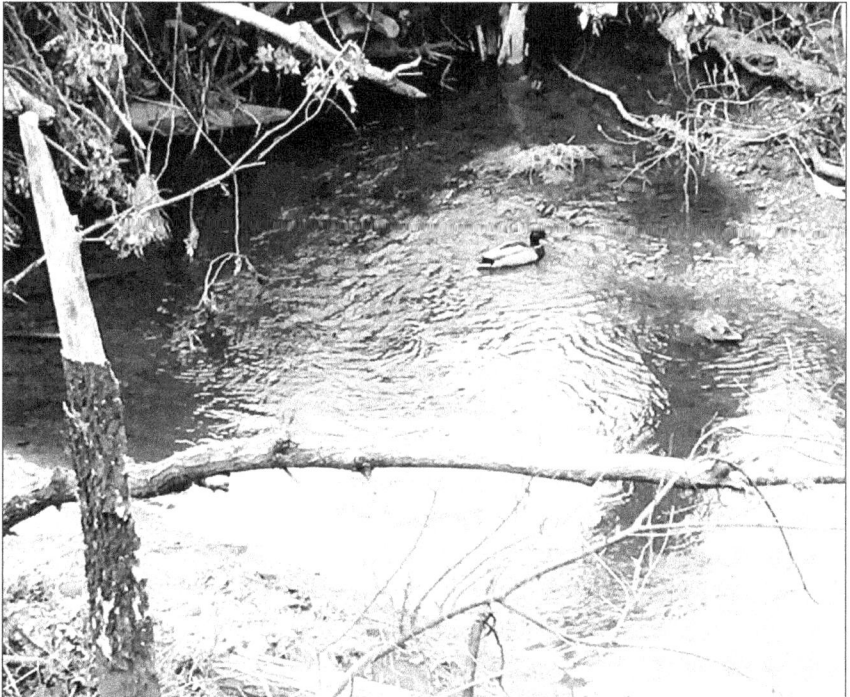

SEEING YOU

I miss you
In all the hustle and bustle of my new life
I'll have moment to pause
And see your face
And hear your voice
As if you were still with me.

You always made me smile
When we were together
And even today
I'll smile for no apparent reason
And make people think
I'm a little silly.

And if I'm sitting by the lake
Or looking out the window
Or walking through our favorite park
I'll cry for no apparent reason
And make people think
I'm a little daffy.

I've always been a collector
I like to rummage through old memories
And wonder what might have been
My friends say I need to forget the past
And put it behind me
Sometimes I wish I could.

WILL YOU LOVE ME?

I look into my bedroom mirror
And practice all my lines.
I need to tell you of my love
That conquers space and time.

The figure that looks back at me
Seems calm and quite serene –
I wish that he could talk to you
And tell you of my dreams!

The fancy clothes I'm wearing
May come as a surprise –
I picked the colors out myself
To match your pretty eyes!

The flowers I hold in my hand
Will get you in the mood –
So when I tell you of my love
I hope that you'll approve!

There's just one thing I'd like to know
Before I risk my pride –
Will you love me back again
Do our stars align?

NATURE'S CALL

I didn't hear the birds chirping –
I was too busy working!
The wind blowing through the trees
Didn't put my mind at ease!

Then one day I was told
That I was getting old!
Even as I slumbered
My days on earth were numbered!

I closed my eyes and meditated –
My world was over-cogitated!
Let the vibes come crashing through –
Fly within the rainbow's hue!

But even as I cried
I saw the clear blue sky!
We're all part of the same frequency –
Feel the earth beneath your feet!

The beauty did astound
As I stopped and slowly looked around –
Perhaps the greatest thing of all
Is simply answer Nature's call!

PATTY LYNN

Patty Lynn
My next of kin
Fought a fight
All through the night!

An active girl
She liked to twirl!
She spun the baton
At her high school prom!

She could sell a house –
On a deal she'd pounce!
Like Mom Maxine –
It was in her genes!

With her sister, Nicki
The two were nifty!
They'd play around
And scout the town!

Her Father Nick
Would play card tricks
And treat the girls
To an ice cream whirl!

Her husband Kevin
Came down from heaven!
As her health declined
He would toe the line!

To breathe was tough –
It made life rough!
Her lung transplant
Was quite a grant!

She fought the fight
To extend her life –
And treated each day
Like a brand new play!

Eternal be her memory
That we might join her reverie –
And like Patty Lynn –
Live life and grin!

GET ME WELL!

I want to run fast –
Be the first in class!
Climb up the monkey bars –
Touch the highest stars!

Swing high, up in the sky
No reason ever to cry!
Going down a slide that never ends –
Waving hello to all my friends!

Being sick is no fun –
I'd really like to laugh and run –
Flying through the air
Without a single care!

Throwing food into the lake
Watching fishes as they take!
Skipping a stone across the water –
Playing on the teeter totter

Playing tag at recess –
Pounding my chest!
Running fast and shouting loud
Playing hopscotch with my old crowd!

Let me show you all my charm –
Take this bandage off my arm!
That's what I'd really like to do –
When my chemotherapy is through!

Printed in the USA
CPSIA information can be obtained
at www.ICGtesting.com
JSHW010018280524
63581JS00001B/1

9 798986 956169